CANCER CHEMOTHERAPY

The Jones and Bartlett Series in Nursing

Basic Steps in Planning Nursing Research,
Third Edition
Brink/Wood

Bone Marrow Transplantation
Whedon

Cancer Chemotherapy: A Nursing Process Approach
Burke et al.

Cancer Nursing: Principles and Practice,
Second Edition
Groenwald et al.

Chronic Illness: Impact and Intervention,
Second Edition
Lubkin

A Clinical Manual for Nursing Assistants
McClelland/Kaspar

Clinical Nursing Procedures
Belland/Wells

Comprehensive Maternity Nursing, Second Edition
Auvenshine/Enriquez

Critical Elements for Nursing Preoperative Practice
Fairchild

*Cross Cultural Perspectives in Medical Ethics:
Readings*
Veatch

Drugs and Society, Second Edition
Witters/Venturelli

Emergency Care of Children
Thompson

First Aid and Emergency Care Workbook
Thygerson

Fundamentals of Nursing with Clinical Procedures,
Second Edition
Sundberg

1991-1992 Handbook of Intravenous Medications
Nentwich

Health and Wellness, Third Edition
Edlin/Golanty

Health Assessment in Nursing Practice,
Second Edition
Grimes/Burns

Healthy People 2000
U.S. Department of Health & Human Services

*Human and Anatomy and Physiology Coloring
Workbook and Study Guide*
Anderson

Human Development: A Life-Span Approach,
Third Edition
Frieberg

Intravenous Therapy
Nentwich

Introduction to the Health Professions
Stanfield

Management and Leadership for Nurse Managers
Swansburg

Management of Spinal Cord Injury,
Second Edition
Zejdlik

Medical Ethics
Veatch

Medical Terminology: Principles and Practices
Stanfield

Mental Health and Psychiatric Nursing
Davies/Janosik

The Nation's Health, Third Edition
Lee/Estes

Nursing Assessment, A Multidimensional Approach,
Second Edition
Bellack/Bamford

*Nursing Diagnosis Care Plans for Diagnosis-
Related Groups*
Neal/Paquette/Mirch

Nursing Management of Children
Servonsky/Opas

*Nursing Research: A Quantitative and
Qualitative Approach*
Roberts/Burke

*Nutrition and Diet Therapy:
Self-Instructional Modules*
Stanfield

Oncogenes
Cooper

Personal Health Choices
Smith/Smith

A Practical Guide to Breastfeeding
Riordan

Psychiatric Mental Health Nursing, Second Edition
Janosik/Davies

Writing a Successful Grant Application,
Second Edition
Reif-Lehrer

CANCER CHEMOTHERAPY
A NURSING PROCESS APPROACH

Margaret Barton Burke, RN, MS, OCN
Pain Rehabilitation Associates
Boston, Massachusetts
Oncology Nursing Consultant
West Roxbury, Massachusetts

Gail M. Wilkes, RN, MS, OCN
Oncology Clinical Nurse Specialist
Boston City Hospital
Boston, Massachusetts

Deborah Berg, RN, BSN
Research Nurse
Division of Clinical Oncology
Dana-Farber Cancer Institute
Boston, Massachusetts

Catherine K. Bean, RN, BA, BSN, OCN
Nurse Educator
formerly Dana-Farber Cancer Institute
Boston, Massachusetts

Karen Ingwersen, RN, MSN, OCN
Clinical Nurse III
Beth Israel Hospital
Boston, Massachusetts

JONES AND BARTLETT PUBLISHERS
BOSTON

Editorial, Sales and Customer Service Offices
Jones and Bartlett Publishers
20 Park Plaza
Boston, MA 02116

Library of Congress Cataloging-in-Publication Data

Cancer chemotherapy : a nursing process approach / Margaret Barton Burke
. . . [et al.].
   p. cm.
  Includes bibliographical references.
  Includes index.
  ISBN 0-86720-434-6
  1. Cancer—Nursing. 2. Cancer—Chemotherapy. I. Barton Burke, Margaret
  [DNLM: 1. Antineoplastic Agents—therapeutics use—nurses'
instruction. 2. Neoplasms—drug therapy—nurses' instruction. 3. Neoplasms—
nursing. WY 156 C213] RC266.C34 1991
  610.73'698—dc20
  DNLM/DLC
  for Library of Congress   91–4654
                             CIP

Typing and Word Processing: Sherry I. Littler
Illustrator: Chris Young
Text and Cover Design: Rafael Millán
Typesetting: Publication Services, Inc.

DISCLAIMER

The drug information presented in *Cancer Chemotherapy: A Nursing Process Approach* has been adapted from manufacturers' current package inserts, standard reference sources, and current research on cancer chemotherapy. As such, it has not been tested, verified, or screened by the publisher or authors. The writers and publisher of this book have made every effort to ensure that the dosage regimens set forth in the text are accurate and in accord with current labeling at the time of publication. However, in view of the constant flow of information resulting from ongoing research and clinical experience, as well as changes in government regulations, readers are urged to check the package insert and consult with a pharmacist, if necessary, for each drug they plan to administer to be certain that changes have not been made in its indications or contraindications or in the recommended dosage for each use. This is particularly important when a drug is new or infrequently employed. While the drugs included in this publication were chosen on the basis of frequency of use and appropriate indications, the publisher and authors do not necessarily advocate, and take no responsibility for, the use of the products described herein.

Printed in the United States of America
95 94 93 92 91   10 9 8 7 6 5 4 3 2 1

CONTENTS

Preface   xi
Acknowledgments   xiii

**PART I.   From the Advent of Chemotherapy to Current Research:
The Cancer Nursing Role**

1. *Cancer Chemotherapy and Nursing Practice: A Unique Blend*   3
   History of Cancer Therapy   3
   Advent of Cancer Chemotherapy   5
   New Frontiers of Therapy   7
   Advances in Chemotherapy   7
   Evolution of Oncology Nursing   9
   Table 1.1   Nursing Approaches to Cancer Care: The Oncology Nursing
      Society Standards   10
   Unique Role of the Nurse in Cancer Chemotherapy   10
   Conclusion   13
   Bibliography   13

2. *Clinical Oncology Research and the Nurse's Role*   15
   Introduction   15
   The Development of the National Cancer Institute and Anticancer Drug
      Research   15
   Clinical Trials   16
   The Phases of Clinical Trials   17
      Phase I Clinical Trials
      Phase II Clinical Trials
      Phase III Clinical Trials
      Phase IV Clinical Trials
   Ethical Issues in Clinical Research   20
   The Roles of Nurses in Clinical Oncology   22
      Clinical Nurse Specialist
      Clinical Research Nurse
      Oncology Nurse
   Summary   25
   Bibliography   25

PART II. Cancer Chemotherapy: Mechanisms and Nursing Care

3. *Cell Cycle Kinetics and Antineoplastic Agents* 29
   The Cell Cycle and Its Importance 29
   Cell Cycle Phase-Specific Agents 31
   Cell Cycle Phase-Nonspecific Agents 32
   Chemotherapy and Cell Kinetics 32
     Tumor Growth
     Cell Kill Hypothesis
     Relevance of Cytostatic versus Cytotoxic Agents in Designing
       Chemotherapeutic Regimens
   Classification of Antineoplastic Agents 34
     Alkylating Agents
     Antimetabolites
     Antibiotics
     Plant Alkaloids (Mitotic Inhibitors)
     Hormones
     Miscellaneous Agents
     Investigational Agents
       Chemotherapeutic Agents
       Biologic Response Modifiers (BRMs)
   Rationale of Single-Agent Therapy versus Combination Therapy 40
   Mechanisms of Drug Resistance 41
   Innovative Uses of Chemotherapy 43
     Autologous Bone Marrow Transplantation
     Colony Stimulating Factors (CSFs)
   Bibliography 47

4. *Potential Toxicities and Nursing Management* 49
   Introduction 49

   **SECTION A. Toxicity to Rapidly Proliferating Normal Cell
   Populations** 50
     I. Bone Marrow Depression (BMD) 50
     Introduction
     Nursing Management of the Patient with Bone Marrow Depression
     Bone Marrow Depression: Thrombocytopenia
     Anemia
     Table 4.6 Standardized Nursing Care Plan for the Patient
       Experiencing Bone Marrow Depression 62
    II. Mucositis 67
     Stomatitis
       Infections
       Nursing Interventions

Esophagitis
Table 4.10 Standardized Nursing Care Plan for the Patient
Experiencing Stomatitis 76
Diarrhea
Table 4.11 Standardized Nursing Care Plan for the Patient
Experiencing Diarrhea 82
III. Alopecia 84
Table 4.12 Standardized Nursing Care Plan for the Patient
Experiencing Alopecia 85
IV. Gonadal Dysfunction 86
Table 4.14 Standardized Nursing Care Plan for the Patient
Experiencing Sexual Dysfunction 90

SECTION B. Nausea and Vomiting 91
Antiemetic Treatment 94
Pharmacology of Antiemetics 96
Phenothiazines
Butyrophenones
Substituted Benzamides
Benzodiazepines
Glucocorticosteroids
Cannabinoids
Antihistamines
Extrapyramidal Side Effects: Assessment and Intervention 100
Table 4.16 Standardized Nursing Care Plan for the Patient Experiencing
Nausea and Vomiting 102

SECTION C. Toxicity to Other Organ Systems 101
Introduction 101
I. Cardiotoxicity of Antineoplastic Drugs 105
II. Pulmonary Toxicity 106
III. Hepatotoxicity 112
IV. Nephrotoxicity 113
Table 4.21 Relative Risks of Chemotherapeutic Agents:
Nephrotoxicity 115
V. Neurotoxicity 121
Central Nervous System (CNS) Toxicity
Neuropathies
Table 4.26 Standardized Nursing Care Plan for the Patient
Experiencing Neuropathy 128
Bibliography 132

5. *Chemotherapeutic Agents: Standardized Nursing Care Plans to
Minimize Toxicity* 139
Introduction 140
Acridinyl anisidide (AMSA, M-AMSA) 141

Adrenocorticoids   145
Aminoglutethimide   149
Androgens   153
5-Azacytidine   156
Aziridinylbenzaquinone (AZQ)   159
Bleomycin sulfate   163
Busulfan   169
Carboplatin (Paraplatin)   171
Carmustine   175
Chlorambucil   179
Cisplatin   183
Cyclophosphamide   188
Cytarabine, cytosine arabinoside   193
Dacarbazine   197
Dactinomycin   203
Daunorubicin hydrochloride   208
Doxorubicin hydrochloride   213
Estramustine phosphate   218
Estrogens   223
Etoposide   227
Floxuridine   233
5-Fluorouracil   238
Flutamide (Eulexin)   242
Hexamethylmelamine   244
Hydroxyurea   247
Idarubicin   251
Ifosfamide   256
L-asparaginase   261
Leucovorin calcium   266
Leuprolide acetate   268
Lomustine (CCNU, CeeNU)   270
Mechlorethamine hydrochloride   273
Melphalan   280
6-Mercaptopurine   285
Mesna   288
Methotrexate   290
Methyl-CCNU (semustine, MeCCNU)   295
Mitoguazone dihydrochloride (methyl-GAG)   299
Mitomycin   305
Mitotane   310
Mitoxantrone (Novantrone)   313
Pentostatin   318
Plicamycin, mithramycin   322
Procarbazine hydrochlorozide   326
Progestational agents   330

Streptozocin   332
Tamoxifen citrate   337
6-Thioguanine   340
Thiotepa   343
Trimetrexate   346
Vinblastine (Velban)   349
Vincristine   355
Vindesine   360
VM-26 (teniposide)   365
Bibliography   370

PART III.   Clinical Application

6. *Principles of Chemotherapy Administration*   375
Chemotherapy Checklist   376
Issues in Chemotherapy Administration in Ambulatory and
   Home Settings   376
Nursing Assessment: Pre- and Postchemotherapy   378
Reactions: Extravasation, Anaphylaxis, and Hypersensitivity   383
   Extravasation
   Hypersensitivity and Anaphylactic Reactions
Bibliography   396

7. *Drug Delivery Systems*   397
Routes of Administration   397
Intravenous Administration   400
   Vein Selection
   Intravenous Therapy Techniques
   Dealing with the "Veinless" Patient
Controversial Issues in Chemotherapy Administration   406
Dose Calculations and Modifications   407
Drug Interactions   408
Drug Delivery Systems   409
   Silastic Catheters
   Implantable Venous Access Ports (VAPs)
   Silastic Catheters Versus Implanted Ports: Choosing the Best System
   Ambulatory Continuous Infusion Systems
   External Pumps
   Implantable Pumps
Conclusion   422
Bibliography   422

8. *The Safe Handling of Cancer Chemotherapeutic Agents*   425
Introduction   425

Toxicity of Antineoplastic Drugs   425
Review of the Literature   427
Exposure Potential   427
Practice Implications   427
The Oncologist's Office   430
The Community   432
Conclusion   432
Bibliography   434

Appendices

Appendix 1: National Cancer Institute's Common Toxicity Criteria   438
Appendix 2: Chemotherapeutic Acronyms   442
Appendix 3: Recommendations for Handling Cytotoxic Agents: OSHA
Guidelines   445
Appendix 4: Cancer Chemotherapeutic Agents Compatibility Chart:
Oncology Drug Compatibilities   449
Appendix 5: Nomograms for Determination of Body Surface Area from
Height and Weight (Adults)   455
Appendix 6: Table of Standard Body Weights   458

Index   459

PREFACE

THE ORIGINAL INTENT of the authors was to develop a quick reference for nurses working with chemotherapeutic agents. The result was a text with an in-depth discussion of side effects, administration techniques, and corresponding nursing diagnoses. The care plans suggested by the authors are intended to be individualized for the patient receiving chemotherapy for cancer. While reading this text, keep in mind that not all interventions are appropriate for all patients.

The care plans in this book are presented to the reader with a specific time focus. By this we mean that both patient care and nursing care should be revised constantly. Individualized care should be adapted to the ever-changing needs of the patient. Thus, the static care plans in this text are intended to be guidelines from which the practitioner builds an individualized care plan for a patient receiving chemotherapy. The care plans are based on the American Nursing Association (ANA)/Oncology Nursing Society (ONS) Standards for Oncology Nursing Practice.

This book supplements other oncology nursing textbooks and provides "hands on" information to assist the nurse in providing comprehensive care to the patients receiving chemotherapy and to their family. It is designed to be used as a quick reference for the more than forty chemotherapeutic agents available in practice settings. The focus of the text is on the chemotherapeutic agents, their side effects, the corresponding nursing diagnoses and care plans, and safe methods of administration and handling of these drugs.

Part I reviews the history of chemotherapy and the role of the oncology nurse in current chemotherapy research. In chapter 1 the authors explore the history of chemotherapy in the treatment of cancer. In addition, the evolution of oncology nursing as a specialty area of practice is discussed. Concluding this chapter is the nursing process theory which blends the science of chemotherapy administration with the art of nursing care provided for the oncology patient population. Chapter 2 looks at the various professional nursing roles that have evolved since chemotherapy became a standard treatment modality for many persons with cancer.

Part II provides the core of the whole text— how the drugs work and nursing care plans on major side effects of individual drugs. Chapter 3 discusses cell cycle kinetics and builds the necessary foundation for the subsequent chapters of the book. Chapter 4 provides an in-depth discussion on the potential side effects of chemotherapy. Standardized nursing care plans are presented which address potential drug toxicities in terms of nursing diagnoses, and recommend nursing interventions and outcome criteria based on ANA/ONS practice guidelines. Chapter 5 is the heart of the textbook, where the reader will find the chemotherapeutic agents and an abridged version of the care plans from chapter 4. Standardized nursing care plans are concise and address the potential toxicities specific to each chemotherapeutic agent. The intent is to enable the practitioner to provide safe and effective nursing care to patients receiving chemotherapy.

Part III reviews technical procedures for administration and safe handling of antineoplastic agents. Chapters 6 and 7 discuss administration techniques, and include safety checklists and recommendations for management of untoward reactions. Chapter 8 covers the safe handling of antineoplastic agents.

Appendices present helpful reference material, such as acronyms for chemotherapeutic drug regimens, standard doses for accepted drug regimens, and a quick reference chart for common drug side effects.

This text is meant to be used by the advanced practitioner and the novice alike. The theoretical framework is based on nursing diagnosis and standards for nursing practice. Most of the nursing diagnoses included in the text are those approved by the North American Nursing Diagnosis Association (NANDA). The ONS standards of practice and guidelines for care of the person receiving cancer chemotherapy are the theoretical framework for the text.

The beginning practitioner will be able to not only use the nursing diagnoses in the text but will be able to review the basic principles of chemotherapy administration and content on chemotherapeutic agents. The advanced practitioner may use the text as a reference guide.

ACKNOWLEDGMENTS

IT APPEARS that when a book is completed the author or authors get the credit for putting the whole thing together. In the case of this book, that is only partially true. We feel it is only appropriate to acknowledge some of the support that was given behind the scenes to the authors.

It is nearly impossible to express in words the appreciation I feel toward my friend and husband, Tom. He provides the coaching, the humor, and the listening ear to all facets of my life, including this book. He and my daughters, Amelia and Whitney, actively participated in all aspects of this book. They attended many planning meetings and several copy-editing sessions. Their patience with me was extraordinary and their demands of my time were minimal during the production of this book. All three have begun actively writing because of this venture.

Special thanks to my sister, Debbie Wilkes, for her administrative advice and word-processing skills.

My gratitude to Denis Hammond, M.D., of New Hampshire Oncology-Hematology Associates, who gave me the first opportunity and courage to share my expertise with my peers, and to Robert J. Mayer, M.D., of the Dana-Farber Cancer Institute, who has always been there for me with encouragement and inspiration. Special thanks to my husband Ed, my best friend, who has always understood and supported my need for a career, even when I was temporarily in doubt. And last but certainly not least, thank you to my coauthors, who were always available with emotional and technical support and inspiration. You made this tremendous project a great learning experience. Margaret and Gail, thank you for inviting me to be a part of your wonderful concept.

To my husband, Leeward, for his love and support.

I offer my thanks and admiration to Ellen Powers, R.N., M.S., nurse manager of the 4 Stoneman Inpatient Oncology Unit, who exemplifies the commitment of Beth Israel Hospital of Boston to the highest standards of nursing practice.

Liz Sorenson was the copy editor for this book. It was with her time, patience, attention to detail, and persistence that made the finished product a book that we are all proud to publish. We thank you for your behind-the-scenes work.

Thank you also to Jones and Bartlett Publishers for working with novice authors. We both had a vision that was realized in this book.

Margaret Barton Burke
Gail M. Wilkes
Deborah Berg
Catherine K. Bean
Karen Ingwersen

PART I

FROM THE ADVENT OF CHEMOTHERAPY TO CURRENT RESEARCH: THE CANCER NURSING ROLE

CANCER CHEMOTHERAPY AND NURSING PRACTICE: A UNIQUE BLEND

CANCER HAS EXISTED as a disease for many centuries, although it is often thought that cancer is a disease of the modern world. The earliest evidence of cancer comes from Egyptian remains, revealing that cancers such as osteogenic sarcoma and nasopharyngeal carcinomas existed in the year 2500 B.C. (Shimkin 1977). In order to understand the development of chemotherapy and the role of the oncology nurse in administering chemotherapy agents, it is helpful to review the history of cancer therapy.

HISTORY OF CANCER THERAPY

The disease of cancer dates back as far as prehistoric times. There is evidence that cancer affected animals long before man was on earth. The studies of the remains of a Cretaceous dinosaur and a Pleistocene cave bear indicate the existence of tumors of the vertebrae (Brothwell 1967). Evidence of malignant neoplasms was documented in Egyptian mummies some 5000 years ago (Wells 1963). The number of cases of these prehistoric and ancient tumors are small, but they support the assumption that cancer is a very old disease, afflicting animals and man long before written history.

As cancer dates back to antiquity, so too is there evidence in the earliest Egyptian writing of medical treatment for benign tumors (such as lipomas and polyps) and for malignant cancers of the stomach and uterus (Breasted 1930). Early treatment of these tumors by the Egyptians consisted of surgical removal of benign lipomas and polyps with a knife or a red-hot iron. Cancer of the stomach was treated with boiled barley mixed with nuts, and cancer of the uterus was treated with a mix of fresh dates and pig's brain which was then introduced into the vagina (Ebbell 1937).

As early as the Greco-Roman Period (500 B.C.–A.D. 500), cancer was recognized and given a grave prognosis. Evidence of cancer was documented in the writings of Hippocrates (the "father of medicine") and other medical authorities of the period, such as Celsus, Artaesus, and Galen (Shimkin 1977). Shimkin's book describes the predominant theory regarding cancer during this period. At this time in history (500 B.C.–A.D. 500), the body of man was defined by the four Humors: blood, phlegm, yellow bile, and black bile. When in proper proportions, in regard to mixture, quantity, and force, man remained healthy. If any Humor was out of proportion (diminished or increased) man became ill. The four Humors were the biological counterparts for Air, Fire, Water, and Earth which in certain proportions produced heat, cold, wet, and dry. Cancer was believed to be the result of an excess of black bile (also called *melanchole*, or *atrabilis*). Cancer was and still is, in many respects, a melancholy disease.

The Medieval Period (A.D. 500–1500) saw little progress in science and medicine. These years were dominated by political and religious struggles. Cancer was still believed to be caused by an excess of black bile. Superficial tumors and ulcers were treated by wide excision and cauterization. Caution was used if tumors were unable to be treated by excision. The more extensive tumors and ulcers were treated with caustic pastes, and treatment included a combination of phlebotomy, herbal potions, diet, powder of crab, and other symbolic charms. Medicine during this time remained a combination of astrology, herbal potions, caustic pastes, excisions and cauterizations, and blood letting. None of the pastes, potions, or symbolic charms had any benefit systemically, but some did have escharotic effects on local tumors. In particular, arsenic paste may have had an antitumor effect. The use of arsenic compositions continued throughout the centuries up to 1865, when marked improvements were observed by Lissauer after a solution of potassium arsenite (Fowler's Solution) was given to a patient with chronic leukemia. A few years later, Billroth demonstrated a dramatic response of lymphosarcoma to Fowler's Solution (Haddow 1970). The Renaissance and Reformation periods (1500–1600) saw a continuation of the treatment of cancer through use of excisions and caustic powders and pastes. Cancer was beginning to be studied more as the field of anatomy began to develop (Shimkin 1977).

Shimkin (1977) continues to describe the evolution of cancer treatments through the centuries. The seventeenth century (1600–1700) saw a change in the theory of cancer. Cancer was no longer thought to be a result of an excess of black bile, but was now seen as a result of stasis and abnormalities of lymph. Surgery continued to be used for local tumors. In breast tumors, the technique of mastectomy was used. Without anesthesia or antiseptic techniques, the breast was removed by a total slice-removal followed by cauterization. In addition, the opinion that cancer was contagious began to develop during this century.

Up to this time in history, the chemotherapy of cancer remained a treatment using caustic pastes and potions which showed little concrete value. An important development occurred in the 1600s that would later encourage the investigation of the chemotherapy of cancer. The success of the chemotherapy of cancers is directly linked to the successful discovery of the chemotherapy of infections. Beginning in 1630, the first real chemotherapeutic *drug* (chemical used to treat disease) was used by the Jesuits who used a tea made from the bark of the chinchona tree to treat malaria. In addition, dysentery was treated by using a drug from the bark of a tree in Brazil. From these crude and simple extracts came quinine and emetine (ipecac), which have become well established in the treatment of malaria and amoebic dysentery respectively (Burchenal 1977). These drugs can be considered the first successful curative chemotherapeutic agents. They were used without knowledge of the etiology of disease, the identity of chemicals, or the action of the drugs (Devita et al. 1982). These successes provided the support that drugs could cure diseases. However, further advances in both the chemotherapies of infectious diseases and cancer would have to wait until the early twentieth century when Paul Ehrlich, the "father of chemotherapy," would make important discoveries that would affect both the course of infectious diseases and the course of cancer treatment.

During the eighteenth century (1700–1800), surgery remained the primary means for treating localized tumors. The theory that cancer was originally a localized, resectable disease caused by inflammation was developed during this time. Attention was being given to the disease known as cancer and the first hospitals specifically for cancer opened in France (1740) and England (1792). The treatment of cancer was emerging, but was still in an embryonic state.

Towards the end of the century it was discovered that environmental carcinogens could be epidemiologically linked to cancer. The use of snuff and the exposure to soot of chimneys was causally related to nasal cancers and scrotal cancers, respectively.

The nineteenth century (1800–1900) was an age of inventions. The field of oncology was ushered into a new era. A better understanding of tumor histology resulted from the invention of the achromatic microscope. The use of anesthesia as well as the introduction of antisepsis allowed for the surgical removal of deeper cancers of internal organs. As mentioned before, the first chemical agent to be used against a malignant disease was arsenic, in the form of potassium arsenite. Another mixture was used against a malignant disease in 1893 by Cooley. This was a mixture of streptococci and bacilli (Cooley's toxins) which demonstrated an objective response in sarcoma. The treatment was dangerous and its results were unpredictable. Still, a few people were cured of cancer in the nineteenth century.

Three discoveries that occurred at the turn of the century were to have a great impact on the treatment of cancer. The first event was the development of the radical "en bloc" mastectomy by Halsted whereby the primary tumor and the draining lymph nodes were surgically removed. Secondly, the discovery of X rays by Roentgen opened up a new modality, besides surgery, to treat tumors that could now be visualized.

Radiation therapy was introduced following the discovery of the radioactivity of uranium in 1896 by Becquerel and of radium in 1898 by Marie and Pierre Curie. Use of radiation therapy in the treatment of cancer first occurred in 1896, and soon, by 1905, the first patient with carcinoma of the uterus was treated with radium. During this time, cancer was seen as an incurable disease (Dangle and Flynn 1987). In 1913, the American Cancer Society (ACS) was established as a voluntary organization dedicated to the control and elimination of cancer in the United States.

ADVENT OF CANCER CHEMOTHERAPY

A third event was to form the backbone for programs that would help develop cancer chemotherapeutic agents. The idea that drugs could be used in the treatment of malignant disease was supported by the great successes seen with the synthetic chemicals and natural products used to cure parasitic and common bacterial infections and tuberculosis in rodent models and man. At the turn of the century, Paul Ehrlich, who coined the term *chemotherapy* and was named the "father of chemotherapy," made tremendous advances in the discovery of chemicals used to control infections (Burchenal 1977). Ehrlich tested these drugs on rodent models, the model most likely to predict the effectiveness of these drugs in humans. It was the theory of using rodent models that led George Clowes of Rosewell Park Memorial Institute in the early 1900s to develop inbred rodent lines that would carry transplanted rodent tumors. These rodent models provided the testing ground for the early cancer chemotherapeutic agents (DeVita et al. 1982). At last, potential cancer chemotherapeutic drugs were being investigated and tested for their effect against tumors in humans. Cancer chemotherapy had come a long way from the ineffective use of metallic salts such as arsenic, copper, and lead by the early Egyptian and Greek civilizations.

The modern era of chemotherapy was initiated by the discovery of the effective use of estrogens in prostate and breast cancer (Shimkin 1977). The alkylating agents were discovered under the cloak of wartime secrecy, when a group of investigators connected to the Chemical Warfare Service were looking at the toxic effects of poison gases. In an accident in Naples Harbor, sailors were exposed to poisonous mustard gas. As a result many developed marrow and lymphoid hypoplasia (Knobf et al. 1984). Looking at these results, it was thought that a derivative of this gas could be useful in treating cancers. Given a code designation of HN2 (and subsequently known as *nitrogen mustard*), this agent was used to treat lymphomas. It was first given to patients with Hodgkin's disease at Yale University in 1943. The patients' tumors responded to treatment (i.e., they became smaller), and soon a cancer chemotherapy program was begun at Sloan-Kettering Institute for Cancer Research in New York. The results of these investigations were not made public until 1946 because of the secret nature of the Chemical Warfare Program (DeVita et al. 1982). The clinical effect of nitrogen mustard caused great excitement among researchers interested in treating cancers but was short-lived as all the patients relapsed. From these studies though came other such derivatives as Myleran and melphalan (Burchenal 1977).

In 1947, a significant discovery by Dr. Sydney Farber was made in the treatment of childhood acute leukemia (Farber et al. 1948). He demonstrated the activity of the antifols as effective cancer agents. A related drug, methotrexate, would later be developed as an effective agent in treating choriocarcinomas (DeVita et al. 1979). Use of chemotherapy agents against solid tumors was disappointing, until 1956, when methotrexate was used successfully against advanced choriocarcinoma, leading to over fifty percent of patients being cured of their disease. Also that year, the first patient with Wilm's tumor was cured using chemotherapy, and the first bone marrow transplant was performed (Dangle and Flynn 1987). As a result of these important discoveries, the development of cancer chemotherapeutic agents began in earnest. It was these dramatic results in the treatment of leukemia and choriocarcinoma that led the U.S. Congress to appropriate $5 million for the development of the Cancer Drug Development Program, established through the National Cancer Institute (NCI). Through this program, many of our known chemotherapeutic agents have been developed (Saunders and Carter 1977).

The appropriations of such funds opened up the more reliable testing and development of cancer chemotherapeutic agents. In the last forty years thirty or more agents were developed that have efficacy against a variety of malignant diseases. Over the years changes have occurred in treatment regimens that have brought dramatic results against certain cancers. Single-agent drug therapy was the accepted treatment regimen in the earlier days of chemotherapy development. Today, combination chemotherapy has resulted in long-term remissions (Krakoff 1977), more effective prevention of resistance, and tolerable side effects with maximal dose (Murinson 1981). Cure is possible in patients with gestational choriocarcinoma, advanced Hodgkin's disease, non-Hodgkin's lymphomas, Burkitt's lymphoma, childhood leukemias, and testicular cancers. Increased survival has been reported in many other lymphomas and leukemias (Stonehill 1978).

Another approach that has shown evidence of increased survival rates and longer disease-free intervals is the use of adjuvant chemotherapy (Groenwald 1987). It is known that, despite surgery and radiation, many cancers recur. This recurrence is believed to be a result of undetectable micrometastases. The modern use of chemotherapy primarily evolved from a need to treat metastatic, disseminated disease. Adjuvant chemotherapy has proved effective in Wilm's tumor, osteosarcoma, Ewing's sarcoma, embryonal rhabdomyosarcomas in children, nonseminomatous testicular cancer, and both premenopausal and postmenopausal breast cancer (Cline and Haskell 1980).

Forty years ago, it was believed that chemotherapy was ineffective against cancer. Fifteen years ago, only hematologic and embryonic tumors were thought to be treatable by cancer chemotherapy. Today, combination chemotherapy and adjuvant chemotherapy have achieved great success in the treatment of malignant disease. However, there is still a long way to go. The prospects for the future lie in several areas that are just now being explored.

NEW FRONTIERS OF THERAPY

Drug therapy, supportive therapy, bone marrow transplantation, and biological response modifiers are in the forefront of cancer treatment methodology. All of these therapies are used in combination to enhance drug effectiveness. New drugs are being tested and developed in a variety of programs through the National Cancer Institute, as well as in programs in pharmaceutical companies. The development of new drugs has been the cornerstone of cancer chemotherapy. New strategies related to a more effective use of chemotherapy and hormones are underway (Frei 1985).

Supportive therapy has improved the survival of cancer patients. With the availability of platelets, hemorrhage is no longer a leading cause of death. Infections still remain a problem for many patients but the development of antibiotic agents has improved the survival rates. Once pathogens are identified, an effective antibiotic regimen should contain more than one drug with known activity against them. The combined antibiotics should have known synergism, as well as the least amount of toxicity to major organs (e.g., kidneys) (Knobf et al. 1984).

Both allogeneic (matched-donor) and autologous (self-donor) *bone marrow transplantations* have shown success in a variety of cancers. This area is just being explored and holds a great deal of promise. Also, the use of growth factors to hasten bone marrow recovery permits more consistent, and perhaps higher, drug dosing.

The field of *biological response modifiers* is just opening up and it would require another chapter to fully address this topic. This area represents an exciting new field for cancer treatment. Monoclonal antibodies are now being combined with powerful, naturally occurring toxins to target specific tumor cells. The monoclonal antibodies become the vehicle for the toxin to enter the specific tumor cell and destroy the cell. This process spares the normal cell from the toxic effects of the drug (Vitetta et al. 1987).

The field of cancer treatments has grown over the years. More than forty chemotherapeutic agents have proven useful in treating malignant diseases. The development of new drugs is slow and not very promising. The prospect for the future lies not only in trying to prevent disease, but in more effective use of established drugs, more intensive supportive therapy, and in exploring the field of immunology (Cline and Haskell 1980).

ADVANCES IN CHEMOTHERAPY

A better understanding of cancer, together with more effective therapies including the use of multimodality therapy, has resulted in improved survival statistics. For example, one in three persons diagnosed with cancer in 1960 survived five years, compared to one in five in 1930. The limited success with single-agent chemotherapy inspired the use of combination chemotherapy (initially applied to leukemias and lymphomas). It is now used for many solid tumors as part of multimodality therapy (Dorr and Fritz 1980). Today, there are well over forty chemotherapy agents, and chemotherapy is considered equally important to surgery and radiation in multimodality therapy. It is currently estimated that chemotherapy may be helpful for two out of every three persons with cancer, offering cure, control, or palliation. As of 1989, sixty-five percent of cancer patients are alive five years after diagnosis.

Figure 1.1 illustrates the time sequence of drug discovery, and it is clear that initial successes have slowed. Research efforts are now being directed toward new ways of combining drugs to optimize the relationship of drug action and tumor biology, such as synchronization of tumor cells in an effort to maximize cell kill in a specific cell cycle phase. Measures to "rescue" the patient from the potentially lethal effects of aggressive chemotherapy on normal bone marrow cells, using autologous bone marrow transplantation or using

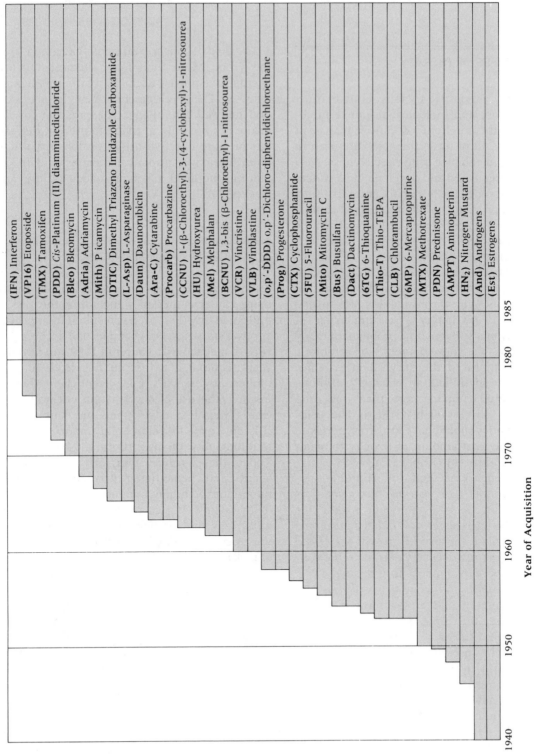

Figure 1.1 Time sequence of anticancer drug discovery

Source: Reprinted with permission from Krakoff IH, Cancer chemotherapy agents, *CA—A Cancer Journal for Clinicians* 37(2):96 (Mar/Apr 1987).

colony-stimulating growth factors to hasten bone marrow recovery are also being explored.

EVOLUTION OF ONCOLOGY NURSING

It is a tremendously exciting time for oncology nurses who care for patients receiving chemotherapy. The challenges to nurses are enormous, but the professional and personal rewards can be of equal magnitude. Oncology nursing has not always offered these opportunities. The nurse caring for the patient with cancer at the turn of this century provided supportive care for patients who felt "isolated and doomed" (Given 1980). As the ability to cure, control, and palliate tumors improved with advances in treatment and supportive measures, the role of the nurse caring for patients with cancer emerged as a specialized role.

In 1955, the National Cancer Institute's Cooperative Clinical Trials Program was initiated, and the nurse on the clinical research team functioned largely as a data collector (Henke 1980). In the 1960s, as the clinical trials became more complex, the research nurse became the liaison to other members of the health care team, answering the questions from the medical housestaff about the research protocol and administering the investigational chemotherapy. Perhaps most importantly, the research nurse was the patient's advocate, providing counsel and support. In addition, the expanded role of the nurse included patient education and monitoring the patient's response to therapy. The clinical research team was seen as the model for optimal cancer care, and nursing departments of hospitals sought nurses with oncology experience (Henke 1980).

The Federal government in 1956 provided educational traineeship grants for cancer nursing education. As the role of chemotherapy as a treatment modality emerged, nurses in large medical centers began administering chemotherapy, sharing the responsibility with physi-

cians (Dangle and Flynn 1987). These nurses became chemotherapy specialists, while chemotherapy in smaller hospitals continued to be the physician's responsibility with the nurse monitoring the patient's responses to drug administration.

In 1971, the National Cancer Act provided funds for cancer nursing education and research (Dangle and Flynn 1987, 387), and in 1973 the American Cancer Society sponsored the First National Conference on Cancer Nursing. As the profession of oncology nursing continued to grow, nurses felt a need for collegial support, education, and networking so that small interest groups around the country gave way to the birth of a national organization, the Oncology Nursing Society (ONS), which was founded in 1974. Annual ONS Congresses provided nursing education, support, and help in remaining current with the rapidly expanding body of knowledge about chemotherapeutic agents, administration techniques, and nursing management of drug side effects and toxicities. Soon, the technical expertise of the early "chemotherapy nurses" had matured to the professional expertise of nurses working to develop the knowledge of the nursing care of patients receiving chemotherapy. Currently, oncology nurses engage in research to determine the best ways of managing drug side effects, such as nausea and vomiting, hair loss, and stomatitis.

This decade has seen most oncology nurses become responsible for the administration of chemotherapy. Chemotherapy educational programs, providing the theoretical principles for practice, have been developed according to Oncology Nursing Society guidelines. These programs are given in concert with a guided clinical practicum, where nurses new to chemotherapy administration can develop skills safely and competently (Welch-McCaffrey 1985).

ONS has developed standards for cancer nursing practice which identify specific nursing behaviors that permit safe, competent, high-quality patient and family care. A summary of ONS Standards, revised in 1987, appears in Table 1.1.

Table 1.1 Nursing Approaches to Cancer Care: The Oncology Nursing Society Standards

ONS Professional Practice Standards, 1987 (Revised)

1. The oncology nurse *applies theoretical concepts* as a basis for decisions in practice.

2. The oncology nurse *systematically and continually collects data* regarding the health status of the client, the data are recorded, accessible, and communicated to appropriate members of the multidisciplinary team . . . collects data in the following high-incidence areas:
   a. prevention and early detection
   b. information
   c. coping
   d. comfort
   e. nutrition
   f. protective mechanisms
   g. mobility
   h. elimination
   i. sexuality
   j. ventilation
   k. circulation

3. The oncology nurse *analyzes assessment data* to formulate nursing diagnoses.

4. The oncology nurse *develops an outcome-oriented care plan* that is individualized and holistic. This plan is based on nursing diagnoses and incorporates preventive, therapeutic, rehabilitative, palliative, and comforting nursing actions.

5. The oncology nurse *implements the nursing care plan* to achieve the identified outcomes for the client.

6. The oncology nurse *regularly and systematically evaluates the client's responses* to interventions in order to determine the progress toward achievement of outcomes and to revise the data base, nursing diagnoses, and the plan of care.

7. The oncology nurse *assumes responsibility for professional development and continuing education* and *contributes* to the professional growth of others.

8. The oncology nurse *collaborates with the multidisciplinary team* in assessing, planning, implementing, and evaluating care.

9. The oncology nurse *participates in peer review and interdisciplinary program evaluation* to assure that high-quality nursing care is provided to clients.

10. The oncology nurse *uses* the CODE FOR NURSES and *A Patient's Bill of Rights* as *guides for ethical decision making* in practice.

11. The oncology nurse *contributes to the scientific base* of nursing practice and the field of oncology *through the review and application of research.*

Source: Adapted from American Nurses' Association 1987, *ANA and ONS: Standards of Oncology Nursing Practice*, Kansas City, Mo. Reprinted with permission.

UNIQUE ROLE OF THE NURSE IN CANCER CHEMOTHERAPY

"Making a nursing diagnosis" is the process of collecting information through assessment, and using this information to make judgments about the patient's need for care (Gordon 1987, 3). "Nursing diagnosis" refers not only to the pro-cess of diagnosing but also to the diagnostic judgment reached and is expressed in a category name (Gordon 1987, 7).

In the practice of oncology, nurses work intimately with physicians and the drugs they prescribe, specifically in chemotherapy. At times the lines become blurred regarding what are dependent, independent, and collaborative responsibilities when discussing patient care, and medical and nursing practice. This text will assist the nurse in understanding and translating the specific information about chemotherapy and the required nursing care necessary for safe practice. The care of patients receiving chemotherapy provides fertile ground for innovative clinical nursing practice, and this practice evolves from accurate patient assessment and identification of nursing diagnoses.

The nursing process is the foundation on which nursing care is based. The process includes the following:

- assessment
- diagnosis
- planning
- intervention
- evaluation

assess the patient will not be obtained. The tool utilized for collecting data does not matter—several assessment tools are available in practice. Many of these tools are institution specific. Some may be based on the functional health patterns identified by Gordon (1987).

This text suggests a manageable structure to evaluate the vast amount of information which is needed in order to assess a patient prior to administering chemotherapy. The chapters offer assessment criteria in relevant domains: 1) Biophysical, as in intravenous site selection, degree of bone marrow suppression, and condition of oral mucosa prior to therapy; 2) Cognitive-affective, as in assessing level of readiness to learn, and what information needs to be taught; and 3) Psychosocial, as in the practitioner's ability to be sensitive to the impact of the diagnosis of cancer and the fear of its treatment for the patient.

Assessment

Many nurses are uncomfortable using nursing diagnosis. Guzzetta, et al., believe this discomfort can be traced to a fundamental gap between assessment and formulation of nursing diagnoses (Guzzetta et al. 1989). An initial objective nursing assessment is needed for care planning. This assessment should be based on standards of practice. Systematic assessment of the patient is the basic tenet of the nursing process and professional nursing practice. Debate continues within the nursing profession as to whether the tool (structure) or the data gathering (process) is the key to successful nursing process. This text is not meant to endorse either the structure or the process. This text does infer that patients must have a comprehensive assessment if a nursing diagnosis is to be made. Guzzetta asserts that if nurses make an incorrect assessment, and collect non-nursing data, they will continue to have problems with nursing perspective, and the appropriate data necessary to

Diagnosis

In 1973, the North American Nursing Diagnosis Association (NANDA), formerly the National Group for the Classification of Nursing Diagnosis, published its first list of nursing diagnoses. Since that time, the interest in nursing diagnosis and its application in clinical settings has grown substantially (Carpenito 1989).

NANDA is continually reviewing and updating the approved list of diagnostic categories. The diagnoses most recently accepted by NANDA tend toward descriptions, such as hypothermia, fatigue, and ineffective breast feeding. NANDA has begun the work of renaming the older, more awkward diagnoses, e.g., "skin integrity, impaired, actual" (Tribulski 1988). The experience with the cumbersome language of nursing diagnosis has taught the profession a valuable lesson in practicality. This text is one more step toward the practical use of nursing diagnosis in care of patients with cancer who are receiving chemotherapy.

Nursing diagnosis was meant to be a shorthand term that helps the nurse make an intellectual jump directly to standards, goals, and interventions. Recently, nursing diagnosis or problem identification in nursing practice has been included in revisions of nurse practice acts. Therefore, accountability for nursing interventions, or a nurse's explicit responsibility to a consumer, should be reflected in the professional practice of a nurse. The definition states that diagnoses are made by professional nurses (Gordon 1987, 8). The recently revised *ANA and ONS: Standards of Oncology Nursing Practice* (American Nurses' Association 1987) clearly delineates the responsibility of nurses caring for patients with cancer to use nursing diagnoses. Commonly used nursing diagnoses for patients with cancer are listed at the end of the *ONS Standards*.

Cancer nursing is described as complex. The complexity of a patient's condition requires that nursing care be comprehensive. Through the language of nursing diagnoses, the beginning practitioner (novice) and the expert alike can diagnose clients' conditions using the same terminology.

Planning

One difference between novice and expert is in the repertoire of experiences from which the practitioner develops a care plan. The care plan serves as a communication tool for the nursing staff. It describes specific problems or needs of the client and prescribes interventions for directing and evaluating care (Carpenito 1987, 52). Carpenito identifies the following purposes for care planning:

- Blueprint to direct charting
- Communication tool (identifying to the nursing staff) what to teach, what to observe for, what to implement
- Specific intervention for the individual, family, and other nursing staff members to implement
- Evaluation and review of prescribed care

The care plan, as prescribed by both the nurse and physician, is goal directed toward the cure, stabilization, or palliation of cancer and optimization of response to treatment. The authors have attempted to establish priorities of care for the patient receiving specific chemotherapeutic agents. In addition, the authors have developed nursing care plans based on dependent, independent, and collaborative nursing orders. The plans in chapter 3 are elaborate in nature but illustrate the maximum care involved with a given diagnosis, and are based on ONS guidelines for care of patients with cancer. In chapter 4, in addition to the fact sheets on chemotherapeutic agents, an abridged edition of the care plans is included. These plans are meant to be used as a quick reference outlining what the nurse needs to know when administering a specific chemotherapeutic agent.

Intervention

Intervention is the actual process of giving care to the patient. The administration of chemotherapy involves knowledge of drug pharmacology and tumor kinetics, patient assessment parameters, and techniques of physical examination. Technical expertise is based on the principles of 1) intravenous therapy and use of venous access devices, 2) drug administration and safe handling of antineoplastic agents, and 3) adult learning.

Most patients receive chemotherapy in an ambulatory setting, so that there are time constraints on the nurse-patient interaction. Nurses administering chemotherapy evaluate their patients' tolerance to past chemotherapy, and make recommendations for changes in antiemetic therapy to prevent or optimize control of nausea and vomiting. Nurses take responsibility for educating patients in self-care measures so that patients and their families are able to care for them(selves) in such a way that tolerance of chemotherapy is optimized.

Evaluation

Evaluation is the final step in the nursing process. When discussing the nursing process, evaluation has different purposes. The first is evaluation of the written care plan. The second is evaluation of the patient's progress, and third, evaluation of the timeliness of the care plan.

The authors remind the reader that the nursing diagnoses and care plans in this book are a "snapshot" picture in time. These care plans provide a framework by which the nurse can understand principles and practice of chemotherapy administration in order to give chemotherapy safely. That is to say, the nurse can know the correct information about the drug in order to administer it safely and be an informed participant in the treatment; diagnose and care for the client effectively; and evaluate the patient's response to nursing care and treatment.

CONCLUSION

The Oncology Nursing Society (ONS) Standards are the framework on which the practice of oncology nursing is built. Reference is made throughout this text to tools published by the ONS, American Cancer Society, and the National Cancer Institute. The suggestion for these tools is to make the reader aware of the fact that standards of practice are available as are similar publications to operationalize these standards and implement them in a practical manner. It is up to the reader of this text to use what is available to provide the optimal care to the patient receiving cancer chemotherapy.

BIBLIOGRAPHY

American Nurses' Association (1987) *ANA and ONS: Standards of Oncology Nursing Practice.* Kansas City, ANA

———— (1980) *Nursing: A Social Policy Statement.* Kansas City, ANA

Breasted JH (1930) *The Edwin Smith Surgical Papyrus.* Chicago, University of Chicago Press

Brothwell D (1967) The evidence of neoplasms, in Brothwell D, and Sanderson AT (eds): *Disease of Antiquity.* Springfield, Ill., CC Thomas, 320–345

Burchenal JH (1977) The historical development of cancer chemotherapy. *Seminars in Oncology* 4(2) (June). Philadelphia, Grune and Stratton

Carpenito LJ (1989) *Handbook of Nursing Diagnosis.* Philadelphia, Lippincott

———— (1987) *Nursing Diagnosis Application to Clinical Practice* (ed 2). Philadelphia, Lippincott

Cline MJ, Kaskell CH (1980) *Cancer Chemotherapy* (ed 3). Philadelphia, Saunders

Craytor J (1985) Highlights in education for cancer nursing. *ONF* 12(1): 19–27

Dangle RB, Flynn K (1987) Historical perspective, chapter 36, in Ziegfeld, CR (ed): *Core Curriculum for Oncology Nursing.* Philadelphia, WB Saunders Co, 375–390

DeVita VT, Hellman S, Rosenberg S (1982) *Cancer: Principles and Practice of Oncology.* Philadelphia, Lippincott

DeVita V, et al (1979) The drug development and clinical trials programs of the division of cancer treatment, National Cancer Institute. *Cancer Clinical Trials* 2: 195–216

Dorr RT, Fritz WL (1980) *Cancer Chemotherapy Handbook.* New York, Elsevier Press

Ebbell B (1937) *The Papyrus Ebers: The Greatest Egyptian Medical Document.* Copenhagen, Levin and Munksgaard

Farber S, et al (1948) Temporary remissions in acute leukemia in children produced by folic acid antagonists, 4-aminopteroyglutamic acid (aminopterin). *New England Journal of Medicine* 238: 787–793

Frei E (1985). Curative cancer chemotherapy. *Cancer Research* 45: 6523–6537

Gilman A (1963) The initial trial of nitrogen mustard. *AM J Surg* 105: 574–578

Given B (1980) The education of the oncology nurse: the key to excellent patient care. *Seminars of Oncology* 7: 71–79

Golbey RB (1960) Chemotherapy of cancer. *AJN* 60: 521–523

Gordon M (1987) *Nursing Diagnosis Process and Application* (ed 2). New York, McGraw-Hill

Groenwald S (1987) *Cancer Nursing: Principles and Practice.* Boston, Jones and Bartlett

Gross J (1986) Clinical research in cancer chemotherapy. *ONF* 13: 56–65

Guzzetta C, et al (1989) *Clinical Assessment Tools for Use with Nursing Diagnoses.* St. Louis, CV Mosby

Haddow A (1970) David A. Kamofsky memorial lecture: thoughts on chemical therapy. *Cancer* 26: 737–754

Haskell CM (1985) *Cancer Treatment* (ed 2). Philadelphia, WB Saunders Co.

Henke C (1980) Emerging roles of the nurse in oncology. *Seminars of Oncology* 7(1): 4–8

Hilkemayer R (1982) A historical perspective on cancer nursing. *ONF* 9: 47–56

Hubbard SM (1981) Chemotherapy and the cancer nurse, in Marino L (ed): *Cancer Nursing.* St. Louis, CV Mosby, 287–343

Hubbard S, DeVita VT (1976) Chemotherapy research nurse. *ATN* 76: 560–565

Hubbard SM and Seipp CA (1985) Administration of cancer treatments: practical guide for physicians and oncology nurses, in DeVita VT, Hellman S, Rosenberg SA (eds): *Cancer Principles and Practice of Oncology.* Philadelphia, JB Lippincott

Janssens PA (1970) *Palaeopathology, Diseases and Injuries of Prehistoric Man.* London, John Baker

Knobf MKT, Fischer DS, Welch-McCaffrey D (1984) *Cancer Chemotherapy: Treatment and Care.* Boston, GK Hall

Krakoff IH (1977) Systemic cancer treatment: cancer chemotherapy, in Horton J, Hill GJ (eds): *Clinical Oncology.* Philadelphia, Saunders

Lind J and Bush NJ (1987) Nursing's role in chemotherapy administration. *Seminars in Oncology Nursing* 3(2): 83–86

Maxwell MB (1982) Research with antiemetics for cancer chemotherapy: problems and possibilities. *ONF* 9: 11–16

McCray ND (1979) Oncology patient assessment tool. *ONF* 6: 15–18

Mundinger MO (1987) Nursing diagnoses for cancer patients. *Cancer Nursing,* June: 221–226

Murinson DS (1981) Clinical pharmacology, in Rosenthal SN, Bennett, JM (eds): *Practical Cancer Chemotherapy.* Garden City, NY, Medical Examination

Oncology Nursing Society. (1988) *Cancer Chemotherapy Guidelines.* Pittsburgh, ONS

Saunders JF, Carter SK (eds) (1977) *USA-USSR Monograph: Methods of Development of New Anticancer Drugs.* National Cancer Institute Monograph 45 (DHEW Publication No. 76–1037)

Shimkin MB (1977) *Contrary to Nature.* DHEW Publication (NIH) 76–720. Washington, US Department of Health, Education, and Welfare, Public Health Service, NIH

Stonehill EH (1978) Impact of cancer therapy on survival. *Cancer* 42: 1008–1014

Tribulski JA (1988) Nursing diagnosis: waste of time or valued tool? *RN:* 30–34

Vitetta ES, Fulton RJ, May RD, Till M, Uhr JW (1987) Redesigning nature's poisons to create antitumor reagents. *Science* 238: 1098

Welch-McCaffrey D (1985) Rationale, development and evaluation of a chemotherapy certification course for nurses. *Cancer Nursing* 8: 255–262

Wells C (1963) Ancient Egyptian pathology. *Journal of Laryngol. Otol.* 77: 261–265

2

CLINICAL ONCOLOGY RESEARCH AND THE NURSE'S ROLE

INTRODUCTION

THE SCOPE OF PRACTICE for the oncology nurse includes "clinical practice, education, administration, and research" (McNally 1985). This book provides theoretical information as well as "hands-on" information to assist the oncology nurse in providing comprehensive cancer care to the client and to significant others. The purpose of this chapter is to provide information on the development of drugs through clinical trials, the use and definition of drug protocols, the phases of clinical trials, and ethical issues that surface during clinical trials. The oncology nurse who works in research may see a variety of nursing roles. These roles are also discussed. As treatments for cancers become more complex, there is a greater likelihood that an oncology nurse may become involved with patients undergoing clinical trials. With the information provided in this chapter, it is the authors' hope that the oncology nurse will be able to provide better care to the patient with cancer.

THE DEVELOPMENT OF THE NATIONAL CANCER INSTITUTE AND ANTICANCER DRUG RESEARCH

The evolution of clinical chemotherapy research began when the U.S. Public Health Service created the Office of Field Investigations in Cancer at Harvard University in the 1930s. In 1939 the Office moved to Bethesda, Md. to become part of the newly formed National Cancer Institute (NCI) (Zubrod 1984). A brief history of cancer research follows:

1949   NCI satellite units at U.S. Public Health Service Hospital, Baltimore; Univ. of Calif., San Francisco; George Washington University Medical School, Washington, DC

1953   Establishment of the Clinical Center at NCI; $1 million appropriated by Congress to leukemia research

1955   Establishment of the Cancer Chemotherapy National Service Center (CCNSC) at NCI

1971   National Cancer Act passed by Congress; $100 million approved for cancer research, leading to the development of the National Cancer Program, and the Division of Cancer Treatment, NCI, National Institutes of Health

1985 $25 million appropriated by Congress to cancer chemotherapy research

The establishment in 1955 of the CCNSC initiated a significant drug development program for cancer research. The CCNSC functioned as a pharmaceutical house run by NCI which would move drugs quickly and safely into clinical trials. In 1965 the program was expanded to review international drugs, which, upon receiving Investigational New Drug (IND) approval, would be moved into clinical trials across the country (Zubrod 1984).

Today, the Division of Cancer Treatment, NCI, National Institutes of Health, plays a major role nationally and internationally in cancer research and anticancer drug development. In the past, pharmaceutical companies had little interest in antineoplastic agents. Now with demonstrated potential for profit of certain anticancer drugs and recent government incentives to pharmaceutical companies, the NCI and the pharmaceutical firms collaborate to share costs in both preclinical and clinical areas (Wittes 1987).

The goal of the NCI and the pharmaceutical industry is to define the activity of new anticancer drugs and make those drugs available to cancer patients as quickly as possible. The objective of the clinical research done through NCI, as well as through the pharmaceutical industry, is aimed at improving the survival and quality of life for clients with cancer. A methodology to test this clinical research is the clinical trial.

CLINICAL TRIALS

The definition of a *clinical trial* is a carefully and ethically designed research study that answers a scientific question (Gross 1986). A clinical trial represents a research study that strives to demonstrate advancements in medical therapy for patients. The aim is that there will be some evidence of therapeutic improvement which ultimately can be extended to all patients (Livingston and Carter 1982). In cancer clinical trials, the ultimate goal is to help improve quality of life for the cancer patient, as well as to improve survival rates.

The success of the development of anticancer agents has increased greatly due to the results of clinical trials (Carter 1977). Although animal studies can give some clues to what can be expected in terms of toxicity or efficiency, it is only through clinical trials that information re-

garding the effects of therapy on humans can be obtained (Reich 1982a). Experiments with drug therapies on humans have gone on since ancient times. It was not until the nineteenth and twentieth centuries that the need for systematic experiments was stressed in the medical community (Bull 1959). Today, it is extremely unusual for any new therapy to be released into the medical community without having gone through multiple clinical studies to determine therapeutic effectiveness (Reich 1982a). The underlying concept for any good clinical trial is that the idea is worth testing. Other practical considerations include statistical advice, ethical considerations, cost considerations, technical feasibility, availability of clinical facilities, competence of the proposed researcher, and other legal considerations (Carter 1977). The ethical considerations in research will be discussed at a later point in this chapter. The following discussion will cover the components of clinical trials including the definition of a protocol, and the various phases of the clinical trial.

An important aspect of a successful study is that the resulting data is *interpretable*. In order to reproduce data that is interpretable, the investigator must carry on "a tentative procedure or policy." The procedure or policy becomes a meaningful clinical trial when the experiment is carried out under controlled conditions in order to achieve the end effect. Critical components of a clinical research study compromise what is referred to as a *protocol* (Carter 1982). There must be a definition of what end effect is sought; a reason why the hypothesis was chosen to be tested. Criteria must be defined for what types of patients are to be included, the size of the group, and how evaluations of these groups will be made. A protocol presents a clear definition of the research study. The protocol is the written guideline that outlines the proposed clinical management and is supplemented by objective information based on scientific findings (Simon 1982). Table 2.1 shows the essential components of any protocol.

Table 2.1 Components of a Protocol

1. Introduction and Scientific Background for the Study
2. Study Objectives
3. Patient Selection
4. Study Design (which includes schematic diagram)
5. Treatment Program
6. Procedures in Event of a Response, No Response, or Toxicity
7. Required Clinical and Laboratory Data (Pretreatment Evaluation)
8. Criteria for Evaluating the Effect of Treatment
9. Statistical Considerations
10. Informed Consent
11. Record Forms
12. References
13. Study Chairperson(s) and Telephone Number(s)

Source: Carter 1977

The importance of the Introduction and Scientific Background in a protocol is that it is the framework of justification for why the experiment is being carried out. Critical to the protocol is the definition of the Study Objectives. The Objectives outline what hypothesis is being tested and the related general observations that are expected to be made. Patient Selection defines the criteria patients must meet in order to be eligible for the study. Outlined in this section should be the type of population to be studied; the prior therapy that is allowable in the study; the number of patients to be selected; and age eligibility. In addition, the definition of those patients who might be ineligible for entry into protocol should also be outlined (Carter 1982). Usually, if a patient is declared ineligible, it is due to a coexisting condition. The general background design of the protocol is included in the Study Design; Treatment Program; Procedures in the Event of a Response, No Response, or Toxicity; and Pretreatment Evaluation of clinical and laboratory data. The section on Criteria for Evaluating the Effect of Treatment is essential to all protocols (Simon 1982). Definitions of responses should be outlined. Estimating the numbers of patients to be studied, as well as whether the patients will be randomized or not, are important elements for the Statistical Considerations of the protocol. Record Forms and References are usually placed in appendixes. Copies of Consent forms may also be in an appendix (Carter 1982) for ready reference. It is mandatory that informed consent be obtained by physicians. The U.S. Department of Health and Human Services has mandated that physicians obtain informed consent to protect human subjects in research.

A clean and descriptive protocol that defines the research question, the scientific data that supports the hypothesis, and the planned testing in humans, and evaluates the response to treatment results in sound clinical trials (Hubbard and Donehower 1980).

THE PHASES OF CLINICAL TRIALS

The development of new drugs is a long complex process. Anticancer agents go through a selection process (drug screen) that has been established through NCI (table 2.2).

An article by Gross (1986) contains a diagram that describes the number of compounds that are initially reviewed compared to the actual

Table 2.2 Steps in Cancer Drug Development

Acquisition
Screening
Production and Formulation
Toxicology
Phase I: Clinical Trials
Phase II: Clinical Trials
Phase III: Clinical Trials
Phase IV: Clinical Trials
General Medical Practice

Source: DeVita 1982, 144. Reprinted with permission.

number of compounds that make it to toxicity studies (clinical trials). As can be seen in figure 2.1, only a small handful of drugs make it to clinical trials after several years of reviewing and screening.

By the time a drug becomes available to the general medical community it has gone through extensive testing for toxicity in both animals and humans. The federal law mandates that any new drug considered for use in humans must undergo thorough toxicity testing in animals first (Carter 1977). If there is an indication that the drug may be used safely therapeutically in humans, then at this point the drug sponsor will apply for Investigational New Drug (IND) approval through the Food and Drug Administration (FDA). Included in the IND is a careful and ethical description of the planned testing in humans. Before the drug can be tested in humans, the sponsor must submit all the results of the animal studies to the FDA. Once the drug has approval, human testing begins (Pines 1981). Human testing is divided into four phases. Table 2.3 defines the four phases of clinical trials.

Phase I Clinical Trials

A phase I clinical trial is the first clinical phase of testing in humans. The purpose of the phase I

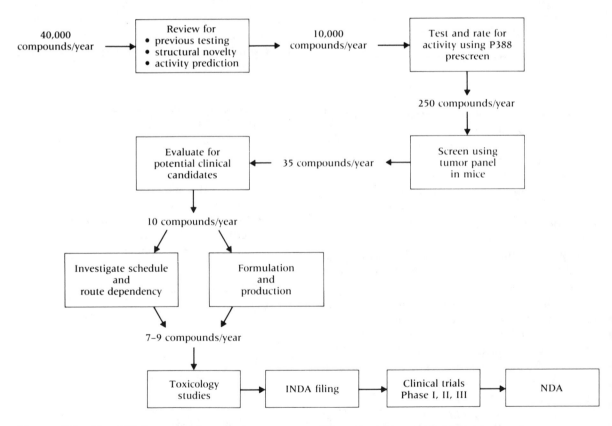

Figure 2.1 The NCI drug development program outlines the phases of study in new drug research. INDA = investigational new drug application; NDA = new drug application.
Source: Gross 1986, 62. Reprinted with permission.

Table 2.3 The Four Phases of Clinical Trials

Phase I:
  Define toxicities of a new chemotherapeutic
    agent
  Determine maximum tolerated dose
  Determine new treatment schedule
  Determine new route of administration
Phase II:
  Determine antitumor activity at given dose and
    schedule
  Further define toxicities
Phase III:
  Compare with conventional treatments
Phase IV:
  Elicit more information about the drug once it
    has been released for commercial use
  Determine the principles for combined modality
    and the associated problems

trial is to define the *maximum tolerated dose (MTD)*. Gross (1986) has defined the MTD as "the dose at which toxicities are reversible, treatable, and not life threatening." In addition to establishing the MTD, phase I trials aim at establishing the optimal schedule and safe administration of a given dose. In phase I, pharmacology of the new drug will be looked at as well (Gross 1986). Phase I studies are usually designed to start at a low dose that is not expected to produce serious side effects. Usually three patients are treated at the initial dose schedule. That initial dose is based on toxicology reports from the animal studies (Simon 1982). There are approximately five dose escalations in a phase I study. Three or more patients are usually enrolled for each dose escalation (Gross 1986).

Careful monitoring and recording of toxicities is essential to this phase of clinical trials. The nurse plays a key role in this phase of investigation. The nurse is often the one who will administer the treatment and therefore is in a prime position to observe for toxicities (Gross 1986). The role of the nurse in clinical research will be discussed at a later point in this chapter.

The completion of the phase I studies is marked by the description of toxicities observed, the extent of severity of the toxicities, and an establishment of doses for further studies.

Patients who are involved in phase I studies have usually exhausted conventional therapy. The purpose of phase I is not to find antitumor activity, but to establish a safe dose in humans. A drug is not considered inactive because it does not show any antitumor activity in phase I. It should always be considered for phase II studies unless it produces unacceptable toxicities (Reich 1982b).

Phase II Clinical Trials

Once a starting dose for several schedules of administration has been established through phase I studies, the new drug moves into phase II testing. The purpose of phase II trials is to determine antitumor toxicity of the agent in a variety of cancers (Hubbard 1985). Carter (1977) describes a twofold approach to phase II studies: drug oriented and disease oriented. In the *drug-oriented approach*, a drug is evaluated when used in a variety of cancers. Although this has been the commonly employed approach in the past, it has certain limitations (Simon 1982). There can be misleading results because of the patient selection. Response rates may be affected for many reasons. Although the number of patients may be large, there may be relatively few patients with a particular disease that has the potential to respond to the drug. Patient status can affect the response to the drug; and prior extensive therapy can alter the ability of the drug response (Carter 1977). Carter (1977) goes on to describe that perhaps the greater danger is not in overestimating the responsiveness of a new drug but rather in underestimating a drug and failing to study it effectively.

The second approach to phase II studies as outlined by Carter (1977) is the *disease-oriented approach*. This approach evaluates a drug in the treatment of a specific type of cancer. Usually these studies fall into two categories: a controlled randomized study or a nonrandomized sequential study. The *nonrandomized* phase II study looks at patients with a specific disease of a subcategory (pancreatic vs. all gastrointestinal cancers or squamous cell cancer of lung vs. all lung cancer). In a *randomized* study, a patient is randomly assigned to two or more therapeutic regimens. One of the reasons for randomizing patients is to hopefully eliminate any conscious or unconscious bias on the part of the researcher.

The goal of phase II and phase I studies is that the benefits must outweigh the risks. Patients must be carefully evaluated for eligibility for phase II trials. Aside from detecting the antitumor activity of a new drug, phase II trials also build on the knowledge obtained through phase I studies. Carter (1977) points out the additional information on drug toxicity, administration, and scheduling may be more clearly defined. At the end of the phase II study, there should be adequate information on efficacy and the nature of toxicities to justify further study. This justification for further study should be based on the concept of risk–benefit ratio.

Phase III Clinical Trials

The goal of phase III is to establish the new drug as an effective treatment by comparing it to conventional treatments (Gross 1986). Patients are randomized in phase III study in an effort to eliminate any conscious or unconscious bias of the investigator. The purpose of evaluating the new treatment is to determine absolute efficacy and safety. The drug may be administered in a variety of ways; it may be administered alone, may be combined with standard therapy, or may be substituted for drugs in standard therapy. The new agent may also be compared to single or combined drugs already known to be effective (Gross 1986). The endpoint of the phase III trials is to determine if the new drug demonstrates 1)

greater usefulness than conventional therapy; 2) equivalent or less toxicity; 3) greater potential in combination; or 4) an improvement in survival and quality of life of cancer patients (Knobf, Fischer, and Welch-McCaffrey 1984).

Phase IV Clinical Trials

Phase IV clinical trials study the new treatments that are combined with other modalities. Patients who are eligible are those who have localized disease with significant incidence of recurrence after surgery or radiation (Hubbard 1985). This phase evaluates adjuvant therapy and the potential for producing long-term survival or cure.

ETHICAL ISSUES IN CLINICAL RESEARCH

Clinical trials have become an integral part of the advancement of quality care for persons with cancer. Clinical trials may involve any disease or treatment but they must include the protocol components described earlier. One of the most important components is a section that carefully outlines how the patients' rights will be protected (Gross 1986).

Basic ethical principles should form the cornerstone of any sound clinical trial. The primary principle of a clinical trial should be that the patient will benefit from the drug (Carter 1977). The benefits of the clinical trial must outweigh the potential harm or risk to the patient (Hubbard 1985). Ethical principles are based on respect for human dignity, autonomy (self-determination), and veracity. Individuals are believed to have dignity and worth, and are not just a means of accomplishing some objective (Lynch 1988).

The basic ethical principles and guidelines involving research subjects evolved from the Nuremberg War Trials in 1945. Social outcry at the abuses of medical experiments performed on prisoners in the Nazi concentration camps prompted the Nuremberg Code. The purpose of the Nuremberg Code of 1947 was to set up ethical guidelines for research involving human subjects (Belmont Report 1978). Subsequent codes followed the guidelines of the Nuremberg Code, for example, the Helsinki Declaration of 1964 and the 1971 U.S. Department of Health, Education and Welfare Guidelines (Belmont Report 1978). These formal doctrines outlined the basic laws and regulations for individuals participating in medical research (Lynch 1988).

The development of federal guidelines for clinical research resulted from the evidence of several abuses of research studies. In 1932, the Tuskagee Syphilis Study looked at the untreated course of syphilis. The subjects were not offered the available treatment of arsenic and mercury. Later, in 1953, when penicillin became the acceptable treatment, the subjects again were not offered the available drug (Bandman 1985). In 1963, in a study of the immune system, unsuspecting patients at the Jewish Chronic Disease Hospital in New York were injected with live cancer cells (Belmont Report 1978). In 1964, in order to secure placement in an otherwise overcrowded facility, the parents of mentally retarded children allowed experiments in hepatitis transmission and immunization to be performed on their children (Bandman 1985). These instances highlighted the fact that violations of human rights existed even after the acceptance of the Nuremberg Code. The need to regulate research and protect research subjects was met with the establishment of the National Research Act of 1974. This act established the National Commission for the Protection of Human Subjects of Biomedical and Behavioral Research. The purpose of this commission was to advise the Secretary of the Department of Health, Education and Welfare (HEW) of the impact of research on ethical, legal, and social issues. Through this commission the basic guidelines for informed consent were developed. The Research Act helped establish the Institutional Review Boards (IRB) which protect research subjects through

monitoring and documenting the adherence to federal guidelines.

In 1978, the National Commission for the Protection of Human Subjects of Biomedical and Behavioral Research published *The Belmont Report: The Ethical Principles and Guidelines for the Protection of Human Subjects of Research*. This report came to be known as the "Belmont Report" and has been universally adopted as policy on the conduct of human research.

From the Belmont Report (1978) evolved three general principles that are particularly relevant to ethical research involving human subjects:

1. *Respect for Persons*
   This principle addresses two ethical issues. The first is that *individuals are autonomous*; capable of self-determination. These individuals make judgments about personal goals. No one should obstruct the autonomous actions by denying the individual the freedom to act on those judgments or by withholding information needed to make those judgments. The second issue addresses the fact that *there are some individuals, who*, due to illness, mental disability, or restricted liberty, have diminished autonomy and *are entitled to protection*. The degree of protection will depend on the risk of harm versus the likelihood of benefit to the individual and should be reevaluated on an ongoing basis.

2. *Beneficence*
   The principle of beneficence is defined as "acts of kindness or charity that go beyond street obligation" (Belmont Report 1978). Two expressions of beneficent action are 1) do no harm, and 2) maximize benefits and minimize risks. The principle of beneficence is an integral component in clinical research involving patients.

3. *Justice*
   The principle of justice is defined as *equals should be treated as equals*. This principle addresses the issue of equal distribution of a

treatment. Sometimes different treatments may be given based on age, experiments, competence, deprivation, and position. Justice demands that treatment be provided to individuals who are likely to benefit from the treatment.

The Belmont Report (1978) also recommends that 1) informed consent, 2) risk/benefit assessment, and 3) selection of subjects involved in research be considered when applying the three basic principles to clinical research.

1. *Informed Consent*
   Informed consent is mandatory in clinical trials (Simon 1982). Informed consent contains three major elements: information, comprehension, and voluntariness. *Information* assures that the individuals are given sufficient information regarding the research procedure, the objectives, risks versus benefits, alternative treatments, and the statement outlining the opportunity for the individual to ask questions or to withdraw from the study without being penalized. *Comprehension* refers to the ability of the individual to understand the information. Provisions must be made to adapt the presentation of the information so that the individual may understand. *Voluntariness* refers to the fact that the individual has given consent without coercion or inducement.

2. *Risk/Benefit Assessment*
   The justification for research is based on the ratio of risk to benefit. The guidelines established in the Nuremberg Code and subsequent federal regulations require that the benefits to the individuals and the benefit to society guided by the research have to outweigh the risks to the subjects involved in the research. The risks and benefits must be thoroughly discussed and included in the informed consent.

3. *Selection of Subjects*
   The ethical principle of justice guides the selection of subjects for clinical trials. The researcher needs to exhibit fairness in the individual selection of subjects. Subjects should not be offered treatment that would not benefit them. There should be no preference in the selection of groups of subjects (e.g., adults before children). There should be no implied benefit for being involved in a given study (e.g., prisoners would not receive any special treatment for agreeing to be a part of a study). Unfair advantage should not be taken of potential subjects (prisoners and other institutionalized people should not be considered a potential study group because they are confined).

Ethical principles are essential components to research involving human subjects. Every clinical trial must address both scientific and humanistic questions. By maintaining ethical standards in clinical trials we ensure that individual rights are protected.

THE ROLES OF NURSES IN CLINICAL ONCOLOGY

In 1950, the American Nurses' Association adopted the Code for Nurses (American Nurses' Association 1985). It defines a code for ethical conduct and principles that help guide and evaluate nursing practice. These ethical guidelines are similar to the ethical principles discussed in the previous section. The Code for Nurses is based on the most fundamental principle—respect for persons. The other principles, which are offshoots of the basic principle, are autonomy (self-determination), beneficence (doing good), nonmaleficence (avoiding harm), veracity (truth telling), confidentiality (respecting privileged information), fidelity (keeping promises), and justice (treating fairly).

The Code for Nurses provides a framework within which ethical decision making can be made. We see this code playing an important role in the field of cancer research. The nurse involved in research plays a vital role in assuring the protection of the integrity, privacy, and rights of the patients involved in research. The nurse who is involved in research should be fully knowledgeable about the intent and nature of the research in order to be able to protect patients' rights (American Nurses' Association 1985).

The nursing care of the cancer patient has been in existence for many years (Henke 1980). It is only recently that specialized units for the care of cancer patients have been developed. Many of these units may be involved in clinical research.

As the treatments for cancer became more complex over the years, the role of nurses in cancer research evolved out of necessity. Today, the nurse involved in clinical research has become an integral part of the research team. As the needs of the cancer patients increase, the nurse provides more complex nursing care. Responsibilities of the nurses involved in cancer research are data collection, education, emotional support, and identification and prevention of serious toxicities (Hubbard and Donehower 1980).

There are different nursing roles in a cancer research setting. These roles have different focuses but some job responsibilities may overlap in some cancer research settings. The roles of nurses in cancer research include:

Clinical Nurse Specialist
Clinical Research Nurse
Oncology Nurse

The two focuses are 1) involvement in the conduction of clinical trials, and 2) care for the patients undergoing cancer research trials (Hubbard 1985).

Clinical Nurse Specialist

Specialization in nursing is a concept that has been evolving since 1943, when Frances Ruter envisioned the role of the "nurse clinician." This nurse clinician was a nurse who had an advanced degree and remained actively involved in clinical practice demonstrating clinical competence (Yasko 1983). During the 1950s and 1960s, the term of *clinical specialist* was applied to the nurse with a master's degree in nursing and a specialization in a particular field of nursing (e.g., oncology, cardiology, neurology) (Crabtree 1979). This role of *clinical nurse specialist* (CNS) grew out of the increasing patient populations requiring specialized care, and the increasing, new, and complex technology and treatment methods (Hart et al. 1987). It is generally agreed upon that the purpose of the CNS is to *improve patient care* (Crabtree 1979) and to *improve the standards of nursing practice* (Yasko 1983).

During the first half of the century, there was no formalized education for nurses who worked with cancer patients. The education was gained through clinical experience. During the 1950s and 1960s efforts to promote graduate education for clinical specialization in cancer nursing were spearheaded by the American Cancer Society and the National Cancer Institute, both of which were early voices for cancer nursing (Spross 1983). These educational programs allowed cancer nurses to develop proficiency in caring for cancer patients. Few entry level nursing programs included any educational content on caring for the client with cancer (Yasko 1983). The development of the Oncology Nursing Society (ONS) in the early 1970s has also helped to develop the role of the oncology clinical nurse specialist (OCNS). Cancer nursing has emerged as a specialty through the activities and rapid growth of the ONS.

The roles of the *oncology clinical nurse specialist* (OCNS) parallel the traditional roles of the clinical nurse specialist (CNS). These roles include clinician, consultant, educator, change agent, and researcher (Spross 1983). These roles are of utmost importance when the OCNS is involved with clinical trials. In order to improve the care of the research patient, the OCNS may become the consultant and educator. As an expert in cancer nursing, the OCNS becomes a resource to the patients and their families, providing them with the appropriate education. These educational interventions evolve throughout the course of the disease and treatment. The OCNS develops an expertise for assessing the learning needs of patients and families involved in research. The assessment of needs may also extend to the nursing staff. Guiding the nursing staff who care for patients undergoing research is another aspect of the role of the OCNS as an educator (Welch-McCaffrey 1986). As a clinician working with research patients, the OCNS helps to safely monitor the research treatment and helps minimize any untoward side effects. As a researcher, the OCNS may actively take part in the design of protocols. The OCNS involved in research can provide important assistance in ensuring that research is conducted safely.

Clinical Research Nurse

The role of the clinical research nurse evolved in the 1970s during a time when clinical trials were being evaluated for their therapeutic potential in treating advanced cancers (Hubbard 1985). One of the first roles that recognized the need for collaboration in clinical research, the role of the clinical research nurse changed the focus of nursing from being task oriented to a focus in which the nurse *shared the responsibility for safe administration of investigational therapies* (Hubbard 1985).

Hubbard and Donehower (1980) pointed out that as an integral member of the research team, the nurse develops a fundamental knowledge of clinical research, as well as of the complex needs of the patient involved in clinical research. The authors also report that the research nurse has the opportunity to participate in patient care rounds and conferences that help the researchers learn more about the biology of cancer, as well as the natural history of a particular cancer.

Recently, through the involvement of clinical research nurses, nursing considerations have become included in research protocols (Hubbard 1985). The research nurse plays a major role in data collection and analysis, and publication of research data, and in some settings, has developed a role as investigator in the clinical trials (Gross 1986).

As the role of the clinical research nurse in clinical trials evolved, oncologists became aware of the value of nursing in improving the quality of clinical trials (Hubbard 1985).

Throughout the phases of clinical trials, the research nurse plays a vital role as care giver and treatment administrator, observer of toxic side effects, monitor and recorder of these side effects, resource for patient, patient advocate, data manager, and coordinator of patient care (Gross 1986).

Direct patient care is not the primary focus of the research nurse; rather the focus is the improvement of patient care through the conduct of safe and ethical clinical trials.

Oncology Nurse

The role of the oncology nurse has evolved over the last decade and has taken various forms. For example, some oncology nurses provide direct patient care, and others may focus on the improvement of care as a result of the safe conduct of the research trials. Although there is a different focus to these roles, they both should attempt to meet the needs of the cancer patient. This section will focus on the role of the oncology staff nurse who concentrates on the delivery of *direct patient care*.

In some research settings, the role of the oncology nurse may overlap with the responsibilities of the research nurse. Although the oncology staff nurse may not be involved in the design of the protocol or analysis of the data, and may not become a co-investigator, the nurse remains a vital member of the research team. As the acuity of patients increases and the complexity of clinical trials increases, the oncology nurse provides sophisticated care to the cancer patient. The oncology nurse may be the administrator of investigational therapies. As the administrator of these therapies, the nurse is often the one to observe and monitor for reactions or side effects to treatments (Gross 1986). The accuracy of these observations and documentation of toxicities are of utmost importance, especially in phase I trials where toxicities are defined. As well as being a backbone of clinical research, documentation serves as legal proof of patient care—medical and nursing. Assessments, judgments, and interventions must be documented. According to Shine (1989), the nurse must chart in an objective, accurate, thorough, and timely manner utilizing institutionally approved abbreviations. Regardless of the quality of care given or toxicity noted, if it is not documented in the medical record, technically it did not happen (Shine 1989).

The oncology nurse becomes a resource for the patient undergoing cancer research. Education of both the patient and family may be provided by the oncology nurse. The oncology nurse becomes both educator and advocate for the patient involved in research. The nurse must constantly assess the patient's understanding of the proposed treatment. Evaluating patient needs, the oncology nurse gives consistent and accurate information to the patient and family. This information needs to be simple and concise. It may contain the very nature of the proposed research, methods of administration of the treatment, and the potential risks from side effects. Oftentimes, this is information that has already been addressed by the physician and the nurse is in the position to constantly reinforce it (Lynch 1988).

As a patient advocate, the oncology nurse helps the patient to be clear about decisions based on individual goals and values. The nurse helps the patient to clearly communicate these goals to the health team. Ensuring that the patient receives and understands the essential information, as well as ensuring that there is adequate time for questions and answers, is a vital aspect of patient advocacy. Listening to a patient's fears and anxieties surrounding the unknown is an essential role for the nurse. Oftentimes, the patient feels more comfortable in discussing particular fears and anxieties with the oncology nurses because of their availability and frequent contact (Lynch 1988). Often, the nurse becomes the liaison between the health care team and the patient. As patient advocate, the nurse is the crucial factor in facilitating communication and collaboration.

The role of the oncology nurse as patient advocate and educator is very important in the research setting. The oncology nurse helps the patients understand the purpose, procedure, risks and benefits, and side effects of the research protocol they are scheduled to receive, as well as the impact it will make on their life style.

SUMMARY

There are several roles that have evolved in cancer nursing in a research setting. Many of the responsibilities may overlap. Of importance is the fact that nurses involved in cancer research have demonstrated, through their respective roles, that they have made a significant contribution to the conduct of safe and ethical clinical trials and have established themselves as invaluable resources in cancer research.

BIBLIOGRAPHY

American Nurses' Association (1985) *Code for Nurses with Interpretive Statements*. Kansas City, Mo, American Nurses' Association

Bandman EL (1985) Protection of human subjects. *Topics in Clinical Nursing* 7(2) 15–23

Belmont Report (1978). *See* National Commission for the Protection of Human Subjects of Biomedical and Behavioral Research

Bull JP (1959) Historical development of clinical therapeutic trials. *Journal of Chronic Disease* 10(3) 218–246

Carter SK (1977) Clinical trials in cancer chemotherapy. *Cancer* 40: 544–557

Carter SK, Glatstein E, Livingston RB (1982) Introduction: cancer treatment and clinical research in perspective, in Livingston RB, Carter SK, Glatstein E (eds): *Principles of Cancer Treatment*. New York, McGraw-Hill Book Co, 3–13

Crabtree MS (1979) Effective utilization of clinical specialists within the organizational structure of hospital nursing service. *Nursing Administration Quarterly* Vol 4, 1–11

DeVita VT Jr (1982) Principles of chemotherapy, in DeVita VT Jr, Hellman S, Rosenberg SA (eds): *Cancer: Principles and Practice of Oncology*. Philadelphia, JB Lippincott 132–153

DeVita VT, et al (1979) The Drug Development and Clinical Trials Program of the Division of Cancer Treatment, National Cancer Institute Cancer Clinical Trials (Fall)

Green SB (1981) Randomized clinical trials: design and analysis. *Seminar in Oncology* 8: 417–423

Gross J (1986) Clinical research in cancer chemotherapy. *Oncology Nursing Forum* 13(1): 59–65

Hart CN, Lekander BJ, Bartels D, Tebbitt BV (1987) Clinical nurse specialists: an institutional process for determining priorities. *Journal of Nursing Administration* 17(6): 31–35

Henke C (1980) Emerging roles of the nurse in oncology. *Seminars of Oncology* 7(1): 4–8

Hilkemayer R (1982) A historical perspective on cancer nursing. *ONF* 9: 47–56

Hubbard SM (1985) Principles of clinical research, in Johnson BL, Gross J (eds): *Handbook of Oncology Nursing*. New York, Wiley and Sons

Hubbard SM, Donehower MG (1980) The nurse in a cancer research setting. *Seminar in Oncology* 7(1): 9–17

Knobf MK, Fischer DS, Welch-McCaffrey D (1984) *Cancer Chemotherapy—Treatment and Care*. (ed 2). Boston, GK Hall Medical Publisher

Lind J, Bush NJ (1987) Nursing's role in chemotherapy administration. *Seminars in Oncology Nursing* 3(2): 83–86

Livingston RB, Carter SK (1982) Experimental design and clinical trials: clinical perspectives, in Livingston RB, Carter SK, Glatstein E: *Principles of Cancer Treatment*. New York, McGraw-Hill Book Co, 34–45

Lynch M (1988) The nurse's role in the biotherapy of cancer: clinical trials and informed consent. *Oncology Nursing Forum* 15(6) (suppl): 23–27

McNally JC (1985) *Guidelines for Cancer Nursing Practice*. Orlando, Fla, Grune and Stratton

National Commission for the Protection of Human Subjects of Biomedical and Behavioral Research (1978) *The Belmont Report: Ethical Principles and Guidelines for the Protection of Human Subjects of Research*. Washington, DC, US Department of Health and Human Services. HEW Publication No. (OS) 78-0012

Pines WL (1981) *A Primer on New Drug Development*. FDA Consumer. US Dept of Health and Human Resources. Public Health Service. Washington, DC, Food and Drug Administration, Office of Public Affairs. HEW Publication No. (FDA) 81-3021

Reich SD (1982*a*) Clinical trials—a review of terms and principles: Part I. *Cancer Nursing* June (5) Vol 3, 232–233

——— (1982*b*) Clinical trials—a review of terms and principles—statistical considerations: Part II. *Cancer Nursing* October (5) Vol 5, 399–402

Shine KN (1989) Areas of liability for nurse defendants. *Forum: Risk Management Foundation of the Harvard Medical Institutions*, 10(1) (Jan–Feb)

Simon RM (1982) Design and content of clinical trials, in DeVita VT Jr, Hellman S, Rosenberg SA: *Cancer: Principles and Practice of Oncology*. Philadelphia, JB Lippincott Co

Spross J (1983) An overview of the oncology clinical nurse specialist's role. *Oncology Nursing Forum* 10(3) 54–58

Vendetti JM (1983) The National Cancer Institute antitumor drug discovery program, current and future perspective: a commentary. *Cancer Treatment Reports* 67(9): 767–772 (September)

Welch-McCaffrey D (1986) Role performance issues for oncology clinical nurse specialists. *Cancer Nursing* 9(6): 287–294

Wittes RE (1987) Current emphasis in the Clinical Drug Development Program of the National Cancer Institute. *NCI Updates* 1(12). (December)

Yasko J (1983) A survey of oncology clinical nursing specialists. *Oncology Nursing Forum* 10(1): 25–30

Zubrod CG (1984) Origins and development of chemotherapy research at NCI. *Cancer Treatment Reports* 68: 9–19

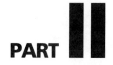

CANCER CHEMOTHERAPY: MECHANISMS AND NURSING CARE

CELL CYCLE KINETICS AND ANTINEOPLASTIC AGENTS

THE CELL CYCLE AND ITS IMPORTANCE

The cell cycle describes a sequence of steps through which both normal and neoplastic cells grow and replicate. This process of cell growth and replication involves five steps, or phases, which are designated by the letters and subscripts G_0, G_1, S, G_2, and M. The phases of the cell cycle are shown in figure 3.1.

The letter G denotes gap phases: time periods in which cells are either preparing for the more active phases of DNA (deoxyribonucleic acid) synthesis and mitosis, or resting. G_1 is referred to as the *first gap*, or *first growth phase*. During this phase, the cell prepares for DNA synthesis by producing RNA (ribonucleic acid) and protein. G_1 includes a *resting phase* called G_0. Cells in G_0 are considered to be out of the cell cycle, that is,

cellular activity does not include replication when the cell is in G_0. Cells can remain in G_0 for varying lengths of time, and can be recruited back into G_1 according to the organism's needs. In this way, cells in G_0 are in a "cellular reservoir": resting cells can be drawn from G_0 to add to the supply of dividing cells in the cell cycle (Bingham 1978).

The *synthesis* of DNA is the major event occurring during the S phase. DNA is the genetic code of information necessary for the growth, repair, and reproduction of the cell. Normal and neoplastic cells differ in the amount of time they spend in the S phase. Many antineoplastic drugs work by causing irreparable disruption in the organization of the DNA code during DNA synthesis. The disruption ultimately results in cell death. The S phase lasts between ten and thirty hours (Brown 1987).

Figure 3.1 Stages in the cell replication cycle. S = DNA synthesis; G_2 = the gap between DNA synthesis and mitosis; M = mitosis; and G_1 = the gap between the end of mitosis and the start of DNA synthesis. (G_0 = resting phase, no replication.)

Source: Groenwald 1987.

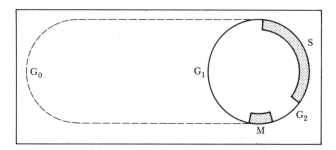

G_2 is the *second growth period*, or *second gap*. The synthesis of RNA and proteins continues as the cell prepares itself for mitosis. Production of the mitotic spindle apparatus (where chromosomes are condensed in preparation for division) also occurs during this phase. G_2 lasts between one and twelve hours.

Actual cell division or *mitosis* occurs during the M phase. The mitotic process consists of four phases: prophase, metaphase, anaphase, and telophase. The major events occuring during the M phase are pictured in figure 3.2.

During the M phase, the cell divides into two daughter cells, each one containing the same number and kind of chromosomes as the parent cell. At the completion of the M phase, the cells will either re-enter the cell cycle at G_1 to undergo further maturation and replication, or await activation by resting in G_0. Normally, cells spend about an hour in M.

The amount of time required to complete the cell cycle (called the *generation time*) varies depending upon the type of cell. While the time from the beginning of S to the end of M seems to be fairly constant, the time the cell spends in G_1 can vary greatly (from twelve to forty-eight hours). The temporal length of G_1 will determine the rate of cell proliferation (Baserga 1981).

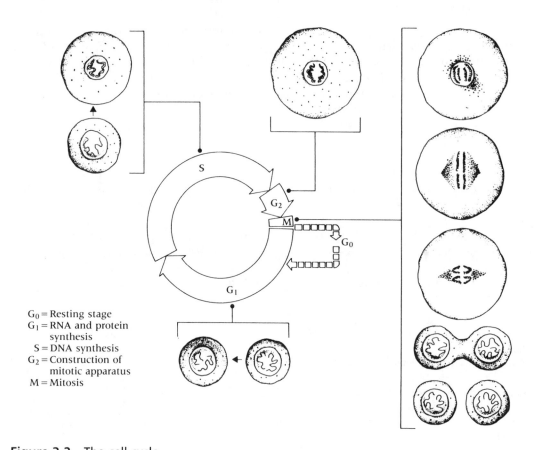

G_0 = Resting stage
G_1 = RNA and protein synthesis
S = DNA synthesis
G_2 = Construction of mitotic apparatus
M = Mitosis

Figure 3.2 The cell cycle

Source: Goodman 1987. Bristol-Myers U.S. Pharmaceutical and Nutritional Group. Reprinted by permission.

Antineoplastic drugs affect both normal and malignant cells by altering cellular activity during one or more phases of the cell cycle. Though both types of cells die as a result of irreparable damage caused by chemotherapy, normal cells have a greater ability to repair minor damage and to continue living than do neoplastic cells. The increased vulnerability of malignant cells is exploited to achieve the therapeutic effects seen with administration of antineoplastic drugs.

Most antineoplastic agents are classified according to their structure or cell cycle activity. Two major classes of chemotherapeutic agents have been established: cell cycle phase-specific and cell cycle phase-nonspecific.

CELL CYCLE PHASE-SPECIFIC AGENTS

Cell cycle phase-specific agents kill proliferating cells only in a specific phase of the cell cycle (phase G_1 through M) (Brown 1987). For example, the vinca alkaloids vincristine and vinblastine are lethal only to cells in the M phase, while hydroxyurea and cytosine arabinoside (cytarabine) inhibit DNA synthesis, and are therefore specific to the S phase. Because phase-specific agents depend on cells being in a specific phase to work, they are most effective against cells that are rapidly cycling. Rapid cycling assures that the cell will pass through the phase in which it will be vulnerable to the effects of the drugs. The antimetabolites and bleomycin are examples of phase-specific agents (see table 3.1).

Some authors (Knopf, Fischer, and Welch-McCaffrey 1984) classify phase-specific agents under a broad class of agents called *cell cycle-specific agents*. These drugs damage both proliferating and resting cells, though they tend to be more effective against actively dividing cells than those in G_0 (Knopf et al. 1984). Therefore, cells that spend most of their time in G_0 will not be affected significantly by cycle-specific agents. For the purposes of simplicity and clarity, and

Table 3.1 Cell Cycle Activity of Chemotherapeutic Agents

Cell Cycle Phase-Specific Agents			
G_1 Phase	**G_2 Phase**	**S Phase**	**M Phase**
L-Asparaginase	Bleomycin	Cytarabine	Vinblastine
Prednisone	Etoposide	5-Fluorouracil	Vincristine
		Hydroxyurea	Vindesine
		Methotrexate	
		Thioguanine	

Cell Cycle Phase-Nonspecific Agents			
Alkylating Agents	**Nitrosoureas**	**Antibiotics**	**Miscellaneous**
Busulfan	Carmustine (BCNU)	Dactinomycin	Dacarbazine
Chlorambucil	Lomustine (CCNU)	Daunorubicin	Procarbazine
Cisplatin	Semustine (MeCCNU)	Doxorubicin	
Cyclophosphamide	Streptozocin	Mitomycin	
Mechlorethamine			
Melphalan			

Source: Goodman 1986.

because the distinctions between classes of anti-neoplastic drugs are often relative, the drugs will be classified as either cell cycle phase-specific or cell cycle phase-nonspecific.

CELL CYCLE PHASE-NONSPECIFIC AGENTS

Cell cycle phase-nonspecific agents do not depend on the phase of the cell cycle to be active. Rather, these agents affect cells in all phases of the cell cycle: resting cells are as vulnerable as dividing cells to the cytotoxic effects of these agents. Consequently, phase-nonspecific agents have been found to be some of the most effective drugs against slow-growing tumors (Knopf, Fischer, and Welch-McCaffrey, 1984). However, because DNA is the target site for these drugs, maximum cell kill is not possible when cells are in the S phase at the time of drug administration. Nitrogen mustard, dacarbazine, and mitomycin are some examples of phase-nonspecific agents.

CHEMOTHERAPY AND CELL KINETICS

A basic understanding of tumor cell kinetics is helpful in comprehending the rationales behind various chemotherapy schedules and regimens.

Tumor Growth

Tumors grow by a progressive, steady expansion. According to Brown (1987), three characteristics of cells should be considered when assessing tumor growth: cell cycle time, growth fraction, and rate of cell loss. *Cell cycle time* is defined as the amount of time needed for the cell to complete an entire cycle from mitosis to mitosis. Cycle times for cancer cells vary from 24 to 120 hours, with most ranging from 48 to 72 hours. It is interesting to note that some of the more rapidly dividing normal cells (e.g., colon

and rectum crypt cells at 39 to 48 hours and bone marrow precursor cells at 19 to 40 hours) have similar, if not faster cell cycle times than cancer cells. It was originally thought that cancer cells cycled and grew faster than normal cells (Brown 1987). It is easily understandable, then, how toxicities to normal cells occur as chemotherapy acts on *all* rapidly dividing cells, not just those that are malignant. The *growth fraction* is the fraction of cells in the tumor that are cycling at a given time. In the early stages of tumor development (i.e., when tumor volume is low), the growth fraction is high and the tumor doubles its volume relatively rapidly. As the tumor grows, however, space becomes restricted and it outgrows its blood and nutrient supply so that the *tumor doubling time* decreases. Common tumor doubling times range from five days to two years.

The last factor influencing net tumor growth is the *rate of cell loss*, which is the fraction of cells that die or leave the tumor mass. Tumor growth will be the net effect of the three factors mentioned above, and will follow a *Gompertzian growth curve* (see figure 3.3).

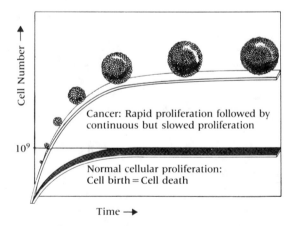

Figure 3.3 Gompertzian growth curve. Tumor growth differs from normal cell growth. Chemotherapy is effective when cell division is rapid.
Source: Goodman 1987. Bristol-Myers U.S. Pharmaceutical and Nutritional Group. Reprinted by permission.

The growth curve is a visual depiction of the idea that, as the tumor mass increases in size, tumor doubling time will slow. The earliest point at which a solid tumor can be detected clinically is when it contains 5×10^8 cells (at this point, it will measure one centimeter in diameter) (Gussack et al. 1984).

Tumor growth characteristics at least partially determine the choice of chemotherapeutic agents used against a tumor. For example, when tumor volume is low, a relatively large percentage of cells are dividing and are thus vulnerable to chemotherapeutic agents that affect dividing cells (cell cycle phase-specific agents). Likewise, when tumor volume is high, fewer cells will be dividing and agents effective regardless of cell division characteristics (phase-nonspecific agents) would be used (Goodman 1986).

Cell Kill Hypothesis

The *cell kill hypothesis* is the theoretical ability of chemotherapeutic agents to kill cancer cells. According to the hypothesis, which was first described in studies by Skipper and Shabel and their colleagues (Skipper, Shabel, and Wilcox 1964; Skipper, Shabel, and Wilcox 1965; Skipper 1968), drugs kill cancer cells on the basis of *first order kinetics*: a certain drug dosage will kill a constant percentage of cells rather than a constant number of cells. Repeated doses of therapy are thus needed to reduce the total number of cells, and the number of cells left after therapy depends upon the results of previous therapy, the time between repeated doses, and the doubling time of the tumor (Belinson 1980). For example, if a therapy has a ninety percent cell kill rate against a given tumor and the tumor is composed of a million cells, one hundred thousand cells would be left living after the first treatment. Repeated treatments should eventually reduce the tumor to a small enough number of cells such that the immune system would be able to kill any remaining cells (Brown 1987).

Unfortunately, cells can mutate over time, causing them to be resistant to chemotherapy. Also, patients with similar tumors can respond to treatment differently, sometimes making therapeutic decisions difficult (Goodman 1986). Consequently, the cell kill hypothesis cannot serve as the only predictor of a host's response to chemotherapy. For further discussion of tumor resistance to chemotherapy, the reader is referred to the end of this chapter.

Relevance of Cytostatic versus Cytotoxic Agents in Designing Chemotherapeutic Regimens

One way in which chemotherapeutic regimens are planned uses the principles of *synchronization* and *recruitment*. *Synchronization* refers to the process of increasing the percentage of tumor cells which are in a specific phase of the cell cycle (Hill 1978). This can be done by administering *cytostatic* agents (those that block or retard cell development in a specific phase of the cell cycle) or by administering *cytotoxic* agents (which kill cells in a specific sensitive phase and lead to a relative increased percentage of cells in the insensitive phases). Also, low doses of antineoplastic agents tend to cause cells to arrest or "block" in certain phases while high doses tend to cause cell death, particularly in certain phases (Gussack, Brantley, and Farmer 1984). According to Hill (1978), the chemotherapeutic purpose of synchronization is to gather cells in a specific phase of the cell cycle so that they are rendered vulnerable to agents that are cytotoxically specific for that phase. For example, cytosine arabinoside's cytostatic properties cause cells to arrest at the boundary of phases G_1 and S (the G_1/S boundary) (Hill 1978). In causing this G_1/S arrest, an increased percentage of cells are "caught" in late G_1-early S, rendering them vulnerable to agents specific for the S phase.

Recruitment is another theoretical construct used to design chemotherapeutic regimens. The term refers to the transformation of resting cells into dividing (or cycling) cells. It can occur as an indirect consequence of cell killing when cell population depletion leads to the recruitment of resting cells back into the cell cycle. Cells that are recruited in this way are more vulnerable to the effects of drugs that work when cells are dividing (i.e., cycle phase-specific drugs) (Gussack, Brantley, and Farmer 1984). The principles of synchronization and recruitment are depicted in figure 3.4.

CLASSIFICATION OF ANTINEOPLASTIC AGENTS

Antineoplastic agents are drugs that are used specifically for the purpose of killing cancer cells. The terms *cancer chemotherapeutic drugs* and *cyto-*

toxic compounds are interchangeable. Cancer chemotherapeutic drugs are generally grouped into seven major classes: alkylating agents, antimetabolites, antibiotics, plant alkaloids, hormones, miscellaneous agents, and investigational agents.

Alkylating Agents

The alkylating agents are members of one of the two primary classes of cytotoxic compounds useful in the treatment of cancer. They are highly reactive compounds that work by interacting chemically with the cellular DNA to prevent replication of the cell. More specifically, by substituting an alkyl group for the hydrogen atoms in

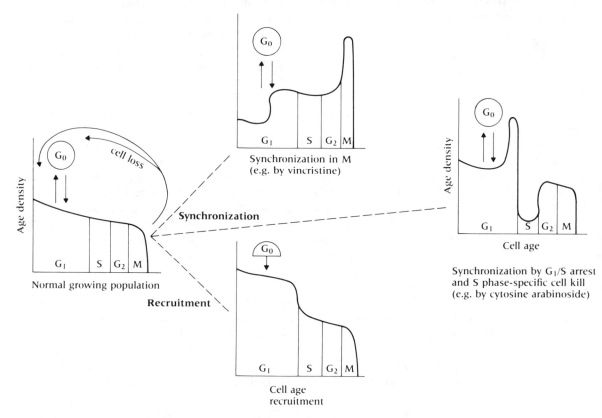

Figure 3.4 Cell synchronization and recruitment

Reprinted with permission from *European Journal of Cancer* 12:79 L.N. van Putten, 1976, Pergamon Press.

cellular molecules, alkylating agents cause single- and double-strand breaks in DNA to cross-link and bond covalently (Chabner and Myers 1985). The DNA strands are thus unable to separate, an action necessary for the replication of cellular genetic material. Alkylating agents also prevent replication by causing a misreading of the DNA code and by inhibiting RNA, DNA, and protein synthesis in rapidly dividing tissues (Chabner and Myers 1985). The nucleic acid base most often involved in the process is guanine, but adenine and cytosine have also undergone alkylation as a result of drug administration. A schematic diagram showing sites and mechanisms of action of all the major chemotherapeutic agents is shown in figure 3.5.

As a class, alkylating agents are considered cycle nonspecific. They exert their lethal effects on cells throughout the cell cycle, but tend to be more effective against rapidly dividing cells. One author postulates that this may be because rapidly dividing cells have less time to repair damage caused in G_1 before they enter the sensitive S phase of the cycle (Chabner and Myers 1985). Because alkylating agents are active against cells in G_0, they can be used to "debulk" (reduce the size of) tumors, causing resting cells to be recruited into active division. At this point, those cells will be vulnerable to the cell cycle specific agents.

The alkylating agents have been proven to be cytotoxically active against lymphomas, Hodgkin's disease, breast cancer, and multiple myeloma.

Unfortunately, patients exposed to high doses of alkylating agents are at higher risk of developing second primary sites of cancer (secondary malignancies) such as bladder cancer (after exposure to cyclophosphamide) and leukemias (after melphalan). Some of the alkylating agents (most notably, cyclophosphamide and AZQ) have a pronounced effect on bone marrow stem cells, producing cumulative myelosuppression after repeated administrations of the drug. The nitrosoureas (BCNU, CCNU, methyl–CCNU) are associated with a delayed myelosuppression with a nadir at three to five weeks after administration

which may continue for several more weeks. Changes in gonadal function have also occurred after treatment with alkylating agents. Oligospermia and azospermia, most often associated with the agents cyclophosphamide and chlorambucil, may be reversible after discontinuation of treatment. Amenorrhea is a common occurrence, but it too may be reversible in some patients.

COMMON ALKYLATING AGENTS

busulfan (Myeleran)

carmustine (BiCNU, BCNU)

chlorambucil (Leukeran)

Cisplatin (*Cis*-Platinum, CDDP, Platinum, Platinol)

cyclophosphamide (Cytoxan, Endoxan, Neosar)

dacarbazine (DTIC-Dome, Imidazole Carboximide)

estramustine phosphate (Estracyte, Emcyt)

ifosfamide (Ifex, IFX, Isophosphamide)

lomustine (CCNU, CeeNU)

mechlorethamine (Nitrogen Mustard, Mustargen, HN_2)

melphalan (Alkeran, L-PAM, Phenylalanine Mustard, L-Sarcolysin)

streptozocin (Streptozotocin, Zanosar)

thiotepa (triethylene thiophosphoramide, TSPA, TESPA)

Antimetabolites

Cells depend on various nutrient products of normal cell metabolism, *metabolites*, for the biologic synthesis of RNA and DNA. The *antimetabolites* are a group of agents that interfere with DNA and RNA synthesis by mimicking the chemical structure of essential metabolites. They prohibit cell replication in one of two ways: antimetabolites deceive cells into incorporating them along certain metabolic pathways essential for the synthesis of RNA or DNA so that a false

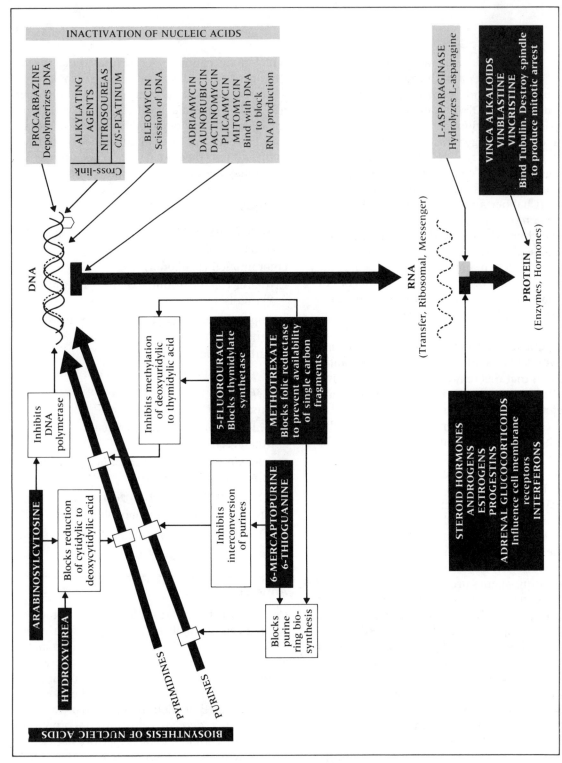

Figure 3.5 Mechanism of action of major chemotherapeutic agents

Reprinted with permission from Krakoff I, Cancer chemotherapeutic agents, *CA—A Cancer Journal for Clinicians* 37(2):96 (Mar/Apr 1987).

genetic message is transmitted; or antimetabolites block the enzymes necessary for the synthesis of essential compounds. The end result is that DNA synthesis is prevented.

Most antimetabolite cytotoxic activity occurs during the synthetic phase (S) of the cell cycle. It logically follows, then, that these agents would be most effective when used against rapidly cycling cell populations. This explains why antimetabolites are more effective against fast-growing tumors than against slow-growing tumors.

The most common toxicities to normal cells occur as a result of the agent's attack on rapidly dividing cell populations. For example, oral mucosal cells, bone marrow stem cells, and cells lining the GI tract are affected by antimetabolite administration. Toxicities that follow such cytotoxic activity include stomatitis, bone marrow depression (myelosuppression), and diarrhea (and other GI sequelae resulting from death of normal cells and tissue sloughing).

Commonly used antimetabolites include folate antagonists (methotrexate, DDMP, trimetrexate), purine antagonists (6-mercaptopurine and 6-thioguanine), fluoropyrimidines (5-fluorouracil, FUDR) and cytosine arabinoside (ARA-C, cytarabine).

COMMON ANTIMETABOLITES

cytarabine (ARA-C, Cytosar-U, cytosine
 arabinoside)

floxuridine (FUDR, 5-FUDR, 5-fluoro-
 2'-deoxyuridine)

5-fluorouracil (fluorouracil, Adrucil, 5-FU)

hydroxyurea (Hydrea)

6-mercaptopurine (purinethol, 6-MP)

methotrexate (Amethopterin, Mexate, Folex)

6-thioguanine (thioguanine, tabloid)

Antibiotics

The antitumor antibiotics are agents that are isolated from microorganisms (Knopf, Fischer, and Welch-McCaffrey 1984). They have both antimicrobial and cytotoxic activity, though the latter predominates. As a class, the antibiotics are cell cycle nonspecific and appear to have several different mechanisms by which they produce their cytotoxic effects. For example, Bleomycin's primary action is to produce single- and double-strand breaks in DNA. The anthracyclines (daunomycin and doxorubicin) intercalate DNA (forming a bond so that DNA is prevented from functioning as a template for RNA and DNA synthesis), cause oxidation-reduction reactions, and react directly with cell membranes at low concentrations to change membrane function (Chabner and Myers 1985).

Mitomycin produces cellular reactions similar to those of the anthracyclines, but also functions as an alkylator. Mithramycin inhibits DNA-directed RNA synthesis, while actinomycin-D's primary action is the intercalation of DNA (Chabner and Myers 1985). Summarizing the above, antibiotics function by either binding or reacting with DNA or by inhibiting the synthesis of RNA or both.

Major dose-limiting toxicities associated with the antibiotics are myelosuppression (all but bleomycin); skin and GI toxicity (actinomycin D); pneumonitis leading to fibrosis (bleomycin); cardiotoxicity and mucositis (doxorubicin and daunorubicin); and hepatic, renal, and blood clotting dysfunctions (mithramycin) (Chabner and Myers 1985).

COMMON ANTIBIOTICS

bleomycin (Blenoxane)

dactinomycin (actinomycin D, Cosmegen)

daunorubicin (Daunomycin, Rubidomycin,
 Cerubidine)

doxorubicin (Adriamycin)

mithramycin (Mithracin, plicamycin)

mitomycin (Mutamycin)

Plant Alkaloids (Mitotic Inhibitors)

The search for new cytotoxic compounds led to the screening of many plant extracts. Four compounds of note (vincristine, vinblastine, etoposide, and teniposide) have survived clinical trials to become recognized as worthwhile antineoplastic agents. Vincristine and vinblastine are called vinca alkaloids and are derived from the shrub *Vinca rosea*. Teniposide and etoposide are derived from products of the mandrake plant.

Plant alkaloids work by crystallizing the microtubular mitotic spindle proteins during metaphase, which arrests mitosis, and causes cell death. At high concentrations of drug, an inhibition of nucleic acid synthesis and protein synthesis has also been noted. The action of plant alkaloids is considered cell cycle phase-specific, occuring during the M phase. Teniposide and etoposide are premitotic in their cytotoxic activity, exerting most of their effect in G_2 (Knopf, Fischer, and Welch-McCaffrey 1984).

Major dose-limiting toxicities of plant alkaloids include myelosuppression (with vinblastine, etoposide, and teniposide) and neurotoxicity (with vincristine, and, to a lesser extent, vinblastine).

COMMON PLANT ALKALOIDS

etoposide (VP 16-213, Vepesid,
   epipodophyllotoxin)
vinblastine (Velban, vinblastine sulfate)
vincristine (Oncovin, vincristine sulfate)
teniposide (VM-26)

Hormones

The growth and development of certain tumors depends to some extent on their existing in a specific hormonal environment (Brown 1987). When that environment is changed, tumor growth is impaired or arrested. Breast, thyroid, prostate, and uterine cancers are examples of solid tumors that are sensitive to hormonal manipulation. With these diseases, the action of hormones or hormone antagonists depends upon the presence of hormone receptors in the tumors themselves (e.g., estrogen receptors in breast cancers). Normally, proteins in the cytoplasm of a cell act as receptors that bind to hormones and transfer them to the nucleus of the cell. Once there, the hormone receptors facilitate the binding of chromatin to the nucleus—a process necessary for the synthesis of messenger RNA which transmits the genetic information necessary for the synthesis of new proteins. The blocking of this process occurs when hormones or their antagonists are administered. Commonly used gonadal or sex hormones are estrogens [diethylstilbestrol (DES), ethinyl estradiol (Estinyl)], progestins [medroxyprogesterone acetate (Provera), megestrol acetate (Megace)], antiestrogens [tamoxifen citrate (Nolvadex)], and androgens [fluoxymesterone (Halotestin, Utadren), testosterone propionate (Oreton)].

Corticosteroids such as prednisone and prednisolone comprise another class of agents useful in the treatment of certain neoplasms. The discovery of their lympholytic action led to their use against lymphatic leukemias, myeloma, and malignant lymphoma. Some evidence exists to suggest that corticosteroids may also recruit malignant cells out of the G_0 phase of the cell cycle and into active division, making them vulnerable to damage caused by cell cycle-specific chemotherapeutic agents (Bingham 1978).

Side effects from hormonal therapy occur as a result of the administering of higher than physiological doses of drug to achieve the desired antineoplastic effects (Brown 1987). For the sex hormones, they include changes in secondary sexual characteristics (e.g., deepening of voice and hirsutism), changes in libido, and fluid retention. For the corticosteroids, side effects include hypertension, fluid retention, hyperglycemia, ulcers, osteoporosis, emotional instability, muscle wasting, increased appetite, Cushingoid features, increased susceptibility to infection, and masking of fevers.

COMMON HORMONAL AGENTS

Adrenocorticoid Agents
cortisone
hydrocortisone
dexamethasone
methylprednisone
methylprednisolone
prednisone
prednisolone

Androgens
testosterone propionate (Neo-hombreol, Oreton)
fluoxymesterone (Halotestin, Ora-Testryl)
testolactone (Teslac)

Estrogens
diethylstilbestrol (DES)
diethylstilbestrol diphosphate (Stilphostrol, Stilbestrol diphosphate)
ethinyl estradiol (Estinyl)
conjugated equine estrogen (Premarin)

Antiestrogens
tamoxifen citrate (Nolvadex)

Progesterones
medroxyprogesterone acetate (Provera, Depo-Provera)
megestrol acetate (Megace, Pallace)

Miscellaneous Agents

Miscellaneous agents are those agents whose mechanisms of action differ from the major classes mentioned above. One of the most commonly used of these agents is L-asparaginase.

Asparagine is a nonessential amino acid required by tumor cells for normal growth and development. The enzymes needed to synthesize asparagine are present in many normal tissues but are lacking in certain tumors, especially those arising from T-lymphocytes (Chabner and Myers 1985). Cells that lack these enzymes derive asparagine from circulating pools of amino acids.

L-asparaginase depletes these pools rapidly and completely. Because normal tissues can synthesize their own asparagine, L-asparaginase has very little toxicity to normal tissues. However, it is a foreign protein, and can cause serious anaphylactic reactions.

COMMON MISCELLANEOUS AGENTS

L-asparaginase (Elspar)
mitotane (Lysodren)
mitoxantrone (Novantrone)
procarbazine (Matulane)

Investigational Agents

CHEMOTHERAPEUTIC AGENTS

Investigational agents are those agents that are currently undergoing clinical trials and are thus not yet approved by the United States Food and Drug Administration (FDA). Such agents include not only new drugs but also approved drugs that are being administered in a manner different from that for which approval was previously obtained. For example, Mitoxantrone has been approved by the FDA in combination with other drugs for the initial treatment of acute nonlymphocytic leukemia (ANLL), but is considered investigational when used against other diseases.

In clinical trials, drugs are procured directly from the National Cancer Institute (NCI) or indirectly through cooperative group protocols (like the Cancer and Leukemia Group B, the Pediatric Oncology Group, etc.), and cancer centers. Though patients generally need to be treated on an NCI-approved protocol to receive investigational drugs, such agents may be obtained in certain circumstances directly from the pharmaceutical company for "compassionate use." This term refers to use of an investigational agent off protocol in a patient for whom no other clinically established treatment options exist. For a thorough discussion of clinical trials, the reader is referred to chapter 2.

BIOLOGIC RESPONSE MODIFIERS (BRMs)

The role of biologic response modifiers in the management of oncology patients has grown dramatically in the last decade. A complete description of their use is beyond the scope of this book. However, because BRMs are being administered with chemotherapy in many clinical trials, they merit a brief discussion here.

According to Mitchell and Bertram (1985), there are six major types of immunotherapy. *Active immunotherapy* refers to a stimulation of the host's intrinsic antitumor activity through *nonspecific* or *specific* means. *Nonspecific active immunotherapy* uses microbial or chemical agents (for example, BCG) to activate macrophages, natural killer cells, and other nonspecific effectors. *Specific active immunotherapy* uses modified antigenic tumor cells or extracted tumor antigens to activate specific effector cells like T cells and "armed" macrophages. Another major type of immunotherapy is *adoptive immunotherapy*. This term refers to the transfer of immunologic cells (e.g., helper T-cells) or information to a host (e.g., lymphokines or monokines like the Interleukins). *Restorative immunotherapy* refers to the repletion of deficient immunologic subpopulations (like T-cells) or the inhibition of suppressor cells (like suppressor T-cells or macrophages). Lastly, *passive immunotherapy* refers to the transfer of antibodies or short-lived antitumor "factors" to the host. An example of passive immunotherapy is the use of monoclonal antibodies against tumor-associated antigens (Mitchell and Bertram 1985).

The future of antineoplastic therapy will inevitably yield numerous combinations of immunologic and chemotherapeutic agents. Some examples of combinations currently under study are Interferon with cyclophosphamide for lymphoma and Interleukin II with dacarbazine for melanoma.

RATIONALE OF SINGLE-AGENT THERAPY VERSUS COMBINATION THERAPY

Single-agent therapy was used often in the early history of cancer chemotherapy. Starting in the 1960s, however, combinations of chemotherapeutic agents were found to produce superior clinical responses with less overall toxicity than single-agent therapy (Knopf, Fischer, and Welch-McCaffrey 1984). With a few exceptions, combination chemotherapy has replaced single-agent therapy in the medical management of cancer.

The major disadvantage of single-agent therapy led to clinical trials with combinations of drugs. Some of the disadvantages noted were: single agents were unsuccessful at achieving long-term remissions; they produced cell lines that were resistant to further drug therapy; and they produced severe or lethal toxicities when given in doses adequate to irradicate the tumor (Hubbard 1981). The most significant of these disadvantages is tumor drug resistance, as this was found to be the most common reason for treatment failure.

The improved therapeutic effects of combination chemotherapy resulted from both the additive and synergistic effects of the drugs used. According to Carter and Livingston (1982), three conceptual approaches have been used in designing drug combinations. The *biochemical approach* asserts that by using drugs that individually produce different biochemical damage, one can attack different sites in the biosynthetic pathways or inhibit processes that are necessary for the normal function of essential macromolecules. The goal of the biochemical approach is to decrease the production and availability of the end products needed by the tumor for normal growth and development.

The *cytokinetic approach* is based on principles of cell cycle kinetics. This approach suggests that drugs should produce changes in cells that render them more vulnerable to cycle-specific agents. For example, it is known that "debulk-ing" a tumor by surgery or chemotherapy causes an increase in the growth fraction (the number of cells undergoing active division) of the re-maining cells. Activating cells in this way would make them vulnerable to cycle-specific agents.

The third approach is the *empirical approach*. Numerous effective combinations of agents have evolved through the use of individual agents that alone have demonstrated antineoplastic activity against a particular tumor. When combined, the mechanisms of action of the different drugs of-ten complement each other to produce maximal cell kill. A distinct advantage of combination chemotherapy is that the toxicities of the indi-vidual drugs often differ, allowing administra-tion of nearly full tolerated doses without severe toxicity. One example of an empirically derived drug combination is MOPP (mechlorethamine, vincristine, prednisone, procarbazine) for the treatment of Hodgkin's disease. The effect on the bone marrow of the drug combination MOPP plus ABVD (Adriamycin, bleomycin, vinblastine, dacarbazine) used against Hodgkin's disease is shown in figure 3.6. A closer look at this drug combination will illustrate some of the principles used in the empirical approach:

PRINCIPLE—*Each drug in the combination should be active against the tumor when used alone.*
Mechlorethamine, vincristine, procarbazine, prednisone, doxorubicin, bleomycin, vinblas-tine, and dacarbazine have all been shown to be active against Hodgkin's disease.

PRINCIPLE—*The mechanisms of action of the dif-ferent drugs should complement each other to pro-duce maximal cell kill.*
The drugs listed above are both cell cycle phase-specific and cell cycle phase nonspe-cific. For example, dacarbazine and mechlore-thamine are alkylating agents and are cell cy-cle phase nonspecific, whereas vincristine and vinblastine are both specific for the S and M phases. Using these drugs in combination the-

oretically assures that cells will be affected regardless of their cycling characteristics at the time of drug administration.

PRINCIPLE—*Drugs that produce toxicities in different organ systems should be combined so that maximal doses of each can be administered without excessive morbidity.*
In the MOPP combination, mechlorethamine is a potent myelosuppressant, whereas vin-cristine's dose-limiting toxicity is often neu-rotoxicity. Prednisone does not affect bone marrow, but sometimes causes imbalances in glucose metabolism and protein breakdown (Knopf, Fischer, and Welch-McCaffrey 1984). Procarbazine's dose-limiting toxicities are nausea and vomiting and myelosuppression, though the myelosuppression occurs much later than that of mechlorethamine (Good-man 1986).

PRINCIPLE—*Drugs should be combined that have tox-icities occurring at different times.*
As mentioned, mechlorethamine's myelosup-pressive nadir occurs at 10–14 days, where-as Procarbazine's is 2–3 weeks after cessation of therapy (Knopf, Fischer, and Welch-McCaffrey 1984). This phenomenon is illus-trated in figure 3.6.

MECHANISMS OF DRUG RESISTANCE

Despite significant advances in the treatment of certain cancers, such as testicular cancer, with curative chemotherapy, for many cancers "cura-tive" chemotherapy is unavailable and develop-ment of effective anticancer drugs for these tu-mors has reached a plateau.

One of the factors preventing the development of curative chemotherapy is the development of tumor resistance to the drug. Laboratory evi-dence has shown that exposure of a cancer cell to a *single* antineoplastic agent can lead to resis-tance to multiple agents, and many of the drugs

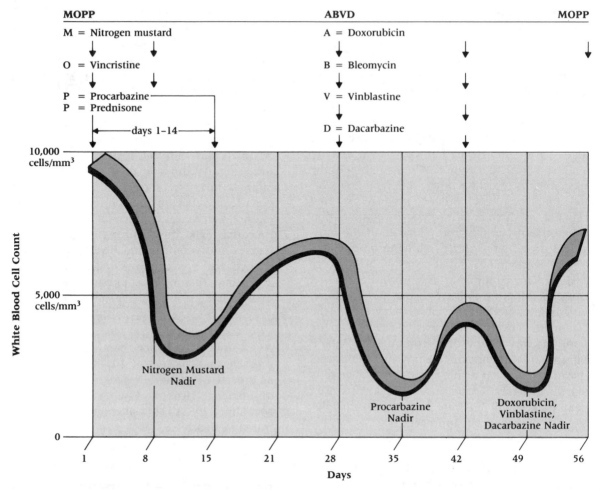

Figure 3.6 The effect of MOPP combined with ABVD on the white blood cell count
Source: Goodman 1987. Bristol-Myers U.S. Pharmaceutical and Nutritional Group. Reprinted by permission.

causing this "multidrug resistance" are natural products, such as vinblastine and Adriamycin (Trent 1989).

The presence of a large cell surface glycoprotein, called p-glycoprotein, on the cancer cells appears to be one of the most important causes of multidrug resistance. Cancer cells with multidrug resistance have a very high number of these cell surface glycoproteins while cells

sensitive to chemotherapy agents have very few if any (Trent 1989).

According to Drs. Kartner and Ling (1989), the p-glycoprotein molecule works like a pump so that chemotherapeutic drugs enter the cell, but are then quickly pumped back out of the cancer cells leaving cells undamaged by the chemotherapy. Certain normal body cells have p-glycoprotein molecules on their surface, possibly as an evolutionary protective mechanism to remove ingested toxins. As might be expected, these normal cells are found in organs frequently resistant to chemotherapy, such as the kidneys, adrenal glands, liver, and parts of the gastrointestinal tract, while cells that are extremely chemosensitive, like blood cells, have almost no p-glycoprotein (Trent 1989).

Genetically, the cells that contain p-glycoprotein and which then demonstrate multidrug resistance (MDR) usually have gene amplification of MDR, or PGY1. According to Goldstein et al. (1989), this amplified gene is transcribed into the RNA that produces the p-glycoprotein molecule. The investigators also found that the highest levels of the gene (cells having the most amplified genes) were found in chemoresistant cancers of the colon, kidney (renal cells), liver, adrenal cortex, and lung (non-small cell with neuroendocrine properties), and in pheochromocytoma, islet cell tumor of the pancreas, carcinoid tumor, and chronic myelegenous leukemia in blast crisis (Goldstein et al. 1989).

Other cellular abnormalities found in cancer cells resistant to chemotherapy include the following (Curt, Clendeninn, and Chabner 1984; Trent 1989):

Defective transport of the drug into the cell with increased drug excretion so that there are decreased intracellular concentrations of drug

Defective drug metabolism

Increased drug inactivation

Altered DNA repair with increased cell efficiency to excise or repair DNA damage caused by drug

Altered drug target, so drug cannot recognize intracellular target (i.e., enzyme, nucleotide)

As more is learned about the mechanisms of drug resistance, models can be developed and tested that target these mechanisms and attempt to make the cancer cells sensitive to chemotherapeutic agents.

Current research efforts include the following:

Identifying agents or drugs that would inactivate the p-glycoprotein molecule in cells (Kartner and Ling 1989)

Identifying agents, such as Tumor Necrosis Factor, that are more effective against resistant tumor cells (Trent 1989)

Identifying chemomodifiers that may be combined with chemotherapy agents to increase their effectiveness, such as the calcium channel blocker agents amioderone and verapamil (Trent 1989)

Some of the advantages of combination chemotherapy are: it allows for maximal cell kill within the range of toxicity tolerated by the patient for each drug, it provides for a broader range of coverage of new resistant tumor cell lines (this seems to be the major reason for the success of combination chemotherapy over single-agent therapy), and it prevents or slows the development of new resistant cell lines (DeVita 1985). An important advance made with the institution of combination chemotherapy was the use of intermittent treatment schedules, which permitted the recovery of normal tissues between treatment cycles.

In summary, combination chemotherapy has replaced single-agent chemotherapy in the medical management of most tumors because of its improved clinical responses and decreased toxicity over that seen with single-agent therapy.

INNOVATIVE USES OF CHEMOTHERAPY

Discovery of new chemotherapeutic agents has slowed in recent years. Instead, the old drugs are being used in new ways. Both autologous bone marrow transplantation and colony stimulating factors are adjuncts to giving chemotherapy in amounts previously not thought to be possible. Both of these treatments augment dose-limiting toxicity, a reason for reducing the dosage of chemotherapy or for stopping treatment altogether.

Autologous Bone Marrow Transplantation

Relatively recent advances in the technology of bone marrow transplantation (BMT) have made it look promising for the present and future treatment of selected malignancies (Freedman 1988). One of the first signs of the potential importance of BMT appeared in an article by Lorenze et al. (1951), where it was reported that the parenteral infusion of bone marrow could save the lives of lethally irradiated mice through the subsequent engraftment of the bone marrow cells. In the following years, BMT was attempted in many human subjects (predominantly oncology patients with end-stage disease). It enabled clinicians to treat tumors with significantly higher (in fact, lethal) doses of chemotherapy or radiation, as the infusion of viable bone marrow "rescued" the patient from life-threatening myelosuppression. Unfortunately, complications related to disease progression, graft versus host disease, lack of adequate blood product support, and other factors led to few successes (Doney and Buckner 1985). Refining the process of BMT and overcoming some of the complications mentioned above has led to its greater use in diseases like acute and chronic leukemia, preleukemic states, lymphoma, multiple myeloma, neuroblastoma, and some solid tumors such as lung and breast cancers as well as nonmalignant hematologic disorders (Doney and Buckner 1985).

Much of the nursing care involved in any bone marrow transplant relates to the management of the side effects of chemotherapy and radiation. For the purposes of illustration, only one type of BMT, autologous, will be outlined here.

Autologous BMT uses a patient's own bone marrow to "rescue" him from the lethal effects of antineoplastic drugs or radiation (Freedman 1988). Autologous BMT is only used in malignant diseases, and the patient is usually in remission when the treatment is given (Gorin 1986; Yeager et al. 1986). To this point, it has been difficult to interpret some of the outcome data related to autologous BMT, as it is unclear whether relapses are due to failure of the treatment to eradicate disease or due to reinfusion of diseased marrow.

There are five major phases of autologous BMT. In the *first phase*, the patient is screened for eligibility for BMT protocols, and educated as to the procedure and implications of consenting to participate in the particular BMT program. A thorough physical exam is performed, as well as several baseline studies. Every patient also undergoes a psychological assessment to determine his potential tolerance to the weeks of isolation necessary to complete the program. During the *second phase*, about one liter of bone marrow is harvested from the patient (usually from the iliac crests) through the use of multiple large-bore needle aspirations. The procedure is generally done in the operating room under general anesthesia, and a central venous access device is placed at the same time (Freedman 1988).

The *third phase*, immunosuppression, involves delivering lethal doses of chemotherapy or radiation therapy to the patient. The purposes of this phase are as follows: to destroy the immune system to decrease the possibility of graft versus host disease, to destroy remaining malignant cells, and to prepare space in the bone marrow for the new cells (Cheson and Curt 1986; Kamani and August 1984). Nursing care in the third phase focuses on management of the symptoms frequently caused by the treatment. For example, cyclophosphamide is often used as an immunosuppressive agent, and frequently causes hemorrhagic cystitis. Nursing care involves monitoring the urine for blood, and regulating the flow rate of the bladder irrigation. The *fourth phase* is the reinfusion of the bone marrow. The bone marrow, which has been filtered to remove bone chips and fat particles, is placed in a preservative and put into cold storage (Freedman 1988). When needed, it is infused as with any blood product via the venous access device or administered "IV push" using large syringes. Though the reinfusion is usually uneventful, complications such as volume overload, pulmonary abnormalities related to fat emboli, and allergic reactions have been noted (Kamani and August 1984; Hutchison and King 1983).

The *final phase*, engraftment, is characteristically a "waiting period," during which the infused marrow cells slowly engraft in the patient's bone marrow. The *physiologic* areas often needing nursing attention during this phase are:

nutrition (nausea and vomiting are sometimes severe and protracted, necessitating constant use of antiemetics; stomatitis also leads to decreased oral intake, requiring the institution of parenteral nutrition and pain relief measures);

potential for infection (monitoring for symptoms of bacterial, viral, and fungal infections, treating them with antibiotics, antifungal agents, etc., and teaching self-care measures to decrease the possibility of infection are common nursing functions); and

potential for bleeding (nursing is usually responsible for monitoring patients for signs of bleeding and anemia, and for administering blood products).

Psychosocial needs are also often addressed by nurses. The BMT process is frequently a long, difficult ordeal for the patient, who must find ways of coping with the social isolation and boredom of confinement to a single hospital room for at least six to eight weeks. The patient and family must adapt to the uncertainty of both daily changes in the patient's physical status and eventual outcome of the treatment. According to Popkin and Moldow (1977), proximity to death is perhaps the major stressor during BMT. Involvement of nurses and social workers is often critical to the effective coping of the BMT patient.

The future of BMT is at least partially dependent upon our ability to prevent or manage more effectively the complications that often arise in the course of the treatment, whether related to the treatment itself or to the patient's underlying disease process (Thomas 1988). For example, cyclophosphamide and total body irradiation are standard immunosuppressive therapies used in BMT with leukemic patients. Studies are currently underway that examine the potential role of different drug regimens and fractionated irradiation as well as different rates of irradiation exposure in causing immunosuppression (Thomas 1988).

Other studies are currently looking at ways in which stem cells might be separated from other marrow components so that the reinfused cells are concentrated and free of malignant cells. For example, marrow purging uses physical, immunologic, or pharmacologic methods to rid the marrow of malignant cells (Schryber, LaCasse, and Barton-Burke, 1987). Peripheral stem cell harvesting (in which stem cells are harvested from peripheral blood) is also being attempted, and has as its advantages no marrow tumor contamination, and no need to use general anesthesia for the harvest. It is also possible that the white blood cells would reconstitute more rapidly, because a greater number of committed progenitor cells are reinfused. Other promising technologies currently receiving attention include: use of Interferon before or after grafting for its antileukemic effect; use of growth factors such as erythropoietin, G-CSF and IL-1 to stimulate a rapid recovery of the bone marrow; use of bone-seeking radioisotopes to deliver high doses of irradiation to the marrow while sparing normal tissues; and the use of monoclonal antibodies attached to radioactive isotopes or chemotherapy which would be directed at target malignant cells (Thomas 1988).

The use of autologous bone marrow transplantation offers new frontiers for cancer chemotherapy. Along with these new frontiers come new challenges for the nurse who cares for the patient receiving this treatment modality.

Colony Stimulating Factors (CSFs)

Though they are still in the relatively early phases of clinical trials, preliminary results suggest that colony stimulating factors will become useful adjuncts to chemotherapy. As such, they deserve brief mention here. For an overview of CSFs and their use in oncology patients, the reader is referred to an article by Haeuber and DiJulio (1989).

Colony stimulating factors (also referred to as hematopoietic growth factors) are a set of humoral glycoprotein factors that stimulate the process of hematopoiesis for all major types of cells produced in the bone marrow (Haeuber and DiJulio 1989; Clark and Kamen 1987; Seiff 1987). Cells in the bone marrow are dependent upon these factors for normal growth and differentiation. CSFs are also partially responsible for maintaining dynamic equilibrium in the marrow. For example, decreased oxygen or hemorrhage might stimulate erythropoietin production, in turn causing an increase in the number of mature red blood cells in the blood. In the same way, thrombopoietin might be released in response to low platelet counts, or either granulocyte colony stimulating factor (G-CSF) or granulocyte-macrophage colony stimulating factor (GM-CSF) might be released as a response to infection (Haeuber and DiJulio 1989). The latter case is perhaps most significant for oncology patients, as neutropenia-related infection is one of the most significant causes of morbidity and mortality in the oncology patient population.

The colony stimulating factors work by attaching to receptors on the membranes of target cells and setting into action the cellular processes involved in the differentiation, maturation, or proliferation of the cells. With neutrophils, the CSFs have also been seen to increase their functional activities. The two types of CSFs that have gained the most attention in the oncology world are granulocyte-macrophage colony stimulating factor (GM-CSF) and granulocyte colony stimulating factor (G-CSF). In addition to stimulating progenitor cells to become granulocytes, macrophages, or eosinophils, GM-CSF has induced such functional changes in mature cells as enhancing phagocytic activity. G-CSF functions in a similar way on the granulocyte line of cells, but seems to be even more involved in determining functional performance of the cells than GM-CSF (Clark and Kamen 1987; Seiff 1987).

According to Haeuber and DiJulio (1989), use of GM-CSF and G-CSF in humans has focused on four subpopulations: leukopenic AIDS patients, cancer patients receiving chemotherapy, bone marrow transplant patients, and patients with myelodysplastic syndromes. In all populations studied, the CSFs have produced a dose-dependent rise in white blood cell subpopulations which fell after treatment was stopped, indicating that the CSFs may reduce the depth and length of postchemotherapy nadirs. This is particularly important, considering that myelosuppression is often a dose-limiting toxicity of chemotherapy which leads to a delay in treatment or a reduction in the dose of the drug. One author also observed that the CSFs seemed to afford a group of bladder cancer patients some protection from chemotherapy-induced mucositis commonly seen with that therapy (Gabrilove, Jakubowski, Scher, et al. 1988).

The side effects and toxicities of the CSFs are similar to those of other biological response modifiers, and tend to be mild. They include fatigue, fever, myalgia, loss of appetite, and transient bone pain. Fortunately, these side effects seldom cause patients enough discomfort to cause them to refuse further CSF treatment.

As CSFs become more widely used, it will be more important for nurses to understand their uses, administration, side effects, and the management of symptoms associated with their side effects. Nurses will need to educate patients and families as to the above, especially as the agents become more common in outpatient settings.

BIBLIOGRAPHY

Chemotherapy

Bakemeier RF (1983) Basic concepts of cancer chemotherapy and principles of medical oncology, in Rubin P (ed): *Clinical Oncology for Medical Students and Physicians: A Multidisciplinary Approach* (ed 6). New York, American Cancer Society, 82–95

Baserga R (1981) The cell cycle. *New England Journal of Medicine* 304(8): 453–459

Becker TM (1981) *Cancer Chemotherapy: A Manual for Nurses.* Boston, Little, Brown and Co.

Belinson JL (1980) Understanding how chemotherapy works. *Contemporary Obstetrics and Gynecology* 21: 2–17

Bingham CA (1978) The cell cycle and cancer chemotherapy. *American Journal of Nursing*, July, 1201–1205

Bonfiglio TA, Terry R (1983) The pathology of cancer, in Rubin P (ed): *Clinical Oncology for Medical Students and Physicians: A Multidisciplinary Approach* (ed 6). New York, American Cancer Society, 20–29

Brown J (1987) Chemotherapy, in Groenwald S (ed): *Cancer Nursing: Principles and Practice.* Boston, Jones and Bartlett, 348–384

Carter S, Livingston R (1982) Principles of cancer chemotherapy, in Carter S, Glatstein E, Livingston R: *Principles of Cancer Treatment.* New York, McGraw-Hill Book Co, 95–110

Chabner BA, Myers CE (1985) Clinical pharmacology of cancer chemotherapy, in DeVita VT, Hellman S, Rosenberg SA: *Cancer: Principles and Practice of Oncology.* Philadelphia, JB Lippincott Co, 287–327

DeVita VT (1985) Principles of chemotherapy, in DeVita VT, Hellman S, Rosenberg SA: *Cancer: Principles and Practice of Oncology.* Philadelphia, JB Lippincott Co

Goodman MS (1988) Concepts of hormonal manipulation in the treatment of cancer. *Oncology Nursing Forum* 15(5): 639–647

――― (1987) *Cancer: Chemotherapy and Care.* Bristol-Myers Oncology Division

Groenwald S (1987) *Cancer Nursing: Principles and Practice.* Boston, Jones and Bartlett

Gussack GS, Brantley BA, Farmer JC (1984) Biology of tumors and head and neck cancer chemotherapy. *Laryngoscope* 94: 1181–1187

Hill BT (1978) Cancer chemotherapy: the relevance of certain concepts of cell cycle kinetics. *Biochimica and Biophysica Acta* 516: 389–417

Hubbard SM (1981) Chemotherapy and the nurse, in Marino LB: *Cancer Nursing.* St. Louis, Mo, Mosby

Knopf MKT, Fischer DS, Welch-McCaffrey D (1984) *Cancer Chemotherapy: Treatment and Care* (ed 2). Boston, GK Hall Medical Publishers

Mitchell MS, Bertram JH (1985) Immunology and biomodulation of cancer, in Calabresi P, Schein PS, Rosenberg SA (eds): *Medical Oncology: Basic Principles and Clinical Management of Cancer.* New York, Macmillan Publishing Co

Skipper HE (1968) In *The Proliferation and Spread of Neoplastic Cells,* 21st Annual Symposium on Fundamental Cancer Research at MD Anderson Hospital and Tumor Institute, Houston, Texas. Baltimore, Williams and Wilkins Co, 213–233

Skipper HE, Shabel FM, Jr, Wilcox WS (1965) *Cancer Chemotherapy Reports* 45: 5–28

――― (1964) *Cancer Chemotherapy Reports* 35: 1–111

Weimann MC, Calabresi P (1985) Pharmacology of antineoplastic agents, in Calabresi P, Schein PS, Rosenberg SA (eds): *Medical Oncology: Basic Principles and Clinical Management of Cancer.* New York, Macmillan Publishing Co

Ziegfeld CR (ed) (1987) Chemotherapy, in *Core Curriculum for Oncology Nursing.* Philadelphia, WB Saunders Co, 225–234

BMT

Cheson BD, Curt GA (1986) Bone marrow transplantation: current perspectives and future directions. *Journal of the National Cancer Institute* 76: 1265–1267

Doney KC, Buckner CD (1985) Bone marrow transplantation: overview. *Plasma Therapy Transfusion Technology* 6: 149–161

Ford R, Ballard B (1988) Acute complications after bone marrow transplantation. *Seminars in Oncology Nursing* 4(1): 14–24

Freedman SE (1988) An overview of bone marrow transplantations. *Seminars in Oncology Nursing* 4(1): 3–8

Gorin NC (1986) Autologous bone marrow transplantation in acute leukemia. *Journal of the National Cancer Institute* 76: 1281–1287

Hutchison MM, King AH (1983) A nursing perspective on bone marrow transplantation. *Nursing Clinics of North America* 18: 511–522

Kamani N, August CS (1984) Bone marrow transplantation: problems and prospects. *Medical Clinics of North America* 68: 657–674

Lorenze E, Uphoff DE, Reid TR, et al (1951) Modification of irradiation injury in mice and guinea pigs by bone marrow injection. *Journal of the National Cancer Institute* 12: 197–201

Miller RA, Maloney DG, Warnke R, et al (1982) Treatment of B-cell lymphoma with monoclonal anti-idiotype antibody. *New England Journal of Medicine* 306: 517–522

Popkin M, Moldow C (1977) Stressors and responses during bone marrow transplantation. *Arch Internal Medicine* 137: 135

Santos GW (1984 suppl) Bone marrow transplantation in leukemia: current status. *CA* 54: 2732–2740

Schryber S, LaCasse CR, Barton-Burke M (1987) Autologous bone marrow transplantation. *Oncology Nursing Forum* 14(4): 74–80

Thomas ED (1988) The future of marrow transplantation. *Seminars in Oncology Nursing* 4(1): 74–78

——— (1985) Chronic leukemias, in DeVita VT, Hellman S, Rosenberg SA: *Cancer: Principles and Practice of Oncology*. Philadelphia, JB Lippincott Co, 1739–1752

——— (1980) Marrow transplantation for marrow failure or leukemia. *Compr Therapy* 6: 69–73

Weiden PL, Zuckerman N, Hansen JA, et al (1981) Fatal graft versus host disease in a patient with lymphoblastic leukemia following normal granulocyte transfusions. *Blood* 57: 328–332

Yeager AM, Kaizer H, Satos GW, et al (1986) Autologous bone marrow transplantation in patients with acute nonlymphocytic leukemia, using *ex vivo* marrow treatment with 4-hydroperoxycyclophosphamide. *New England Journal of Medicine* 315: 141–147

Mechanisms of Drug Resistance

Curt GA, Clendeninn NH, Chabner BA (1984) Drug resistance in cancer. *Cancer Treatment Reports* 68: 87–99

Gerlach JH, Kartner N, Bell DR, Ling V (1986) Multidrug resistance. *Cancer Surveys* 5(1): 25–46

Goldstein LJ, Galaski A, Fojo M, et al (1989) Expression of a multidrug resistance gene in human cancers. *Journal of the National Cancer Institute* 81(2): 116–124

Kartner N, Ling V (1989) Multidrug resistance in cancer. *Scientific American* 260(3): 44–51

Pastran I, Gottesman M (1987) Multiple drug resistance in human cancer. *New England Journal of Medicine* Vol. 316: 1388–1393

Trent JM (1989) Mechanisms of drug resistance, in *Proceedings, Advances in Clinical Oncology*, Snowbird, Utah, March 1989, 33–35

CSFs

Clark S, Kamen R (1987) Hemopoietic colony stimulating factors. *Science* 236(805): 1229–1237

Gabrilove JH, Jakubowski A, Sher H, et al (1988) Effect of granulocyte colony stimulating factors on neutropenia and associated morbidity due to chemotherapy for transitional-cell carcinoma of the urethelium. *New England Journal of Medicine* 318(22): 1414–1422

Haeuber D, DiJulio JE (1989) Hemopoietic colony stimulating factors: an overview. *Oncology Nursing Forum* 16(2): 247–255

Seiff C (1987) Hematopoetic growth factors. *Journal of Clinical Investigation* 79: 1549–1557

4

POTENTIAL TOXICITIES AND NURSING MANAGEMENT

INTRODUCTION

Cancer is a disease of the cell. Cancer chemotherapeutic agents, or antineoplastic agents, are intended to interfere with cell replication to bring about either tumor cell kill (via cytotoxic drugs) or cessation of growth (via cytostatic drugs). However, as yet, we are unable to target chemotherapy agents directly against tumor cells exclusively, sparing normal, rapidly dividing cells. As a result, we see temporary damage in normal frequently dividing, or proliferating, cell populations such as bone marrow, gastrointestinal mucosa, gonads, and hair follicles. Damage to normal cells is usually temporary, because normal cells have better repair mechanisms than malignant cells.

In addition, certain drugs may have an affinity for specific organ(s) in the body, and cause organ toxicity over time. For example, doxorubicin, an anthracycline drug, may cause myofibril damage in the heart, leading to increased risk of cardiomyopathy with cumulative drug doses over 450 mg/m^2–550 mg/m^2.

As nurses, we are taught to monitor patient tolerance of drugs, and to discuss drug discontinuance with the physician when signs or symptoms of drug toxicity are observed (Levine 1978). As oncology nurses caring for patients receiving chemotherapy, we *expect* certain toxicities such as neutropenia, that would otherwise not be tolerated with other medications. Our role as patient educators is to teach patients and families self-care, and our competent assessment and intervention to minimize complications and optimize patient tolerance of therapy are crucial for patient safety and quality of life. We work closely with other members of an interdisciplinary team to accomplish this. In order to better understand chemotherapy-related toxicities, it is important to understand the timing and mechanism of occurrence.

Perry and Yarbro (1984) have classified common toxicities by time of occurrence, whether onset is immediate, early, or late. These include the following:

1. *Immediate onset, hours to days after administration:* nausea/vomiting, phlebitis, hyperuricemia, renal failure, anaphylaxis, skin rash, teratogenicity. Specific drugs may cause: hemorrhagic cystitis (Cytoxan), radiation recall (actinomycin D), fever/chills (bleomycin), hypertension (procarbazine), and hypotension (etoposide).

2. *Early onset, days to weeks:* leukopenia, thrombocytopenia, alopecia, stomatitis, diarrhea, megaloblastosis. Specific drugs may cause: paralytic ileus (vincristine), hypercalcemia

49

(estrogens, antiestrogens), hypomagnesemia (cisplatin), pancreatitis (L-asparaginase), fluid retention (estrogen, steroids), pulmonary infiltrates (methotrexate, bleomycin), and ototoxicity (cisplatin).

3. *Delayed onset, weeks to months:* anemia, aspermia, hepatocellular damage, hyperpigmentation, pulmonary fibrosis. Specific drugs may cause: peripheral neuropathy (vincristine, cisplatin), cardiac necrosis (Adriamycin, cyclophosphamide), SIADH (cyclophosphamide, vincristine), and hemolytic-uremic syndrome (mitomycin C).

4. *Late onset, months to years:* sterility, hypogonadism, premature menopause, second malignancy. Specific drugs may cause: hepatic fibrosis/cirrhosis (methotrexate), encephalopathy (methotrexate; CNS radiation), and cancer of the bladder (cyclophosphamide).

This chapter will focus on common toxicities, and examine pathophysiologic mechanisms, nursing management, and patient teaching strategies to minimize complications and optimize patient tolerance of treatment.

The first section addresses chemotherapy-induced damage to rapidly proliferating normal cell populations: the bone marrow, the gastrointestinal tract epithelium, the hair follicles of the scalp, and the gonads.

Following this, the next section deals with specific organ toxicities, drugs implicated, and specific principles the interdisciplinary team uses to monitor for or prevent toxicity. Appendix 1 supplies a table that quantifies common toxicities, and provides a mechanism to define, compare, and evaluate toxicity in chemotherapy regimens. This table was developed in 1988 by the National Cancer Institute together with cooperative groups such as the CALGB (Cancer and Leukemia Group B), SWOG (Southwest Oncology Group), and ECOG (Eastern Cooperative Oncology Group). It is suggested that the reader review this table prior to reading this chapter.

SECTION A. TOXICITY TO RAPIDLY PROLIFERATING NORMAL CELL POPULATIONS

I. BONE MARROW DEPRESSION (BMD)

Introduction

The bone marrow is an organ that is constantly active, responding to the human body's need for white blood cells to protect against infection, red blood cells to carry oxygen to the body's cells, and platelets to prevent bleeding. Chemotherapy works by interfering with cell division of frequently dividing cells, so the bone marrow stem cells, which divide frequently to provide the formed blood cell elements as needed by the body, are often temporarily injured by chemotherapy. In fact, bone marrow depression may become the dose-limiting toxicity for many drugs. In order to understand the potential damage of chemotherapy on the bone marrow, it is helpful to review the normal development of blood cells in the bone marrow. It is believed that all cells develop from a pluripotent stem cell, which has the ability to differentiate and mature into the formed blood cell elements seen in the peripheral blood (see figure 4.1).

Leukocytes, or white blood cells, are composed of five different cell types (McConnell 1986), which can be separated into two groups: those with granules in their cytoplasm (*granulocytes*), and those without. Most important of the granulocytes are the *neutrophils*, which are the body's first line of internal defense against infection or invading microorganisms. These cells represent the largest number of white blood cells, and converge at the site of infection. Thus, when the infection is severe, so many neutrophils are needed to halt the infection that the bone marrow releases immature neutrophils, called *bands*

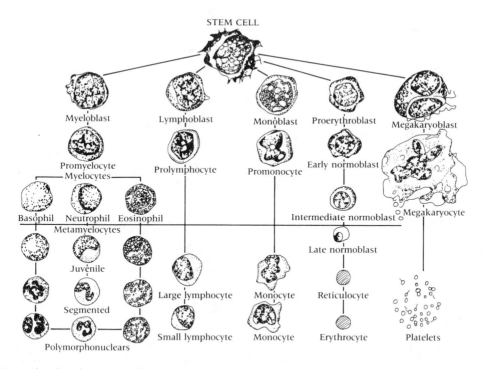

Figure 4.1   The development of the various formed elements of the blood from bone marrow cells

or *stabs*, or perhaps even more immature cells, into the peripheral bloodstream. This is called a *shift to the left*. There is an increased percentage of neutrophils and usually an increased number of white blood cells overall (leukocytosis) in a left shift. Bacterial infections in general cause a rise in the percentage of neutrophils, whereas viral infections may decrease the neutrophil count (McConnell 1986). Other granulocytes are the *eosinophils*, which are active against allergens and parasites, and *basophils*, which have a role in histamine production and fibrinolysis, and are released during chronic inflammation. The white blood cells without granules are the *lymphocytes*, which provide cell-mediated immunity (T-cells), and antibody production (B-cells), and the *monocytes*, which represent the body's second line of defense, destroying remaining microorganisms and removing debris from the site of infection.

Monocytes are helpful in phagocytosing both mycobacteria and fungi.

Chemotherapy does not affect circulating, mature blood cells because they are no longer dividing. Rather, chemotherapy damages stem cells which have a cell generation time of 6–24 hours (Brager and Yasko 1984), decreasing the bone marrow's ability to replace the body's used blood cell elements, in particular the neutrophils and platelets. Because all blood cells have a fixed life span (white blood cells—6 hours, platelets about 10 days, and red blood cells about 120 days), the effect in lowering the blood counts occurs at a predictable time *after* the chemotherapy is administered, usually 7–14 days depending on the specific drug. The *lowest* point reached in the peripheral blood count after chemotherapy is administered is called the *nadir* (see table 4.1).

Table 4.1 Bone Marrow Depression: Expected Time of Drug Nadirs

Drug Class	Nadir	Recovery
I. Alkylating Agents		
a. mechlorethamine (nitrogen mustard)	7–15 days	28 days
b. melphalan (Alkeran)	10–12	42–50
c. busulfan (Myleran)	11–30	24–54 days
d. chlorambucil (Leukeran)	14–28	28–42
e. cyclophosphamide (Cytoxan)	8–14	18–25
f. ifosfamide	mild	after 2 weeks
g. cisplatin (Platinol)	14	21
h. carboplatin	18–24	4–6 weeks
i. dacarbazine (DTIC)	21–28	28–35
j. nitrosoureas		
carmustine (BCNU)	26–30	35–49
lomustine (CCNU)	40–50	60
semustine (MeCCNU)	28–63	82–89
streptozocin (Zanosar)	as single agent not myelosuppressive	
II. Antimetabolites		
a. cytosine arabinoside (Ara-C)	12–14	22–24
b. fluorouracil (5-FU)	7–14	16–24
c. methotrexate (MTX)	7–14	14–21
d. mercaptopurine (6MP)	7–14	14–21
e. hydroxyurea (Hydrea)	18–30	21–35
f. 5-Azacytadine	14–17	28–31
III. Vinca Alkaloids		
a. vincristine (VCR)	4–5 but relatively nonmyelosuppressive	7
b. Velban (Vlb)	5–9	14–21
c. vindesine	5–10	10 days
IV. Podophyllotoxins		
a. etoposide (VP-16)	9–14	20–22
b. VM-26	3–14	28
V. Antibiotics		
a. bleomycin (Blenoxane)	nonmyelosuppressive	
b. daunorubicin (Daunomycin, Cerubidine)	10–14	21
c. doxorubicin (Adriamycin)	10–14	21–24
d. actinomycin (actinomycin D)	14–21	22–25
e. mitomycin C (Mutamycin)	28–42	42–56
f. mithramycin (mithracin)	14	21–28
VI. Steroids (do not cause myelosuppression)		
VII. Miscellaneous		
a. mitoxantrone (Novantrone)	8–10	after 2 weeks
b. procarbazine (Matulane)	25–36	36–50
c. asparaginase (Elspar)	not myelosuppressive	

Source: Modified from Dorr RT, Fritz W (1980) *Cancer Chemotherapy Handbook*, New York, Elsevier Press, 103–104

Certain alkylating agents, such as mechlorethamine (nitrogen mustard) and the nitrosoureas (e.g., lomustine (CCNU)) cause direct stem cell suppression (Dorr and Fritz 1980). Fortunately, many cells in the bone marrow are not actively dividing, with as many as 15–50% of stem cells in the G_0 or resting stage, so that the stem cells can escape from cell cycle phase specific agents. As shown in table 4.1, phase-specific agents, such as the antimetabolites, cause fairly rapid nadirs (7–30 days) with brisk recovery, followed by cell cycle nonphase specific agents such as doxorubicin with nadirs occurring 10–14 days, and recovery in 21–24 days. Finally, the cell cycle nonspecific agents such as the nitrosoureas produce delayed and prolonged bone marrow depression, with nadirs occurring 26–63 days, and recovery in 35–89 days (Bergsagel 1971) (see figure 4.2). Thus, in combination chemotherapy, a drug with an early nadir and recovery in 21–28 days can be administered every 3–4 weeks, in contrast to those with delayed bone marrow depression which can be administered only every 6–8 weeks. In addition, agents like the nitrosoureas may have a cumulative effect, causing severe and less reversible damage to the bone marrow, decreasing bone marrow reserve, and resulting in protracted bone marrow depression (leukopenia and thrombocytopenia). Certain chemotherapeutic agents do not cause significant bone marrow depression: these are vincristine, bleomycin, cisplatin in moderate doses, L-asparaginase, and steroid hormones.

The degree of bone marrow depression is also influenced by other host factors, as seen in table 4.2.

Nursing Management of the Patient with Bone Marrow Depression

Infection occurs frequently in the course of cancer illness and treatment. It is a very serious complication, and is the most common cause of cancer deaths (Brandt 1984). Thus, nursing care is directed toward the prevention of infection if possible, or early identification and intervention

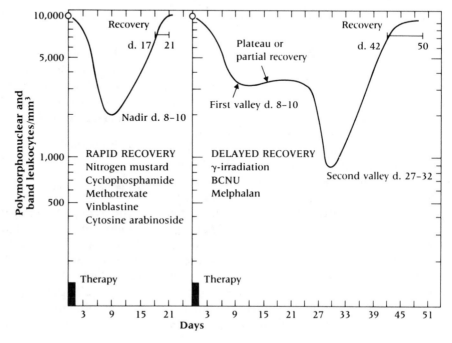

Figure 4.2 Times to recovery of peripheral granulocyte counts following administration of antitumor drugs

Source: From Bersagel DE, An assessment of massive-dose chemotherapy of malignant disease. Originally published in *Canadian Medical Association Journal*, Vol. 104, 1971. Reprinted with permission.

RAPID RECOVERY
Nitrogen mustard
Cyclophosphamide
Methotrexate
Vinblastine
Cytosine arabinoside

DELAYED RECOVERY
γ-irradiation
BCNU
Melphalan

Table 4.2 Factors Affecting the Degree of Bone Marrow Depression

Factor	Influence
1. Age	Advancing age is often associated with reduced functional bone marrow reserves so recovery may be delayed. Studies have shown that many elderly patients are able to tolerate full doses, however (Blesch 1988).
2. Drug dose	The higher the dose of a myelosuppressive drug, the greater the degree of bone marrow suppression. Of greatest importance is the depression of the granulocytes (see figure 4.3).
3. Nutritional state	Protein-calorie malnutrition may reduce the ability to repair normal cells damaged by chemotherapy.
4. Bone marrow reserve	When reserve is limited, bone marrow recovery is delayed with prolonged neutropenia or thrombocytopenia, and a subsequent need to delay treatment or reduce drug dosage. Reserves may be reduced in individuals who have histories of significant alcohol abuse (fatty marrow), and those with tumor invasion of the bone marrow (myelophthisic), with bone marrow failure.
5. Ability to metabolize drug	Renal or hepatic dysfunction can decrease drug metabolism and elimination, resulting in prolonged, elevated circulating blood levels of drug with consequent increased toxicity.
6. Prior treatment	Radiation to sites of bone marrow production (ends of long bones, skull, sternum, ribs, vertebrae, sacrum, upper and lower limb girdles) or prior chemotherapy may cause bone marrow atrophy or fibrosis and decreased bone marrow reserves (hypocellularity).
7. Sequestration of drug	Drugs such as methotrexate are sequestered in physiologic effusions, then slowly released into the systemic circulation with prolonged toxicity.

to prevent further injury. *The single most important risk factor for bacterial infection is a decreased number of neutrophils* (Fox 1981), so it is essential to be familiar with the calculation of the absolute neutrophil count in caring for patients receiving chemotherapy. Normal values for the elements in a white blood cell differential are shown in table 4.3. In determining the numbers of cell elements, 100 cells are examined, and the differential shows how many of the 100 cells are each type of white blood cell. Because the immature neutrophil, called the *band*, is effective in fighting against infection, the number of bands is added to the number of neutrophils first. This figure is easily converted to a percentage by dividing by 100. Thus, to calculate the absolute number of neutrophils in the total white blood count, the number of neutrophils and bands in 100 white

blood cells examined is converted to a percentage, then this index is multiplied times the total number of white blood cells because it is known that this percentage of them should be neutrophils. The formula looks like this:

$$\frac{\textit{Number of neutrophils/mm}^3}{\textit{(absolute neutrophil count)}} = \frac{\textit{white blood cell count}}{\textit{(number of cells/mm}^3)} \times$$

$$\frac{\textit{\% of neutrophils}}{\textit{(including band forms)}}$$

For example, your patient has a total white blood count of 10,000/mm^3. He has no clinical signs of infection, and the differential shows that there are 65 neutrophils, 2 bands, 1 eos, 3 monos, and 29 lymphs. This number should total 100. Because you are interested in the number of neutrophils that fight against infection, you add the neutrophils (65) and the bands

Table 4.3 Normal Values of the White Blood Count Differential

Cell Element	Percentage of Total	Absolute Count
Total WBC Leukocytes	100	5000–10,000/mm³
Neutrophils	50–70	2500–7000/mm³
Lymphocytes	20–40	1000–400/mm³
Monocytes	2–6	100–600/mm³
Eosinophils	1–4	50–400/mm³
Basophils	0.5–1	25–50/mm³

Source: Modified from McConnel EA March *Nursing '86.* © 1986. Springhouse Corporation, 1111 Bethlehem Pike, Springhouse, Pa 19477. All Rights Reserved.

(2), arriving at 67. Thus, 67 of the 100 cells are able to fight against bacterial infection. This number is converted to a percentage: 67 ÷ 100 = 0.67, then multiplied by the total white blood count to approximate the total or absolute number of neutrophils in the body. This equals 6700/mm³, which falls within the normal range of table 4.3.

Normally, leukocytes number 5000–10,000/mm³ cells, and of these, neutrophils represent roughly 50–70%. A normal neutrophil count is 3150–6200/mm³, with polymorphonuclear cells (segs) accounting for 3000–5800/mm³, and bands 150–400/mm³. *Neutropenia* is defined as a neutrophil count less than 2500/mm³. It is easy to understand why *neutropenia is the single most important risk factor in bacterial infection:* there are inadequate numbers of these protective cells to phagocytose and wall off invading microorganisms, and if immature cells are released, they are limited in their effectiveness. The relative risk of bacterial infection *increases* as the absolute neutrophil count *decreases:* there is no significant risk when the absolute neutrophil count is 1500–2000/mm³; there is minimal risk 1000–1500/mm³; moderate risk 500–1000/mm³; and severe risk when the absolute neutrophil count is less than 500/mm³ (Fox 1981).

Bacterial infections are most often related to gram-negative microorganisms (Rodriguez and Ketchel 1981). The longer the duration of neutropenia the greater the risk for infection. In a study by Bodey et al. (1966), the risk was 60% if neutropenia lasted 3 weeks; if the absolute neutrophil count (ANC) was < 100/mm³ during this time, the risk was 100%. Further compromise may occur with lymphopenia occurring 1–2 days after chemotherapy, with recovery in 2–3 days, and corticosteroid-induced T-cell lymphocyte and macrophage dysfunction if steroids are used in treatment (Brager and Yasko 1984). Invasion by microorganisms and infection can be reduced in the neutropenic patient by maintaining intact skin and mucous membrane barriers, eliminating exposure to infecting organisms such as those on the hands of health care workers, and maintaining a well-nourished state which promotes immunocompetence with functioning lymphocytes and antibody formation.

Studies have shown that it is the patient's own normal flora that causes approximately 85%

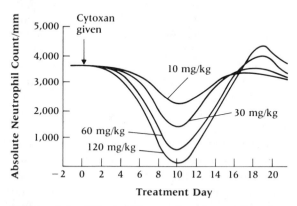

Figure 4.3 Effect of increasing doses of cyclophosphamide on peripheral blood granulocyte counts

Source: From Braine HG, Infectious complications of granulocytopenia after cancer therapy, in Abeloff, Martin D., ed., *Complications of Cancer: Diagnosis and Management,* The Johns Hopkins University Press, Baltimore/London, 1980, Fig. 6-3, p. 152. Reprinted with permission.

of infections in the neutropenic patient. Fever is usually the first sign of infection, and because of the absence of significant numbers of neutrophils, other signs are absent, such as pus formation or consolidation on a chest X ray. Fever (101°F or 38.3°C) in a neutropenic patient, if untreated, can result in death within 48 hours in up to 50% of patients, because sepsis can develop so quickly (Carlson 1985). Thus, infection becomes a medical emergency. Although 40% to 60% of patients with fever never show a culture-proven infection (Pizzo 1983), cultures of potential sites of infection are done, a chest X ray is taken, and empiric broad spectrum antibiotic coverage is started to suppress colonizing organisms. If fever persists, then antifungal therapy is usually instituted.

The most common infective organisms are the gram-negative bacilli such as *Pseudomonas aeruginosa, Klebsiella pneumoniae,* and *Escherichia coli;* next common are fungi, such as *Candida albicans* and *C. aspergillus* (Pizzo 1983), and the increasing incidence of fungi appears related to the widespread use of prophylactic antibiotics. Also, gram-positive organisms are becoming more common, such as *Staphylococcus aureus* and *Staphylococcus epidermidis* (Pizzo 1983). The most common sites of infection are the upper and lower respiratory tract (i.e., pneumonia), and the blood (bacteremias); other less commonly occurring sites are pharynx (pharyngitis or stomatitis), esophagus (esophagitis), perianal region, skin, urinary tract, and central nervous system (Rodriguez and Ketchel 1981).

It is important to look at potential routes of exposure that may lead to colonization of organisms in the neutropenic patient. These are shown in figure 4.4, and include health care providers who do not wash their hands and carry microorganisms from one patient to another, fresh fruits or leafy vegetables which may contain klebsiella or pseudomonas, standing water which may contain pseudomonas, fresh flowers or plants, and the air. In order to reduce the acquisition of new potential pathogens, patients

with an ANC of 500 or less are placed on neutropenic precautions. Scrupulous handwashing with soap, water, and friction prior to entering the patient's room, and between contact with different parts of the patient's body, is the most effective method to prevent spread of microorganisms (Pizzo and Schimpff 1983). If possible the patient should be placed in a private room, but research has shown that there is no significant difference in infection rates between neutropenic patients receiving standard hospital care and those on simple protective isolation as long as scrupulous handwashing was used (Golden 1971; Neuseff and Maki 1981). Total protected environments using laminar flow rooms and GI decontamination have significantly reduced the incidence of infection in neutropenic patients; because of the cost and availability of these environments, they are used primarily for patients undergoing bone marrow transplants (Bodey 1984).

The standardized nursing care plan for the patient experiencing bone marrow depression, with the potential for neutropenia and injury related to infection, is shown at the end of this section. Nursing interventions are aimed at prevention of infection by maintaining intact skin and mucous membranes, and minimizing exposure to environmental sources of infection, as well as early diagnosis and intervention if infection occurs. Because most chemotherapy is administered to ambulatory patients in outpatient settings, patient and family education to prepare the patient for self-care, and specifically for protection from infection and self-assessment if infection occurs, should begin before chemotherapy is initiated.

Bone marrow depression, and neutropenia specifically, often represent the dose-limiting toxicity of chemotherapy. To attempt to increase bone marrow recovery after chemotherapy administration, thus protecting against the dangers of neutropenia, and permitting increased drug doses to be delivered, research is currently exploring the use of Granulocyte-Macrophage Colony Stimulating Factor (GM-CSF), a glycoprotein

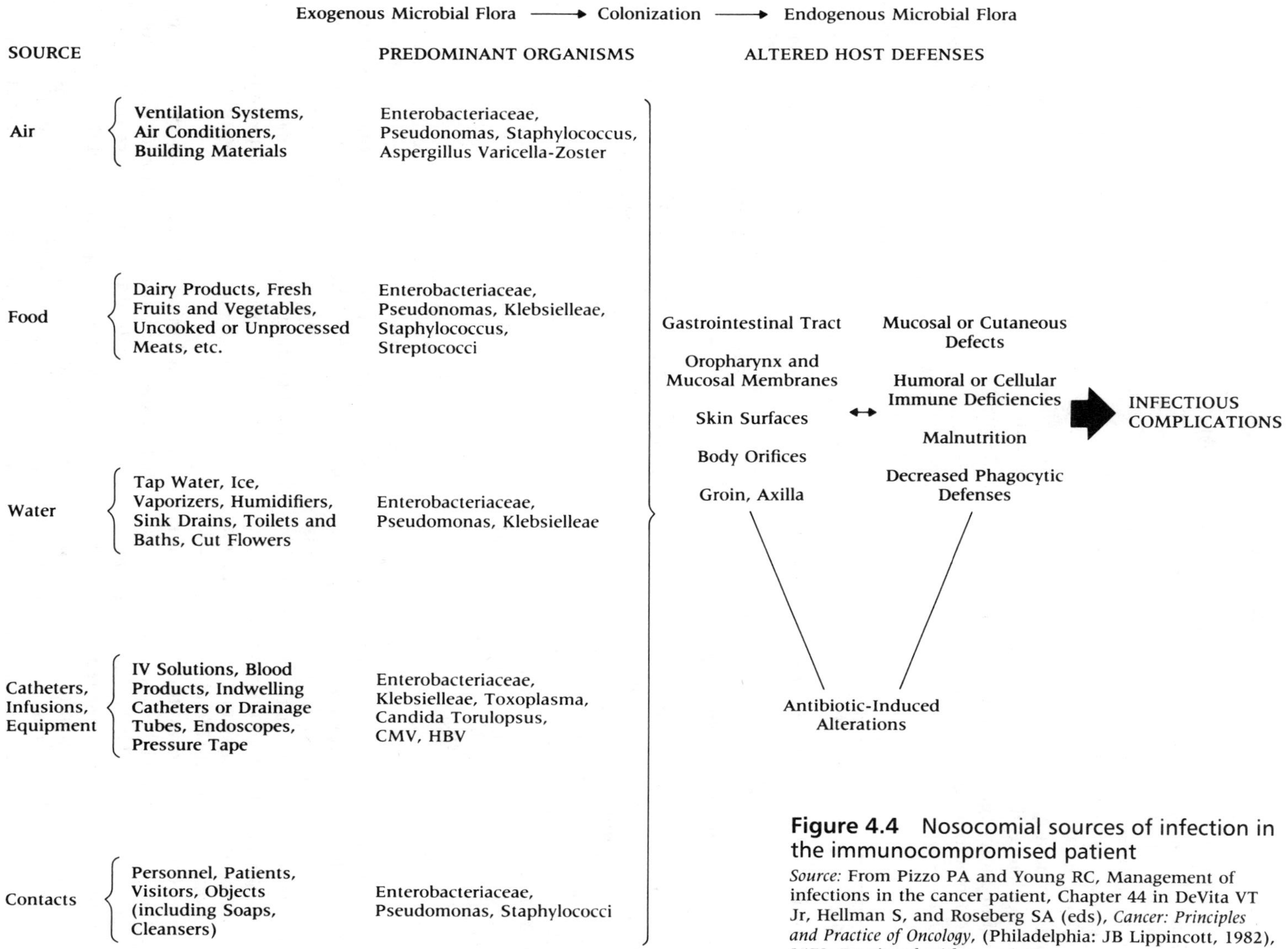

Figure 4.4 Nosocomial sources of infection in the immunocompromised patient

Source: From Pizzo PA and Young RC, Management of infections in the cancer patient, Chapter 44 in DeVita VT Jr, Hellman S, and Roseberg SA (eds), *Cancer: Principles and Practice of Oncology,* (Philadelphia: JB Lippincott, 1982), 1679. Reprinted with permission.

that controls the production, differentiation, and function of the granulocytes and monocyte-macrophages. GM-CSF not only appears to speed the recovery of myelopoiesis after chemotherapy, but also permits higher dosing and more frequent administration of myelosuppressive chemotherapy. In addition, GM-CSF appears to enhance the effectiveness of 1) granulocyte infection fighting, and 2) tumoricidal activity of macrophages (Antman, Griffin, Elias et al. 1988).

Bone Marrow Depression: Thrombocytopenia

Platelets are formed in the bone marrow, and as shown in figure 4.5, arise from megakaryocytes. As they are released from the bone marrow, the megakaryocytes break into tiny fragments called *platelets*. Platelets are important in blood coagulation and represent a key element in hemostasis. Platelets are important in maintaining capillary (vascular) integrity: platelets will adhere to sites of injury in the blood vessel wall, creating a plug that stops blood loss; also, platelets release Factor 3 which initiates clot formation, and also participate in clot retraction (Wroblewski and Wroblewski 1981).

As has previously been discussed, chemotherapy does not damage mature, circulating formed blood cell elements. Rather, the damage to the rapidly dividing progenitor stem cells prevents the platelets from being replaced once they have completed their usefulness in the body. This decrease in platelets is gradual because the life span of a platelet is about ten days, with a nadir that often occurs after that of the white blood cell. Recovery of the white blood cell count usually occurs first, followed by the platelets, and lastly, the red blood cell count. Bone marrow depression of the platelet stem cells may result in *thrombocytopenia*, a decrease in platelet count of less than 100,000/mm³, and increased risk of bleeding. The normal platelet count is 150,000–350,000/mm³. Risk of serious bleeding

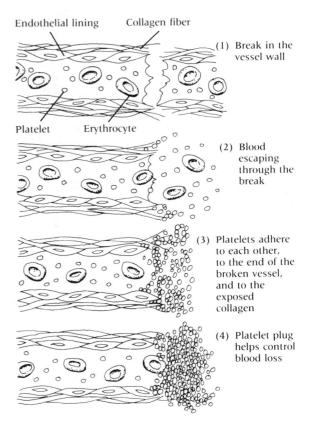

Figure 4.5 Platelet formation

(1) Break in the vessel wall

(2) Blood escaping through the break

(3) Platelets adhere to each other, to the end of the broken vessel, and to the exposed collagen

(4) Platelet plug helps control blood loss

increases as the platelet count decreases: it is mild when the platelet count is 50,000–100,000/mm³; moderate when 20,000–50,000/mm³; and severe when the platelet count is less than 20,000/mm³, with increased risk of spontaneous bleeding. This risk further increases as platelets fall below 10,000/mm³, especially for GI or CNS hemorrhage, and usually requires platelet transfusion.

Drugs that inhibit prostaglandin synthesis, or that interfere with platelet function or production, increase the risk of bleeding. These medications should be avoided if possible, and include all aspirin-containing drugs and nonsteroidal antiinflammatory drugs (NSAIDs) (see table 4.4). Other factors that increase the risk of bleeding are: bone marrow infiltration by tumor (such as leukemia or metastatic cancer which crowd out the normal cell elements in the bone marrow and decrease the number of precursor megakaryocytes); and radiation-induced depression of bone marrow stem cells when the radiation port includes active marrow sites of skull, ribs, sternum, vertebrae, pelvis, and ends of long bones. Nursing care is directed at prevention of bleeding, or if this is not possible, early identification and intervention to minimize bleeding, and this is described in the standardized nursing care plan for care of the patient with bone marrow depression at the end of this section.

Bone marrow depression causes several changes in a patient's physiological and psychosocial functioning. Figure 4.6 illustrates the potential patient problems associated with bone marrow depression and their interrelatedness. These changes will be discussed in the care plan for bone marrow depression.

Initial patient education prior to chemotherapy administration includes avoidance of medications that increase the risk of bleeding, self-assessment for signs of bleeding, and avoidance of injury (table 4.5). Assessment by the nurse of injury potential (bleeding) includes laboratory

Table 4.4 Medications that May Interfere with Platelet Function

Nonprescription products containing aspirin			
Product	(Manufacturer)	**Product**	(Manufacturer)
Alka-Seltzer Effervescent Tablets	(Miles Laboratories)	**Ecotrin Tablets**	(Smith Kline Consumer)
Alka-Seltzer Plus		**Empirin Tablets**	(Burroughs Wellcome)
Cold Medicine Tablets	(Miles Laboratories)	**Excedrin Tablets & Capsules**	(Bristol-Myers Products)
Anacin Tablets and Capsules,			
Maximum Strength	(Whitehall)	**4-Way Cold Tablets**	(Bristol-Myers Products)
Arthritis Pain Formula Tablets	(Whitehall)		
Arthritis Strength Bufferin Tablets	(Bristol-Myers Products)	**Goody's Headache Powder**	(Goody's)
Arthropan Liquid	(Purdue Frederick)		
A.S.A. Tablets/Aspirin Tablets		**Maximum Bayer Aspirin**	(Glenbrook)
A.S.A. Enseals	(Lilly)	**Measurin Caplets**	(Winthrop Pharmaceuticals)
Ascriptin Tablets	(Rorer Consumer)	**Midol Caplets**	(Glenbrook)
Ascriptin Tablets, Extra Strength	(Rorer Consumer)	**Mobigesic Tablets**	(Ascher)
Aspergum	(chewing gum)	**Momentum Muscular**	
		Backache Formula Tablets	(Whitehall)
Bayer Aspirin Tablets	(Glenbrook)		
Bayer Children's Aspirin Tablets	(Glenbrook)	**Os-Cal-Gesic Tablets**	
Bayer Children's Cold Tablets	(Glenbrook)		
Bayer Timed-Release Aspirin Tablets	(Glenbrook)	**Pabalate**	(Robins)
Bufferin Tablets	(Bristol-Myers Products)	**Pepto-Bismol Tablets & Suspension**	(Proctor & Gamble)
Bufferin, Arthritis Strength Tablets	(Bristol-Myers Products)		
Bufferin, Extra Strength Tablets	(Bristol-Myers Products)	**St. Joseph Aspirin for Children**	(Plough)
		St. Joseph Cold Tablets for Children	(Plough)
Cama Arthritis Pain Reliever	(Sandoz Consumer)	**Sine-Off Sinus Medicine Tablets—**	
Congesprin Chewable Tablets	(Bristol-Myers Products)	**Aspirin Formula**	(Smith Kline Consumer)
Cope Tablets		**Supac Tablets**	(Mission)
Coricidin "D" Decongestant Tablets	(Schering)	**Synalgos Capsules**	(Wyeth-Ayerst)
Coricidin Tablets	(Schering)		
Cosprin 325 Tablets	(Glenbrook)	**Triaminicin Tablets**	(Sandoz Consumer)
Cosprin 650 Tablets	(Glenbrook)	**Trigesic**	(Squibb)
Dasin Capsules	(Beechum Labs)	**Vanquish Caplets**	(Glenbrook)
Doan's Pills	(CIBA Consumer)		
Duradyne Tablets			

(continued)

Table 4.4 *(continued)*

Prescription products containing aspirin		
Axotal Tablets	(Adria)	
		Methocarbamol with Aspirin Tablets (Par)
		Micrainin Tablets (Wallace)
B-A C Tablets and Capsules	(Mayrand)	Mobidin Tablets (Ascher)
Bufferin with Codeine No. 3 Tablets		
		Norgesic & Norgesic Forte Tablets (3M Riker)
Darvon with A.S.A Pulvules	(Lilly)	
Darvon Compound Pulvules	(Lilly)	Pabalate-SF Tablets (Robins)
Darvon Compound-65	(Lilly)	Percodan & Percodan-Demi Tablets (DuPont
Darvon-N with A.S.A.	(Lilly)	Pharmaceuticals)
Disalcid Capsules	(3M Riker)	Propoxyphene Compound 65 (Lemmon)
Easprin	(Parke-Davis)	Robaxisal Tablets (Robins)
Empirin with Codeine Tablets	(Burroughs Wellcome)	
Equagesic Tablets	(Wyeth-Ayerst)	Synalgos-DC Capsules (Wyeth-Ayerst)
Fiorinal Tablets	(Sandoz Pharmaceuticals)	Talwin Compound Tablets (Winthrop Pharmaceuticals)
Fiorinal with Codeine	(Sandoz Pharmaceuticals)	Trilisate Tablets and Liquid (Purdue Frederick)
Magan Tablets	(Adria)	Zorprin Tablets (Boots-Flint)
Magsal Tablets	(U.S. Pharmaceuticals)	

Important note: Not a complete list. Other products may also contain aspirin or similar ingredients. Always ask your doctor or pharmacist before taking *any* medication.
Adapted from: *1990 Physicians' Desk Reference, 44th edition,* Oradell, NJ: Medical Economics Company, Inc.

platelet count and its relationship to the expected nadir for specific chemotherapy drugs received, past nadir counts, and medications that may interfere with platelet function. Patient assessment is directed to the systems where most frequent bleeding due to thrombocytopenia occurs (Spross 1985):

gastrointestinal: guaiac emesis, feces; monitor orthostatic vital signs if bleeding suspected and patient can tolerate it

skin and mucous membranes: inspect for *petechiae* (pinpoint capillary hemorrhages on distal extremities; presence of *ecchymoses* or oozing of blood from gums, nose; prolonged oozing from venipuncture sites

genitourinary: hemestick urine, assess for heavy or prolonged menses

respiratory: assess for blood in sputum

central nervous system (intracranial): monitor for any changes in neuro vital signs—blurred

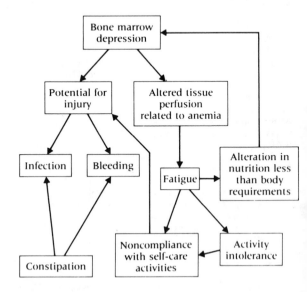

Figure 4.6 Schema for potential patient problems associated with bone marrow depression

Table 4.5 Patient Instructions to Avoid Injury Related to Thrombocytopenia

1. Use soft toothbrush or sponge-tipped applicator.
2. Use electric razor rather than blade razor.
3. Have regular bowel movements (prevent constipation).
4. Avoid vaginal douches, rectal suppositories, enemas.
5. Avoid aspirin, aspirin-containing drugs, and other medications that interfere with platelet function. Avoid alcohol.
6. Blow nose gently, don't bend over so that head is below shoulders.
7. Use water-based lubricant prior to sexual intercourse; avoid anal intercourse.
8. Avoid use of dental floss and toothpicks.
9. Avoid cutting toenails and fingernails; use nailfile.
10. Avoid bumps or falls.
11. If taking corticosteroid medication, make certain you take medication with food, and eat in-between meal snacks.
12. Avoid tight-fitting or constrictive clothing.
13. Report any signs of bleeding or changes in neurologic status.

vision, headaches, disorientation, loss of co-ordination, changes in mental status, irritability, changes in pupil size, reactivity to light

If the platelet count is less than 50,000/mm³, then platelet precautions should be instituted. Intervention is aimed at preventing injury by maintaining intact skin and mucosal membrane barriers. Intramuscular injections, rectal manipulation, deep endotracheal suctioning, and urinary catheterization should be avoided because bleeding may occur secondary to damage to mucosal surfaces or injury to the skin. Pressure should be applied to venipuncture sites for at least five minutes so that an effective platelet plug can form, and venipunctures should be minimized. If the female patient has prolonged menses, or menses occur during thrombocytopenia, discuss with the physician use of medro-xyprogesterone or other hormones to delay menses (Spross 1985) or induce amenorrhea. A safe environment should be maintained for the patient at all times.

Hemorrhage is a life-threatening complication of thrombocytopenia. Early GI bleeding may be detected by testing emesis and stool for occult blood. In order to reduce the risk of intracranial hemorrhage, discourage patient from heavy lifting and use of the Valsalva maneuver (Wroblewski and Wroblewski 1981).

Platelet transfusion is usually administered if there are signs or symptoms of bleeding, or in some cases if the platelet count is less than 20,000/mm³. A transfusion of 10 units will usually increase the platelet count 70,000–90,000/mm³, unless the patient is sensitized, febrile, or there is HLA incompatibility. The most common allergic reactions to platelet transfusion are fever and chills resulting from sensitization to previously transfused platelets, and these are treated with diphenhydramine (Benadryl R) and acetaminophen (Tylenol). However, because fever and chills destroy circulating platelets, future platelet transfusions should be preceded by prophylactic diphenhydramine and acetaminophen or Solucortef (Brager and Yasko 1984).

Anemia

Red blood cells (RBC), or *erythrocytes*, by virtue of hemoglobin, carry molecules of oxygen to the tissues to meet their metabolic needs, and remove carbon dioxide to the lungs for elimination. Red blood cells also help in acid-base buffering of the blood. When the number of circulating red blood cells declines, decreased amounts of oxygen are delivered to the cells, with consequent signs and symptoms of impaired tissue oxygenation. The severity of symptoms is a function of the severity of the anemia.

Anemia resulting from bone marrow depression (see table 4.6) related to chemotherapy occurs rarely, or considerably later than the nadirs for

Table 4.6 Standardized Nursing Care Plan for the Patient Experiencing Bone Marrow Depression

Nursing Diagnosis	Expected Outcome	Nursing Interventions

I. A. Potential for altered health maintenance	I. A. Pt will manage self-care as evidenced by verbal recall or return demonstration of instructions for self-assessment of oral temperature, examination of skin and mucous membranes, signs and symptoms of infection and bleeding, measures to avoid exposure to infection, measures to avoid injury and bleeding, and when and how to notify health care provider	I. A. 1. Assess baseline knowledge, learning style, level of anxiety of pt and significant other
		2. Develop and implement teaching plan:
		  a. Purpose and goal of chemotherapy
		  b. Specific drugs
		    1) mechanism of action
		    2) potential side effects, including bone barrow suppression as appropriate
		  c. Self-care measures
		    1) assessment and care of skin, oral mucosa to prevent infection, trauma
		    2) assessment of temperature BID, or if feels as if fever, and instructions to call health care provider if temperature is over 101°F (38.5°C)
		    3) signs and symptoms of infection (fever, sore throat, cough, painful urination)
		    4) signs and symptoms of bleeding (nose or gum bleeding, capillary or large "black and blues")
		    5) measures to minimize exposure to infection and trauma as described in NCI booklet *Chemotherapy and You: A Guide to Self-Help*
		  d. Provide written information to reinforce teaching, such as the booklet above, free from the NCI

B. Potential for noncompliance with self-care activities	B. Pt and significant other will comply with prescribed measures 90% of the time	B. 1. Reinforce teaching prior to treatment as nurse does prechemo assessment, and prior to pt leaving clinic or hospital after treatment administration 2. Evaluate compliance through telephone call to pt following treatment or discharge, or visiting nurse home visit 3. If pt or significant other is having difficulty with managing self-care activities, consider visiting nurse referral or hospitalization if pt is neutropenic or thrombocytopenic and unable to safely care for self

II. Potential for altered nutrition: less than body requirements

II. A. Pt will maintain within 5% of pretreatment weight

B. Recovery from nadir will approximate expected time based on specific chemotherapy agents

II. A. Assess food preferences

B. Encourage foods high in proteins, calories, and iron

C. Discourage excessive alcohol intake

D. Review dietary instructions with pt, person responsible for preparing food

E. Review teaching material with pt and family from NCI booklet *Eating Hints* for patients receiving chemotherapy, a free publication

III. Potential for injury: infection and bleeding related to bone marrow depression

III. A. Pt will remain free of infection, bleeding and tissue hypoxia

III. A. Assessment of potential for injury related to bone marrow depression:

1. Expected nadir from specific agents administered, nadir from prior treatment cycle if appropriate
2. Major life stressors and coping ability
3. Sexual history and self-care habits re: hygiene
4. Sleep pattern
5. Elimination pattern
6. Nutritional pattern
7. History and physical exam:
   a. Symptoms of infection: fever, pain (swallowing, with elimination, etc.), erythema, presence of exudate
   b. Symptoms of bleeding: dizziness, presence of blood in excretia
   c. Symptoms of anemia: fatigue, dyspnea on exertion, angina
   d. Skin, mucous membranes: are they intact, color, evidence of petechiae or ecchymoses, or exudate
   e. Breath sounds, pulmonary exam
   f. CNS exam
   g. Laboratory data: complete blood count, WBC differential, and absolute neutrophil count

(continued)

Table 4.6 (continued)

Nursing Diagnosis	Expected Outcome	Nursing Interventions

	III. B. Pt will experience minimal complications of bone marrow suppression as evidenced by return to normal temperature and neutrophil count, and absence of major bleeding	III. B. Institute neutropenic precautions for absolute neutrophil count <500/mm^3
		1. Protect pt from exposure to microorganisms:
		  a. Provide private room if possible
		  b. Place sign on door requiring *all* persons who enter to wash their hands meticulously prior to entering the room, that persons with colds or infections should not enter, and that no flowers or fresh fruit or vegetables should be brought into the room
		  c. Place card in nursing cardex instructing that NO intramuscular injections, rectal temperatures, or medications should be administered
		  d. Plan scrupulous hygiene with pt for oral care, daily bath, and meticulous perineal hygiene
		  e. Inspect all intravenous sites, and change dressings using aseptic technique; sites should be changed every 48 hours or earlier if there is any indication of phlebitis
		  f. Avoid invasive procedures such as urinary catheterization if possible
		  g. Wash hands meticulously prior to entering room, and between each physical contact with the pt; monitor that *all* other persons wash their hands prior to entering; ensure that the nurse caring for the pt does not care for any other pt that is infected
		2. Continually assess for presence of infection:
		  a. Monitor vital signs every 4 hours, or more frequently if temperature elevated
		  b. Monitor absolute neutrophil count
		  c. Inspect potential sites of infection: mouth and pharynx, rectum; wounds; intravenous sites, and others, remembering that usual signs of infection such as pus and erythema may be absent
		  d. Monitor for changes in character, color, amount of excretia (sputum, urine, stool)
		  e. Report signs and symptoms of infection to physician and obtain cultures, administer antipyretics and antibiotics as ordered
		3. Instruct pt in stress-reducing activities to promote relaxation and satisfactory sleep/rest patterns

III. C. Institute platelet precautions for pt with platelet count less than 50,000/mm^3:

1. Protect pt from trauma and potential bleeding

   a. Place sign in nursing cardex that no IM or rectal medications should be administered, no aspirin or prostaglandin-inhibiting medications should be administered, and no rectal temperatures should be taken

   b. Minimize number of venipunctures, and apply pressure to site at least 5 minutes until bleeding stops

   c. Avoid invasive procedures such as deep endotracheal suctioning, enemas, douches

   d. Teach pt to brush teeth with soft brush or sponge applicator to prevent trauma to gums; avoid flossing

   e. Provide safe environment, padding side rails when in use, and removing clutter and obstructing furniture from room

   f. Prevent constipation by administering stool softeners as ordered, and encourage fluid intake of 3 liters per day

2. Continually monitor for signs and symptoms of bleeding:

   a. Minor bleeding such as petechiae, ecchymoses, epistaxis, occult blood in stool, urine, emesis

   b. Major bleeding such as hematemesis, melena, heavy vaginal bleeding, changes in orthostatic vital signs >10 mm Hg in blood pressure, or increase in heart rate >10 beats per minute, changes in neuro vital signs

   c. Monitor platelet count, hematocrit daily

   d. Notify physician re signs and symptoms of bleeding, and transfuse platelets as ordered

(continued)

Table 4.6 *(continued)*

Nursing Diagnosis	Expected Outcome	Nursing Interventions
IV. Potential for altered tissue perfusion related to anemia	IV. A. Pt will be without signs and symptoms of severe anemia	IV. A. Assess signs and symptoms of anemia 1. Hematocrit: mild (31–37%), moderate (25–30%), or severe (<25%) 2. Presence of symptoms of mild anemia (paleness, fatigue, slight dyspnea, palpitation, and sweating on exertion); moderate anemia (increased severity of symptoms of mild anemia); and severe anemia (headache, dizziness, irritability, angina, dyspnea at rest, and compensatory tachycardia and tachypnea) B. Encourage pt to change positions gradually, slowly moving from lying to sitting position, and sitting to standing position. Encourage slow, deep breathing during position changes C. Reassure pt that fatigue is related to anemia, and hopefully will improve with transfusion D. Replace red blood cells as ordered, expecting that the 1 unit of RBC will increase the hematocrit. Washed or leukocyte-poor red blood cells are used to prevent antibody formation if the pt is planning to go for a bone marrow transplant E. Assess activity tolerance, and need for oxygen for activity or at rest F. Review foods that are high in iron, and encourage pt to include these in the diet
V. Potential for constipation	V. A. Pt will move bowels at least once every day	V. A. Provide pt education about the goal and means of preventing constipation, such as stool softeners, oral fluids to 3 quarts per day, high fiber diet, and adequate exercise B. Discuss a bowel regime with physician to promote soft, regular bowel movements, especially if the pt is receiving narcotic analgesia
VI. Potential for activity intolerance related to fatigue of anemia, malaise	VI. A. Pt will maintain minimal activity	VI. A. Teach pt to increase rest and sleep periods and to alternate rest and activity periods B. Encourage pt to incorporate foods high in iron in diet, such as liver, eggs, lean meat, green leafy vegetables, carrots, and raisins C. Assess need for homemaker, home health aide, and visiting nurse at home

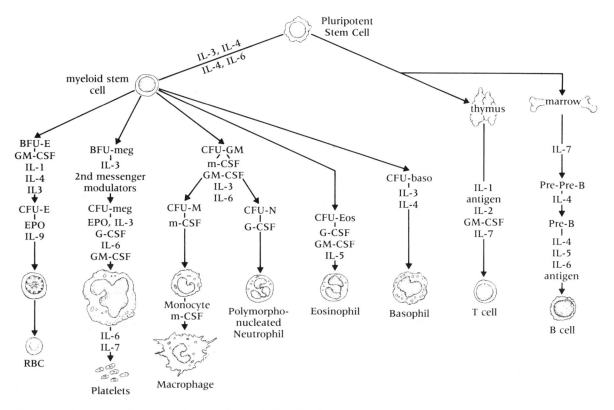

Figure 4.7   Normal maturation of the red blood cell.
From *Oncology Times* xii(10):26 (Sept 1987). Reprinted with permission.

white blood cells and platelets because the life span of the red blood cell is approximately 120 days. Certain chemotherapeutic agents can cause anemia over time, and these include cisplatin. Other factors influencing the development of anemia are as follows: decreased red blood cell precursors by tumor infiltration of the bone marrow; concomitant or previous radiation to active bone marrow with resulting fibrosis; or active bleeding such as with severe thrombocytopenia. The red blood cell development is shown in figure 4.7. The red blood cells are released from the bone marrow as *reticulocytes*, and the cells mature in the blood with the help of Vitamin B12.

Classifications of anemia are shown in table 4.7.

Physical assessment of the patient with anemia may show compensatory changes in vital signs with increased heart rate, and depth of respiration in an effort to try to increase the oxygenation of the tissues. Skin may be blanched, nailbeds pallid, and mucous membranes pale, especially the conjunctiva. Nursing interventions are directed at replacing red blood cells through transfusions when the hematocrit is 25 or less, usually, and patient teaching to minimize fatigue and facilitate early identification of symptoms.

II. MUCOSITIS

Mucositis refers to an inflammation of the mucous membranes, and occurs as a sequela of chemotherapy administration because of damage

Table 4.7 Degrees of Anemia

	Hemoglobin (G/100 ml)	Hematocrit (%)	Symptoms
NORMAL male	14–18	42–52	
NORMAL female	12–16	37–47	
Mild ANEMIA		31–37	Pale, fatigue, slight dyspnea on exertion; palpatation and sweating with exertion
Moderate ANEMIA		25–30	Increased severity of symptoms of mild anemia
Severe ANEMIA		< 25	Headache, dizziness, irritability. Dyspnea on exertion and at rest; angina, compensatory tachycardia, tachypnea.

Modified from Brager and Yasko 1984.

to the frequently dividing cells in the mucosal epithelium which lines the gastrointestinal tract. Mucositis is further specified as to its anatomic location: when it occurs in the oral cavity, it is called *stomatitis*; in the esophagus, *esophagitis*; in the intestines, mucositis is usually manifested by *diarrhea*; and in the rectum, *proctitis*.

The epithelial cells lining the gastrointestinal (GI) mucosa are subjected to "wear and tear" by chemical, mechanical, and thermal factors as the ingested food is chewed, swallowed, digested, and expelled. Thus, there is demand for frequent replacement of the mucosal epithelium cells so that cell birth equals cell death.

Stomatitis

The stem cells of the oral mucous membranes are found in the deep squamous epithelium which lies above the basement membrane. These cells have a lifespan of 3–5 days with the outer epithelial layer being entirely replaced every 7–14 days (Beck and Yasko 1984). Stem cell replication is rapid, taking about 32 hours, with estimated phases of the cell cycle as follows: mitosis (8 hours), G_1 (14 hours), S (10–11 hours), G_2 (10–19 minutes) (Lavalle and Proctor 1978). Unfortunately, chemotherapy agents can-

not distinguish between malignant and normal frequently dividing cells, so the mucosal stem cells are injured *directly*. No longer can these stem cells replace oral mucosal cells lost through normal sloughing, and the decreased renewal of epithelial cells results in thinning of the mucosa (Frattore et al. 1986). There is evidence of beginning tissue damage in 5 to 7 days after chemotherapy administration: pale, dry mucous membranes, burning sensation, dry tongue with raised papillae, and ridging of buccal mucosa. This damage may progress to severe inflammation and ulceration with pain, as shown in figure 4.8, and then recovery occurs within 2–3 weeks without scarring (Engleking 1988).

Figure 4.8 illustrates the development of stomatitis utilizing a stress response model. The phases of Alarm, Resistance, Exhaustion, and Recovery are represented over a span of 21 days.

An objective evaluation of the degrees of stomatitis was developed by Capizzi et al. (1970), and used in Oncology Nursing Society *Guidelines for Cancer Nursing Practice* (McNally et al. 1986). The degrees of stomatitis were labeled Grades I–IV:

Grade I	Erythema of oral mucosa
Grade II	Isolated small ulcerations or white patches. Patient able to eat and drink.

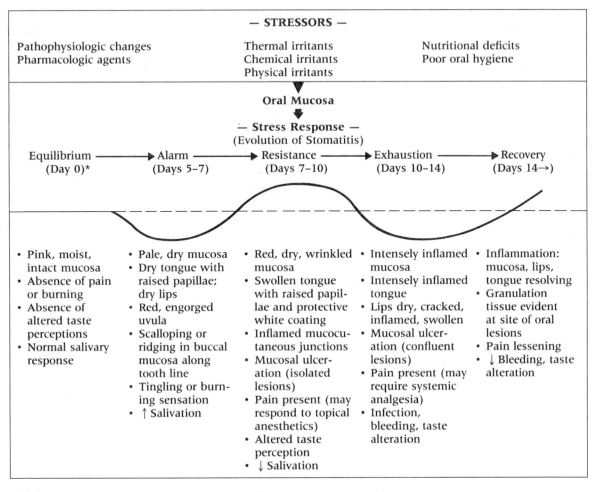

Figure 4.8 Mucosal response to physiological stressors
Adapted from Engleking 1988.

Grade III   Confluent ulceration or white patches covering >25% of oral mucosa. Patient only able to drink fluids.

Grade IV   Hemorrhagic ulceration, ulceration covering >50% of oral mucosa. Patient unable to drink fluids or eat.

According to Frattore, Larson, and Mostofi (1986), the nonkeratinized surfaces of the buccal and labial mucosa, ventral and lateral tongue surfaces, soft palate, and the floor of the mouth are the areas most commonly affected.

Factors that aggravate the degree of stomatitis are drug dose, nutritional deficits, poor oral hygiene, and concurrent radiotherapy to the head and neck (Yasko 1983). The incidence of stomatitis is approximately 40%, and is associated with the antimetabolites (especially methotrexate and 5-fluorouracil), antibiotics (especially bleomycin and doxorubicin), and the plant alkaloids (Dreizen et al. 1975).

Taste alterations are another effect of *direct* cell injury. There are about 10,000 taste buds located on the papillae which cover the tongue. The taste cells that comprise each taste bud are renewed every 5–7 days, and are often damaged by chemotherapy. Thus, mild or more severe stomatitis may be accompanied by taste alterations, and this can be a very distressing side effect. Pain resulting from erythema and ulceration often lead to dysphagia and difficulty speaking. Nutritional deficits are intensified, and further aggravate the damaged mucosa and delay healing.

Indirect injury to the oral mucosa is related to bone marrow suppression as there is increased risk of infection and bleeding. Severe stomatitis usually precedes the drug-induced nadir by 2–3 days. As the nadir occurs, neutropenia increases the risk of superinfection by normal oral flora. Once injury to the mucosa has occurred, infection by bacterial, fungal, or viral organisms can occur. Also, the mucosal barrier is no longer intact, so that a portal of entry for microorganisms into the systemic circulation now exists. Adult patients often have periodontal disease with chronic oral infection (Peterson 1984), and with drug-induced mucosal disease, ulcerative lesions often spread with surface necrosis (Frattore, Larson, and Mostofi 1986).

INFECTIONS

When bacterial infections occur, they are most commonly streptococcal; when the patient is immunosuppressed, the organisms are predominately gram negative, such as pseudomonas, *Escherichia coli*, klebsiella, and proteus (Beck and Yasko 1984). Cultures of suspicious areas should be obtained to determine the causative organism and the proper antibiotic regime.

Fungal infections related to *Candida albicans* are frequently encountered and appear as soft, white, cottage-cheese like patches containing candida and epithelial cells, often overlying red, raw, or bleeding mucosa (Beck and Yasko 1984). This fungus is responsible for one-half of all oral infections during antileukemic therapy, and for almost ⅔ of oral infections in patients receiving chemotherapy for solid tumors (Frattore, Larson, and Mostofi 1986). Risk for fungal infection in-

creases for patients on corticosteroid therapy or prolonged antibiotic therapy with broad spectum agents (Frattore, Larson, and Mostofi 1986). Antifungal treatment begins with topical application of clotrimazole troches (1 troche 5 times/day) or nystatin (up to 500,000 u 3–4 times/day) (Engleking 1988). If candida persists, then systemic treatment with ketoconazole or amphotericin B is required (see table 4.8).

A newly developed oral rinse, chlorhexirine 0.12% mouthrinse (Peridexoral Rinse, Proctor & Gamble), has shown promise in reducing oral mucositis and candida infections (Ferretti et al., *JADA* 114:461, 1987). This was prospectively studied in a double-blind, five-week study of 49 inpatients receiving intensive chemotherapy, and the group using chlorhexidine 0.12% had an 11% incidence of mucositis compared with 50% in the placebo group (Ferritti et al., *JADA*, 1987). In addition, chlorhexidine 0.12% may decrease the incidence of oral candidiasis.

Viral infections, especially those caused by herpes simplex virus I, may occur, and appear as a cluster of vesicles or lip ulcerations (Beck and Yasko 1984). The lesions are initially painful and itching, then rupture within 12 hours, and a crusty exudate forms (Frattore, Larson, and Mostofi 1986). Application of topical acyclovir 5% ointment every 3–6 hours may be helpful, and the nurse should be careful to wear gloves to prevent auto-innoculation (Engleking 1988). The lesions usually regress in 7–10 days (Adrian, Hood, and Skarin 1980).

NURSING INTERVENTIONS

Nursing interventions begin prior to chemotherapy administration with a thorough patient assessment of the oral cavity, and risk factors such as cigarette smoking, alcohol use, periodontal disease, poor oral hygiene, poor nutritional status, and concurrent radiotherapy to head or neck. Dental work may need to be performed prior to chemotherapy. In order to effectively examine the oral cavity, a flashlight, tongue blade, gauze pad, and gloves are needed. Inspect the upper inner lip and gums, dorsal and ventral tongue surfaces, lateral borders of the tongue, inner cheek (buccal mucosa), hard and soft palate, floor of mouth, and oropharynx for: color, moisture, presence of debris, and presence of lesions. A normal mucosa is pink, moist, intact, without debris.

Once a patient is identified as having the potential to develop stomatitis, nursing care is aimed at 1) teaching the patient oral cleansing and self-care, 2) preventing oral infection, 3) identifying early dysfunction, and 4) promoting comfort and optimal nutrition.

The goal of oral cleansing is to keep the mucosa moist, clean, and without debris so that the mucosal barrier remains infection-free. Patients should be taught to perform oral cleansing after meals and at bedtime, brushing with a soft toothbrush, flossing with unwaxed dental floss, and using a mouthwash that does *not* contain alcohol, as this will dry the mucosa (Goodman and Stoner 1985). The Bass technique of toothbrushing is recommended by many nurses: the soft bristled toothbrush is held at a 45-degree angle between the gingiva and teeth, and brushing is in short horizontal strokes (Dudjak 1987; Yasko 1983).

If the patient is edentulous, or has an oral lesion, soft, sponge-tipped applicators can be used. There is considerable debate in the oncology nursing community about the best oral cleanser, and it appears that it is the frequency and consistent practice of oral care rather than the agent that minimizes oral complications (Dudjak 1987). In general, however, the purpose of the cleanser is to remove debris without irritation or damage to the oral mucosa.

Normal saline is nonirritating but does not remove debris or formed crusts. Sodium bicarbonate in moderate doses dissolves thick mucous, decreases oral acidity thus discouraging bacterial growth, and loosens debris; however, some patients do not like the taste (Bersani and Carl 1983). Hydrogen peroxide is a powerful mucosolvent, oxidizing crusted blood and debris, deodorizing the oral cavity, and providing

antimicrobial action (Engleking, 1988). Unfortunately, though, peroxide can break down granulation tissue, and has an unpleasant taste for some patients, despite rinsing after use. Lemon glycerine swabs should not be used for the following reasons: they are drying to mucosa, may decalcify teeth, and create an acid environment which encourages bacterial growth and plaque formation (Poland 1987; Daeffler 1985; Goodman and Stoner 1985).

Most nursing experts agree that patients who have the *potential* to develop stomatitis, but no evidence of stomatitis, should practice oral care after meals and at bedtime with soft toothbrush and paste, and gargle with normal saline or a mouthwash *without* alcohol. Dentures should be removed to cleanse the oral mucosa. If saliva is thick, if the patient has oral cancer, or if the patient has thick mucous, an oxidizing or mucolytic agent should be used such as sodium bicarbonate (1 tsp in 8 oz water) or 1:4 peroxide/normal saline followed by a saline or water rinse. If the patient experiences Grade I (erythema) or Grade II (small ulceration or white patches), the *Oncology Nursing Society Guidelines for Cancer Nursing Practice* recommend cleansing every 2 hours with normal saline, or cleansing every 4 hours with an oxidizing/mucolytic agent if crusts or debris are present, alternating with warm saline gargles. Analgesics such as viscous xylocaine or Benadryl/xylocaine/kaopectate gargles may be required. If white candidal patches are present, an antifungal agent such as clotrimazole troches or nystatin is used for topical control, and this should be administered *after* the patient has cleansed his/her mouth. For Grade III stomatitis (confluent ulcerations with white patches covering >25%) or Grade IV (hemorrhagic ulcerations), cleansing should be practiced every 2 hours: warm saline gargles alternated every 2 hours with an antifungal or antibacterial suspension, unless the patient has thick mucous or saliva. In that case, an oxidizing/mucolytic agent such as sodium bicarbonate or hydrogen peroxide, followed by a saline rinse is used every 4

Table 4.8 Potential Oral Infections Seen in Patients with Stomatitis

Infectious Organism	Appearance	Management		Comments
		Drug	Dose	
Fungi:				
Candida albicans (moniliasis; thrush)	Soft, whitish or cream-colored strands or patches covering all or part of tongue, lips, or buccal mucosa; patches adhere to underlying mucosa; when removed, mucosa is bright red and moist underneath (Daeffler 1985)	clotrimazole 10 mg (Mycelex) troche	dissolve slowly in mouth 5 troches/day for 2 weeks	All topical drugs are applied to clean mucosa, then NPO for 15–30 min
aspergillosis	Lesions often on palate: painful, yellowish ulcers, surrounded by black border (Frattore, Larson, and Mostofi 1986)	nystatin (Mycostatin) suspension	Swish 500,000 u q 4–6 hr, keep in mouth for 2 min, then discard/swallow	Topical drug
		ketoconazole 200 mg/da (Nizoral)	1 tablet daily for 1–2 wks	Systemic therapy if topical treatment ineffective
Bacteria:				
Staphylococcus aureus	Exudative, purulent, and encrusted erosions; less commonly encountered; in the neutropenic patient, lesion is smaller with less pus, and appears as dry, raised, yellow-brown plaque (Frattore, Larson, and Mostofi 1986)	Antibiotic therapy		Antibiotics based on organism sensitivity
Gram Negative bacteria	Raised, creamy, moist, glistening site of infection; nonpurulent; smooth edges; seated on painful, red superficial ulcers			
pseudomonas aeruginosa	Raised lesions enclosed by a red halo; initially, dry, yellowish center turning purple-to-black with necrosis; necrotic core sloughs off disclosing bright red granulation tissue (Frattore, Larson, and Mostofi 1986)			

Virus:			
herpes simplex	Activated by stress of disease and treatment; vesicle is painful and itchy; ruptures within 12 hours, and becomes encrusted with dry exudate; yellowish-brown membrane easily dislodges, causing severe pain; regresses in 7–10 days.	acyclovir 5% ointment	q 3–6 hours while awake	Apply with gloves (topical application)
		acyclovir 200 mg capsules	1 capsule 5 times/day	Systemic therapy for diffuse herpes, until shedding completed
		acyclovir 5 mg/kg IV	Administer over 1 hour, q 8 hours, for 7 days (Zinner, Belcher, and Murphy 1988)	

Modified from Daeffler, RJ (1985) Protective Mechanisms: Mucous Membranes, Chapter 9B, p. 253–274. In *Handbook of Oncology Nursing*, ed. BL Johnson and J Gross. New York: John Wiley and Sons.

hours. Soft sponge-tipped applicators instead of a soft toothbrush prevent pain or trauma to the fragile mucous membranes. If candida persists after topical treatment, then systemic therapy with ketoconazole or amphotericin B is used.

Flossing should be discontinued if bleeding occurs, or if the platelet count is less than 50,000/mm³ or the white blood count is less than 1000/mm³. Also at this time, soft, sponge-tipped applicators should be used instead of a toothbrush.

Comfort is promoted by the use of topical anesthetics such as viscous xylocaine, or "cocktails" such as diphenhydramine/xylocaine/kaopectate gargles, but systemic analgesics may be required including morphine infusions for severe mucositis pain. Sucralfate suspension as described by Ferraro and Mattern (table 4.9) theoretically promotes healing of oral ulcers much as it does with duodenal and gastric ulcers by binding to the proteinaceous exudate of the ulcer, and providing protection for healing (Ferraro and Mattern 1984). Although the use of sucralfate suspension has not been studied prospectively to evaluate oral ulcer healing, when applied 4 times a day after meals and cleansing of the oral cavity, patients have reported decreased pain and discomfort (Wilkes 1986).

Table 4.9 Sucralfate Suspension

To prepare a concentration of 1 Gm/15 ml, 120-ml bottle:

Place 8 sucralfate tablets in a clean 120-ml glass bottle. Add 40 ml sterile water for irrigation: allow tablets to dissolve then shake well. Add 40 ml of Sorbitol 70%, and shake well. Separately, mix 1–3 Ensure® Vari Flavor Pacs with 10 ml sterile water for irrigation and add to the drug mixture. Add sufficient sterile water for irrigation to complete 120 ml. Label: refrigerate, expires in 14 days. Instructions for use: 3 tsp, swish for 2 minutes, then swallow, after posteating mouth-cleansing, and at bedtime.

Source: Ferraro and Mattern (1984).

In addition, misoprostol, a synthetic prostaglandin analogue recently approved by the Federal Drug Administration (FDA) for prevention of gastric ulcers related to nonsteroidal anti-inflammatory drugs, has shown promise in pilot studies in decreasing the severity of mucositis following bone marrow transplantation (Siena et al. 1988).

Esophagitis

Esophagitis is inflammation of the esophageal mucosa caused by injury to basal epithelial cells of the mucosa, similar to that of the oral cavity. Histologically the same, with similar growth rates, esophagitis occurs in about the same time frame as oral stomatitis. Cell replacement is interrupted as the basal stem cells are damaged, and the mucosa lining the esophagus becomes thin and atrophied. Painful ulceration, secondary infection, and hemorrhage may occur. Oral candidiasis can spread to the esophagus by swallowing fungal organisms, and can progress to septicemia by penetration of the esophageal mucosa (Frattore, Larson, and Mostofi 1986). Mucosal healing occurs as the bone marrow recovers, and the white blood count rises (Nunnally and Donoghue 1986).

Risk factors include chemotherapy with antimetabolite drugs, and others which cause stomatitis, and concurrent or subsequent radiation therapy of the neck, chest, or upper back. Esophagitis is usually dose-limiting, and therapy is interrupted until esophagitis resolves.

Early signs and symptoms of esophagitis include discomfort or pain on swallowing (odenophagia), dysphagia of solid foods, and a sensation of having a "lump" in the throat when swallowing (Nunnally, Donoghue, and Yasko 1983). Patient problems are similar to those encountered in patients with stomatitis, and nursing care is directed toward maintaining optimal nutrition for healing, minimizing patient discomfort, and preventing secondary infection.

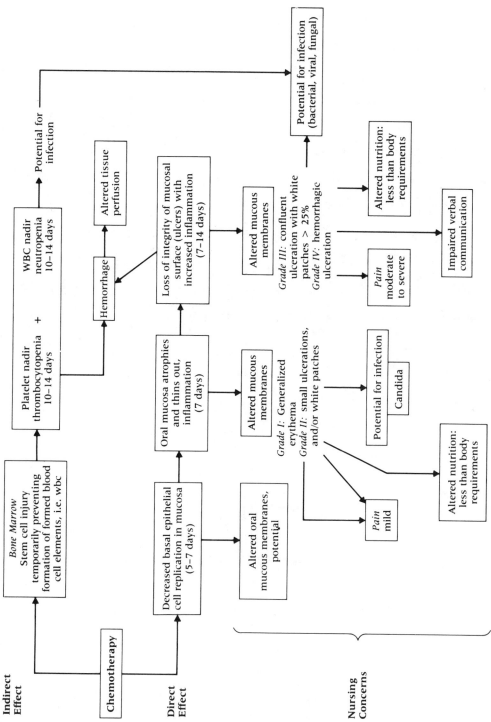

Figure 4.9 Sequelae of mucositis

Table 4.10 Standardized Nursing Care Plan for Patient Experiencing Stomatitis

Nursing Diagnosis	Expected Outcome	Nursing Interventions

I. Potential for altered oral mucous membranes	I. A. Oral mucosa will remain pink, moist, intact, without debris	I. A. Assess oral mucosa (baseline)
		1. Assess history of alcohol use, smoking
		2. Assess history of dental problems, oral hygiene practices, and prior or concurrent radiation to head or neck
		3. Perform oral exam
		  a. Lips
		  b. Upper inner lip and gums
		  c. Tongue (dorsum, lateral borders, ventral surface)
		  d. Inner cheeks (buccal mucosa)
		  e. Hard and soft palate
		  f. Floor of mouth
		  g. Oral pharynx
		4. Assess amount, consistency of saliva
		5. Assess condition of teeth
		B. Assess nutritional status
		C. Initiate and discuss dental referral as needed prior to therapy
		D. Instruct in oral hygiene self-care measures (see IV. Knowledge deficit)

II. Altered oral mucous membranes, *Grade I* (generalized erythema) *Grade II* (small ulceration or white patches)	II. A. Oral mucosa is pink, moist, intact, and painless within 5–7 days	II. A. Assess oral mucosa q shift or at each clinic visit; document size and location of abnormality, and intervention B. Assess comfort, and ability to eat, drink C. Institute oral hygiene q 2 hrs during day and q 6 hrs during night 1. Warm normal saline rinses *unless* crusts, debris, thick mucous or saliva; then use sodium bicarbonate (1 tsp in 8 oz water) q 4 hrs alternating with warm saline rinses q 4 hrs 2. (Warm) sterile normal saline rinses if WBC <1000/mm^3 (Daeffler 1985, p. 268) 3. Reserve hydrogen peroxide (1:4 strength) for *resistant*, thick secretions or white patches (candida), resistant debris, and rinse afterwards with water D. Encourage flossing qd, and brushing with soft bristled brush pc and hs unless plt <40,000/mm^3 or WBC <1500/mm^3 (Beck 1979, p. 44) E. Encourage pt to remove dentures during oral hygiene rinsing, and if irritating mucosa

		F. Encourage pt to moisten lips with medicated lip ointment, water-soluble lubricating jelly, or lanolin
		G. Encourage pt to avoid citrus fruits and juices, spicy foods, hot foods, and to eat bland, cool foods
		H. Discuss use of antifungal therapy if candidiasis present
III. Altered oral mucous membranes, *Grade III* (confluent ulcerations with white patches >25% or *Grade IV* (hemorrhagic ulcerations)	III. A. Oral mucosa will heal within 10–14 days and white patches (candida) will be absent	III. A. Assess oral mucosa q 4 hrs for evidence of infection, response to therapy
		B. Assess ability to eat, drink, communicate
		C. Assess level of comfort, discomfort
		D. Culture ulcerated areas that appear infected
		E. Cleanse mouth q 2 hrs while awake, q 4 hrs during night
		1. Alternate warm saline mouthrinse with antifungal or antibacterial oral suspension q 2 hrs
		2. Use sodium bicarbonate solution for thick secretions, debris; if ineffective in removing debris, use 1:4 hydrogen peroxide followed by water or saline rinse
		F. Suggest soft, sponge-tipped applicator to cleanse teeth, mouth pc and hs
		G. Apply lip lubricant q 2 hrs
		H. After cleansing, sucralfate suspension 15 mins after meals and mouth cleansing—discuss with physician and obtain order. (See table 4.9 for preparation guide.)
IV. Potential for knowledge deficit, re risk for stomatitis and self-care management	IV. A. Pt will verbally repeat steps of self-assessment	IV. A. Instruct pt in stomatitis as potential side effect of chemotherapy as appropriate

(continued)

Table 4.10 (continued)

Nursing Diagnosis	Expected Outcome	Nursing Interventions
	IV. B. Pt will demonstrate self-care techniques (mouth rinse, brushing, flossing)	IV. B. Instruct pt in daily oral exam 1. Use of mirror and self-exam 2. Signs and symptoms to report (burning, redness, blisters, ulcers; difficulty swallowing; swelling of lips, tongue; pain) C. Instruct pt in oral care 1. Remove dentures, wash and rinse mouth, then replace 2. Floss daily with unwaxed dental floss 3. Brush with soft toothbrush and nonabrasive toothpaste pc and hs 4. Rinse with water, saline, dilute sodium bicarbonate solution, or mouthwash without alcohol 5. Avoid oral irritants (tobacco, alcohol, poorly fitting dentures, mouthwashes containing alcohol) D. Instruct pt in self care q 2 hrs if actual stomatitis occurs 1. Cleansing solution of warm normal saline or sodium bicarbonate solution unless resistant thick secretions, debris; then may use 1:4 hydrogen peroxide with water rinse following 2. Medication application as indicated 3. High-calorie, high-protein, cool, bland foods 4. Small, frequent feedings; fluids to 3 L/day
V. Pain related to stomatitis	V. A. Pt states relief from oral pain	V. A. Use mild analgesic q 2 hrs, timing 15 mins ac; gargles must be swished 2 min 1. Viscous zylocaine 2% gargles, 10–15 cc swish/spit q 3 hrs, duration 20 mins (max 120 mg/24 hrs, Brager and Yasko 1984) 2. Orabase emollient for local relief 3. 1:1:1 viscous zylocaine:diphenhydramine HCl (12.5 mg/ml): kaopectate swish and swallow q 2–4 hrs 4. Benzocaine 20%—apply directly or swish and spit (duration 20 mins) 5. Dyclonine HCl (Dyclone) 0.5%–15 mins ac; 5–10 cc swish for 2 mins, gargle and spit, onset 10 min, duration 1 hr B. Parenteral analgesics may be necessary, including morphine infusion

Nursing Diagnosis	Goal	Interventions
VI. Impaired verbal communication related to pain, increased or thickened saliva	VI. A. Pt will communicate needs effectively	VI. A. Assess pt's ability to communicate B. If secretions thick, copious, instruct pt in tonsil-tip suctioning technique C. Develop satisfactory communication tool if pt unable to talk, i.e., magic slate, writing message D. Respond promptly to pt call light
VII. Potential for altered nutrition: less than body requirements related to pain of mucositis	VII. A. Pt will regain baseline weight within 5%	VII. A. Premedicate with analgesics 15 mins ac B. Encourage high-calorie, high-protein, small, frequent feedings with cool, bland liquid or pureed foods; also, creative popsicles, custards C. If inability to eat persists, discuss with physician need for enteral, parenteral nutrition D. Encourage popsicles, ice creams as desired E. Discourage citrus juices, fruits, hot and spicy foods; rough, hard foods
VIII. Potential for infection	VIII. A. Pt will be free of infection B. Infection will be detected early and treated	VIII. A. Assess oral mucosa q 4–8 hrs for s/s infection—culture any suspicious sites B. Monitor vs, T q 4 hrs; if outpatient, teach pt to monitor temp at least BID C. Encourage pt to cleanse oral mucosa prior to administration or antibiotic or antifungal medication—keep NPO for 15–30 mins p medication administration D. Consider administration of antifungal or antibiotic or antibiotic as frozen popsicle if extreme pain as this will decrease discomfort E. Administer systemic antibiotics if ordered
IX. Potential for altered tissue perfusion, related to hemorrhage	IX. A. Pt will be without oral bleeding	IX. A. Assess for s/s bleeding in gingiva, mucosa

(continued)

Table 4.10 (continued)

Nursing Diagnosis	Expected Outcome	Nursing Interventions
IX.	IX. B. Bleeding will be detected early and terminated	IX. B. Remove dentures, partial plates
		C. If *bleeding*, monitor platelet count, hematocrit
		1. Transfuse platelets as ordered
		2. Topical thrombin, aminocaproic acid, or microfibrillar collagen may be ordered (Peterson 1984)
		3. Leave clots undisturbed—discontinue mechanical oral care
		D. Use sponge-tipped applicator rather than toothbrush if platelets <50,000/mm^3 to minimize trauma to gingiva, mucosa
		E. Encourage liquid, cool or cold, high calorie, high protein supplements as tolerated; pt should be NPO if bleeding
X. Xerostomia (uncommon) (especially with Adriamycin)	X. A. Pt will have moist mucosa with thin secretions	X. A. Encourage frequent mouth moisturizing with ice chips, artificial saliva (containing carboxymethyl cellulose)
		B. Oral hygiene pc and hs
		C. Encourage fluids as tolerated, offering fluids every 1–2 hrs
		D. Discourage mucosal irritants (smoking, alcohol)
		E. Encourage soft, moist foods with sauces
		F. Encourage use of sugarless candy or gum to stimulate saliva production
		G. Increase air moisture as needed by humidifier or vaporizer
		H. Q Day do oral assessment as xerostomia may precede stomatitis (erythema)

Diarrhea

Diarrhea is defined by Brager and Yasko (1984) as the passage of three or more soft or liquid stools in a 24-hour period which may occur during or after therapy. The mucosal epithelial cells lining the intestines (villi and microvilli) are characterized by rapid cell division (high mitotic rate) and a cell generation time of 24 hours so that they may replace the cells damaged by the trauma of digestion (Brager and Yasko 1984). It is estimated that between 20–50 million epithelial cells are normally shed *every hour* (Culhane 1983). If these cells are not replaced, the mucosal cells atrophy and become inflamed; the villi and microvilli shorten and become denuded; and the inflamed mucosa produces large amounts of mucous which stimulate accelerated peristalsis. The damaged villi and microvilli, together with the rapid transit time of intestinal contents, prevents absorption of nutrients, water, and electolytes (Brager and Yasko 1984).

Diarrhea is a common and potentially severe side effect of 5-fluorouracil (5-FU). It may precede severe bone marrow depression and usually requires interruption of therapy. Diarrhea occurring during methotrexate therapy is not as common but *requires* interruption of therapy to prevent hemorrhagic enteritis or perforation (Dorr and Fritz 1980). Besides the previously mentioned antimetabolites, other drugs that can cause diarrhea are actinomycin-D, doxorubicin, daunomycin, cisplatin, hydroxyurea, and the nitrosoureas (Perry and Yarbro 1984; Daeffler 1985).

Potential sequelae of diarrhea include malnutrition, fluid and electrolyte imbalance, abdominal discomfort (pain), irritated perianal mucosa or skin, activity intolerance, and fatigue (see figure 4.10). Nursing interventions are directed toward 1) patient teaching regarding high calorie, high protein, low residue diet, elimination of irritating foods, and high fluid intake; 2) monitoring of fluid and electrolyte values, and replacement as needed; 3) providing scrupulous perianal skin

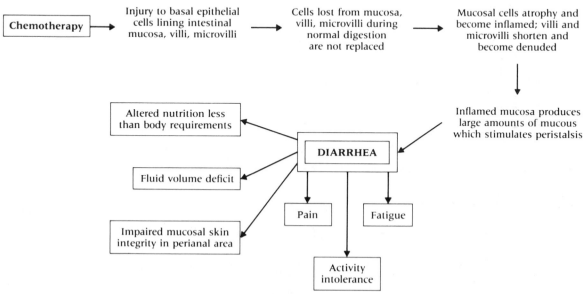

Figure 4.10 Potential sequelae of diarrhea

Table 4.11 Standardized Nursing Care Plan for Patient Experiencing Diarrhea

Nursing Diagnosis	Expected Outcome	Nursing Interventions
I. Potential for altered nutrition: less than body requirements	I. A. Pt will maintain baseline weight within 5% B. Serum electrolytes will be within normal limits	I. A. Assess pt's usual weight, dietary preferences, and usual pattern of bowel elimination B. Monitor intake/output, daily weight, calorie count as appropriate C. Encourage high-calorie, high-protein, low-residue diet in small, frequent meals (cottage cheese, cream cheese, yogurt, broth, fish, poultry, custard, cooked cereals, peeled apples, macaroni, cooked vegetables) D. If diarrhea is severe, recommend liquid diet E. Discourage foods that stimulate peristalsis (bran, whole-grain bread, fried food, fruit juices, raw vegetables, nuts, rich pastry, caffeine-containing foods and drinks) F. Encourage foods high in potassium as appropriate (bananas, baked potatoes, asparagus tips); monitor serum potassium, other electrolytes
II. Potential for fluid volume deficit	II. A. Pt's skin will have normal turgor B. Mucous membranes will be moist	II. A. Encourage 3 liters of fluid/day, especially bouillon, Gatorade B. If nutritional supplements are needed, recommend lactose-free or low-osmolality products C. Monitor intake/output
III. Diarrhea A. Mild/ moderate (4–6 stools/ day) B. Severe (>6 stools/ day)	III. A. Pt will have <4 stools per day	III. A. Assess bowel sounds, and abdomen for ridigity B. Assess frequency, consistency, and volume of stooling, and document. Have pt maintain diary if an outpatient C. Administer antidiarrheal medication as ordered; assess response to therapy; assess need for antispasmodics, antianxiety (anxiolytic) medications D. Instruct pt in self-care measures 1. Self-administration of medications 2. Low-residue diet, fluids to 3 L/day 3. Perianal skin care 4. Alternate rest/activity periods E. Discuss interruption of chemotherapy with physician

IV. Potential for impaired mucosal and skin integrity, perianal skin, related to diarrhea	IV. A. Skin and perianal mucosa will remain intact
	IV. A. Assess perineal, perianal skin, and mucous membranes for integrity and for s/s irritation
	B. Recomment sitz baths p̄ each stool, if diarrhea severe
	C. Provide skin cleansing with water and mild soap p̄ each stool, and application of skin barrier as needed, if patient unable to perform care; otherwise instruct pt in self-care
	D. Apply topical anesthetic as needed
	E. Use absorbent pads under pt to prevent maceration of skin
V. Potential for pain	V. A. Pt will verbalize decreased pain
	V. A. Symptomatic treatment will be given to minimize or alleviate pain
VI. Potential for fatigue	VI. A. Pt will verbalize decreased fatigue
	VI. A. Assess energy level, and help pt to plan activities when energy level is maximal
	B. Assess for changes in life-style necessitated by diarrhea
	C. Encourage pt to alternate rest and activity periods
	D. Provide care that pt is unable to perform; encourage pt to involve family if pt is at home; consider/refer community agencies as needed (for homemaker, home health aide) if diarrhea is severe and resistant to treatment
	E. Assist pt in determining activity priorities and measures to conserve energy
VII. Potential for activity intolerance	VII. A. Pt will participate in activities important to him/her
	VII. A. Activities will be consistent with pt's level of well-being

care, and teaching patient to use sitz baths; and 4) administering medications as ordered to provide relief or cessation of diarrhea. Medications that may provide relief include Pepto-Bismol or Kaopectate every 4–6 hours around the clock or after every loose stool, or Lomotil, loperamide (Imodium) if diarrhea persists (Brager and Yasko 1984). Trials are currently underway to evaluate a new medication, enkephalin BW 942, to control chemotherapy-induced diarrhea (Kris, Gralla, Clark, et al., 1988).

III. ALOPECIA

Another rapidly proliferating normal tissue population is the hair follicles. *Alopecia*, or loss of hair, can range from hair thinning to total loss of scalp hair. The hair follicles have a growth cycle, characterized by a period of active growth (*anagen*, lasting 2–6 years) followed by a resting period (*telogen*, lasting about 3 months), then repeating the cycle (Dunagin 1984). Approximately 90% of hair follicle cells are in active growth at any one time, and exposure to chemotherapy results in destruction of the rapidly dividing epithelial cells of the hair follicle. The stem cells at the base of the hair shaft are damaged, leading to atrophy of the hair follicle, and the subsequent production of a thinner and weaker hair shaft that can break off at the scalp surface (Dunagin 1984) or that is spontaneously released from the hair follicle (Chernecky and Yasko 1986).

Hair loss usually begins 1–2 weeks after a single pulse chemotherapy dose, and becomes maximal 1–2 months later (Dorr and Fritz 1980). The loss is temporary, and regrowth may begin during or shortly after therapy ends, when the drug no longer interferes with active growth. Hair regrowth may be softer in texture, more curly, and slightly different in color. The degree and duration of hair loss depends on the drug dose and length of drug exposure (Chernecky and Yasko 1986). Drugs responsible for alopecia

include alkylating agents, antimetabolites, and antibiotics (Dorr and Fritz 1980). Specifically, Keller and Blausey (1988) list the following:

bleomycin	methotrexate
cyclophosphamide	mitomycin-c
dactinomycin	mitoxantrone
daunorubicin	melphalan
doxorubicin	etoposide
5-fluorouracil	vincristine
hydroxyurea	

Drugs with long halflives of active metabolites, such as doxorubicin, the nitrosoureas, and cyclophosphamide produce severe hair loss (Dorr and Fritz 1980). Other factors influencing the likelihood and severity of alopecia are dose and schedule of administration. Weekly administration of lower dose doxorubicin causes less alopecia than *pulse* doses every 3 weeks (Brager and Yasko 1984), or prolonged continuous infusion therapy (Keller and Blausey 1988). Hair follicles elsewhere on the body do not provide long hair because of a short growth phase, and a long resting phase. Also, at any given time, 90% of these cells are in the resting phase so that chemotherapy does not greatly affect this growth (Dunagin 1984). If the duration of drug exposure is long, cells in the resting phase are lost, and there are no new cells in the growth phase to replace them (Dunagin 1984).

Hair preservation techniques that have been investigated over the years include peripheral scalp hypothermia and constriction. Theoretically, both prevent the chemotherapy drug from reaching the hair follicle by decreasing superficial blood flow to the hair follicle stem cells, and should prevent alopecia. A scalp tourniquet decreases blood flow to the hair follicles, thus decreasing delivery of chemotherapy agent(s). Cold temperatures used in hypothermia cause vasoconstriction and subsequent decrease in blood flow to the scalp; also, hypothermia decreases the metabolic rate of hair follicles in active growth phase, and may inactivate or decrease

Table 4.12   Standardized Nursing Care Plan for Patient Experiencing Alopecia

Nursing Diagnoses	Defining Characteristics	Expected Outcomes	Nursing Interventions
I. Potential body image disturbances related to alopecia	I. A. Chemotherapy agents attack rapidly dividing normal as well as abnormal cells. The cells and tissues responsible for hair growth have a high mitotic rate and are sensitive to the effects of chemotherapy. The potential depends on the activity of the drug in specific phases of replication. The drugs most commonly implicated in causing alopecia because they effect the S phase of the cell cycle are cyclophosphamide dactinomycin daunorubicin doxorubicin vincristine cytosine arabinoside hydroxyurea 5-fluorouracil methotrexate B. Doxorubicin causes alopecia in greater than 80% of patients treated, usually within 21 days. Alopecia caused from cyclophosphamide depends on dose (occurs more frequently with higher doses). Alopecia from methotrexate is also dose related. With 5-fluorouracil, thinning of eyebrows and loss of eyebrows may be observed in addition to loss of scalp hair. Range of alopecia may be from thinning of hair to a total body hair loss. C. Regrowth depends on schedule of treatments and doses administered. Usually regrowth begins 2–3 months after cessation of therapy. D. Whole brain radiation (5,000–7,000 rads) usually results in permanent alopecia as a result of permanent damage to hair follicles. Radiation to lower levels of brain may not cause permanent alopecia.	I. A. Pt, significant other, or family member will verbalize an understanding of factors that cause alopecia (chemotherapy, radiation therapy). B. Pt will discuss the impact of alopecia on his or her lifestyle. C. Pt will demonstrate knowledge of appropriate measures to minimize alopecia.	I. A. Assess pt for being at risk for developing alopecia. B. Instruct pt about hair loss, temporary or permanent, and the effects of chemotherapy on hair follicles. C. Instruct pt on the potential for regrowth and for the potential change in color and texture. D. Assess the impact of alopecia on the pt. E. Encourage verbalization of feelings. F. Encourage pt to cut long hair short so as to minimize the shock of alopecia. G. Discuss various measures to take during hair loss: wigs, scarves, hats, turban, use of makeup to highlight other features, baseball caps, cowboy hats. H. Encourage support groups with people experiencing alopecia. I. Encourage pt to help maintain personal identity by wearing own clothes in hospital and retaining social contacts. J. Instruct pt on proper scalp care: 1. Use baby shampoo or mild soap 2. Use soft brush to minimize pulling at hair 3. Use mineral oil or Vitamin A&D ointment to reduce itching 4. Always use a sunscreen when exposed to sun (SPF 15 or higher) K. If pt loses eyelashes or eyebrows instruct pt to use methods for protecting eyes (eyeglasses, hats with wide brim)

the uptake of temperature-dependent drugs, such as doxorubicin (Keller & Blausey 1988). Hypothermia, with or without a scalp tourniquet may decrease hair loss when doxorubicin doses are less than 40–50 mg/m² (Dean, Griffith, Cetus, et al. 1983). However, patients may feel chills, headache, and a feeling of pressure, and require premedication with acetaminophen 650 mg po prior to the procedure. Cooling is applied 15–20 minutes before treatment, and afterwards for at least 30 minutes.

Because both hypothermia and scalp constriction decrease drug concentration in the scalp, a sanctuary for micrometastatic malignant cells occurs. Therefore, patients with primary tumors that may metastasize to the skin are not appropriate candidates, and these include: patients with leukemia, lymphoma, sarcoma, mycosis fungoides, cancers of the breast, lung, kidney, or stomach. Scalp constriction or tourniquet is contraindicated in patients with hypertension or thrombocytopenia < 50,000/mm³ (Chernecky and Yasko 1986).

Body image concerns may result from alopecia. Baxley, Erdman, Henry, et al. (1984) studied forty male and female patients receiving chemotherapy and found that patients experiencing alopecia had lower body image scores than those who did not lose their hair. Alopecia may adversely affect perceived sexual attractiveness, self-esteem, and social activities, and for many is a visible reminder of cancer and its treatment.

Initially, prior to beginning chemotherapy, nursing assessment should determine the patient's self-perception and interaction with significant others to determine adaptive abilities (Keller and Blausley 1988). Patient teaching and emotional support help the patient first anticipate hair loss, talk about its potential impact, and learn self-care techniques, such as purchase of a wig prior to beginning therapy. Once therapy begins, ongoing support is often necessary to help the patient grieve his or her loss, working through the grief reactions of shock or denial, anger, depression, and finally acceptance. Patients can support each other, with the nurse acting as a facilitator of discussion (Keller and Blausey 1988). It is important to reassure the patient that this is a temporary loss, and hair will grow back. Some men prefer to shave their head once the hair has started falling out, and wear baseball caps. Women may choose scarfs or wigs. In cold climates, because up to 25% of body heat is lost through the scalp, patients should be advised to wear caps at night. Other self-care measures to reduce the mechanical damage to the hair shaft are: avoid excessive brushing or shampooing of hair; avoid electric curlers, hot dryers, and hair dyes; and use a mild, protein-based shampoo every 3–5 days (Chernecky and Yasko 1986). Finally, resources are often available to help the patient purchase a wig: local American Cancer Society (1-800-ACS-2345), some insurance plans if the wig is prescribed by a physician, and for the Internal Revenue purposes, a wig is a tax-deductible expense (Chernecky and Yasko 1986). Patient information materials are available from the Cancer Information Service, Room 307, 550 North Broadway, Baltimore, MD 21205, 1-800-4-CANCER (*Hair Care: Helpful Hints for Chemotherapy Patients*), or may be developed by enterprising nurses, as documented by Keller and Blausey (1988).

IV. GONADAL DYSFUNCTION

The reproductive tissues are composed of rapidly dividing gonadal cells in men, while women are born with their full complement of ovarian follicles. Damage from chemotherapy can result in temporary or permanent sterility, irregular menses, amenorrhea, premature menopause, and alteration in libido. Which, if any, reproductive change occurs depends on the age of the patient when treated, the intensity (dose and duration) of treatment (Perry and Yarbro 1984) and in some cases, on the drug(s) involved. In addition, many chemotherapeutic agents are *mutagenic*, causing changes in the DNA in the ova or sperm, and *teratogenic*, causing alterations in the developing fetus (Brager and Yasko 1984).

Issues of reproduction and sexuality are important because they represent basic human needs. If unaddressed they can lead to dysfunction and a decrease in self-esteem. Cancers that may be cured by chemotherapy often occur in children and young adults, such as acute lymphoblastic leukemia, Hodgkin's disease, and testicular carcinoma (Yarbro and Perry 1985). Thus, even though gonadal injury from chemotherapy does not pose a lethal threat, it is critical to address problems of reproduction and sexuality to help patients and their significant others achieve a high quality of life.

Female changes in reproductive function following chemotherapy treatment appear largely age related, but are also influenced by drug dose intensity, duration of treatment, and previous reproductive health. Women are born with a full complement of primordial ovarian follicles, which number about 448,000 at the ages 6–9, and decrease in number to 8300 at ages 40–44 (Block 1952).

Early studies on women receiving chemotherapy for Hodgkin's disease have shown that ovarian damage is more severe and permanent as the age of the woman increases. Women aged 35 and over are more apt to develop ovarian fibrosis and failure (Yarbro and Perry 1985), whereas younger women are better able to tolerate chemotherapy. However, it is not clear if these women may experience early menopause. In addition, amenorrhea in young women in their 20s is usually reversible, but becomes irreversible after age 30 (Yarbro and Perry 1985). It appears that the ovarian damage is progressive, and women aged 20–30 receiving aggressive chemotherapy often develop complete ovarian failure in their 30s (Chapman 1984). Alkylating agents are the most threatening agents, and cause a loss of ova, and an increase in mutation rate of ova (Kaempfer 1981). Women with ovarian failure

experience symptoms of premature menopause such as "hot flashes," amenorrhea, vaginal dryness, and dyspareunia (Yarbro and Perry 1985). Other events that may occur are atrophy of the endometrial lining of the uterus, irregular menses or amenorrhea, temporary sterility, spontaneous abortions, and stillbirths (Yasko 1983). However, normal-appearing children have been born to mothers who have received chemotherapy, but these children require close follow-up by pediatrician and oncologist (Yasko 1983; Kreuser, Hetzl, Hert et al. 1988).

German investigators, studying reproductive and endocrine gonadal function in young adults receiving chemotherapy for acute lymphoblastic or acute undifferentiated leukemia, found that all male patients (aged 14–38 years old) had azoospermia, with recovery of spermatogenesis in the second year of maintenance therapy. Women in this study (aged 14–36) did not show any reproductive dysfunction as evidenced by intact ovarian follicle function and ovulation, or endocrine dysfunction, as evidenced by normal serum levels of gonadal steroids and gonadotrophins. Drugs administered during induction, consolidation, and maintenance therapy were prednisone, vincristine, daunorubicin, L-asparaginase, cyclophosphamide, mercaptopurine, dexamethasone, vincristine, doxorubicin, thioguanine, and methotrexate. However, the median age of women studied was 23, most of the drugs used were antimetabolites which have less gonadal toxicity, and the total cyclophosphamide dose was 2.6 gm/m^2 versus the higher doses used in treatment of Hodgkin's disease of 6–12 gm (Kreuser et al. 1988).

Chemotherapy-induced gonadal dysfunction in men manifests as damage to the germinal epithelium and stem cell depletion of the seminiferous tubules. This results in severe oligospermia (few sperm) or azoospermia (absence of sperm) (Yarbro and Perry 1985), occurring 90–120 days after initiation of chemotherapy (Yasko 1983). Some drugs, such as the antimetabolites, are relatively nontoxic to gonadal cells while others, such as the alkylating agents, are very toxic. Damage from alkylating agents is reversible up to a certain threshold (i.e., chlorambucil 400 mg, cyclophosphamide 6–10 gm), and becomes irreversible beyond this (Perry and Yarbro 1984). However, for many patients, damage is reversible, with recovery of spermatogenesis occurring within 2 years of cessation of therapy (Drasga et al. 1983; Kreuser et al. 1988).

In advanced Hodgkin's disease, it was found that the risk of gonadal damage using MOPP [mechlorethamine hydrochloride (nitrogen mustard), Oncovin, prednisone, procarbazine] was quite high: at least 80% of men were likely to develop azoospermia, germinal aplasia, and testicular atrophy (Sherins and DeVita 1973). More recently, researchers have determined that apparently equal tumor response with less gonadal dysfunction can be achieved using ABVD (Adriamycin, bleomycin, vinblastine, and dacarbazine) (Bonfante et al. 1985). Patients receiving combined pelvic radiation and alkylating chemotherapy appear to have a high incidence of gonadal failure (Chapman 1984). Finally, treatment for prostate cancer using estrogen is likely to result in impotence.

In summary, whether a patient receiving chemotherapy will develop sterility is unpredictable. The risk in females appears to be largely age-related with women older than age 30 at greatest risk of developing ovarian failure. Failure is also related to specific drug and dose intensity.

In men, damage to the germ cells, and stem cells of the seminiferous tubules may induce temporary sterility. If damage is not permament, normal spermatogenesis returns within two years of termination of therapy. Nursing care focuses initially on accurate patient assessment of coping strategies, body image changes, self-esteem, self-concept issues, sexual identity, role relationships, and support of both the patient and significant other. More obvious drug side effects, such as alopecia, nausea and vomiting, and weight loss or gain can alter one's body image and alter normal sexual patterns. Nursing

interventions to explore the impact on the individual, to encourage the patient to verbalize feelings, and to provide emotional support are helpful, as well as specific suggestions for coping with altered sexuality.

The role of the nurse as an educator is a critical one, as this will help the patient "live" with the treatment. The patient should be taught the actual and potential risks of chemotherapy as they relate to sexual and reproductive health. Male patients may choose to use a sperm bank, and referral should be made *prior* to the initiation of chemotherapy so that functional, dense, sperm can be collected. A list of Human Semen Cryobanks can be obtained from the American Fertility Society, 1608 13th Ave S, Birmingham, Alabama 35256. Costs usually begin at $100 for 1 specimen with a $30–$70 yearly fee for storage. Some patients may have depressed sperm counts prior to therapy, related to disease such as testicular, lymphoma, or hematologic malignancies, and be unable to produce an adequate specimen for preservation. Kaempfer et al. (1985) surveyed cancer patients who had banked sperm for a 10-year period (1974–84): of 24 patients, 3 had withdrawn samples for artificial insemination, and there was 1 confirmed pregnancy with delivery of healthy twins. One patient had fathered two children after discontinuing chemotherapy.

Birth control practices are recommended by most practitioners for 2 years following chemotherapy (Kaempfer et al. 1985) as this provides for evaluation of disease response, avoidance of possible teratogenic drug effects, and in male patients, recovery of spermatogenesis. An assessment of the patient's current birth control practices should be explored, and alternatives discussed as necessary, i.e., patients with hormonally dependent tumors should not use oral contraceptives (Kaempfer et al. 1985).

Smith recommends use of the PLISSIT model for sexual rehabilitation, developed by Jack Annon (Smith 1989), and describes the levels as follows:

Table 4.13 Sexual and Reproductive Dysfunction Caused by the Administration of Chemotherapeutic Agents

Dysfunction	Gender	Causative Factors
I. ALTERED SEXUALITY PATTERNS related to body image changes and decreased level of sexual excitement	Male and Female	A. Side effects of chemotherapy: *alopecia, weight loss* related to nausea/vomiting, *diarrhea, fatigue*; decreased libido.
II. ALTERATIONS IN the ability to achieve SEXUAL FULFILLMENT	Female	A. Side effects of chemotherapy: *dryness of vaginal mucosa* secondary to decreased estrogen levels, *inflammation and ulceration* of vaginal mucosa (mucositis) secondary to stem cell injury B. Other possible factors: altered role function, *fear, fatigue, anxiety, lack of privacy, anger, medications/alcohol/analgesics*.
	Male	A. Side effects of chemotherapy: *temporary impotence* possibly related to fatigue, pain B. Other possible factors: altered role function, *fear, fatigue, anxiety, lack of privacy, anger*, medications/alcohol/analgesics.

III. SEXUAL DYSFUNCTION	Female	A. Side effects of chemotherapy
		  1. *Temporary or permanent sterility*
		    a. *Ovarian fibrosis* with decrease in estrogen levels, decrease in number of available ova, especially with higher dose alkylating agents, and age over 30
		    b. *Atrophy* of endometrial lining of uterus
		    c. *Irregular menses* or *amenorrhea* (may be reversible under 30 years of age)
		  2. *Potential for mutation of available ova* (especially by alkylating agents)
		    a. Spontaneous abortion, stillbirth, birth defects
		    b. May have normal children who should be followed by pedi-oncologist

	Male	A. Side effects of chemotherapy
		  1. *Temporary or permanent sterility*
		    a. Damage and destruction of testicular germ cells, and epithelium of seminiferous tubules
		    b. Oligospermia or azoospermia 90–120 days after treatment begins; normal sperm levels may be achieved several years after therapy
		    c. Testosterone levels not altered
		  2. *Possible sperm mutation*
		    a. Spontaneous abortion, stillbirths, birth defects
		    b. Normal children have been fathered; child should be closely followed by pedi-oncologist.

IV. ALTERATIONS IN FETAL DEVELOPMENT		A. Possible side effects of chemotherapy
		  1. Drugs cross placental barrier
		  2. Antimetabolites (e.g., MTX) and alkylating agents most harmful
		  3. 1st Trimester: Drugs can cause cellular damage and destruction leading to spontaneous abortion
		  4. 2nd, 3rd Trimester: Cellular destruction leads to low birth weight or premature infant, stillbirth, birth defects, great potential for development of malignancy; there may be mutation of ova of female child.

Modified from Yasko 1983.

Table 4.14 Standardized Nursing Care Plan for the Patient Experiencing Sexual Dysfunction

Nursing Diagnoses	Defining Characteristics	Expected Outcomes	Nursing Interventions
I. Sexual dysfunction related to disease process, treatment, or infertility	I. A. Cancer pts often experience some sexual alteration as a result of physical or psychological insults by the disease process, diagnosis, side effects of chemotherapy, surgical intervention, or radiation. B. Some chemotherapy causes sexual infertility: chlorambucil cyclophosphamide doxorubicin cytarabine procarbazine vinblastine C. Dimensions altered by cancer therapy may affect behavior used to express sexual identity.	I. A. Pt will demonstrate knowledge of factors that may potentially affect sexuality. B. Pt will verbalize the potential impact of diagnosis on sexual activity. C. Pt will maintain satisfying sex role and sexual self image. D. Pt will identify strategies used to minimize sexual dysfunction. E. Pt or significant other will identify other measures used for sexual expression.	I. A. Establish a trusting relationship with the pt. B. Assess pt's knowledge regarding the effects of the disease and treatment on sexuality. C. Provide a comfortable, relaxed environment in which to discuss with the pt the effects of disease and treatment on sexuality. D. Allow pt and significant other to verbalize perceptions of how disease and treatment will affect sexual function and sexuality. E. Discuss strategies to minimize sexual dysfunction: 1. Alternative forms of sexual expression 2. Alternative positions to decrease pain and prevent injury 3. Encourage sexual activity when energy levels are highest (in morning, after naps) 4. Help pt to recognize sexual feelings and urges 5. Include sexual partner in counseling and teaching 6. Explain effects of drugs and treatment on fertility 7. Refer for further counseling, if necessary F. Discuss options regarding alternative methods of family planning: 1. Foster parenthood 2. Adoption 3. Provide information on sperm banking

1. Permit the patient to express sexual concerns (95% of problems can be dealt with at this level)
2. Provide limited information regarding the consequences of disease or therapy on sexual functioning
3. Provide specific suggestions for alternative methods of sexual expression
4. Refer for intensive therapy, either surgical or psychosexual

Glasgow, Halfin, and Althausen (1987) suggest that couples who have satisfactory sexual relationships prior to cancer diagnosis and treatment are able to find a satisfactory relationship afterward, while those experiencing problems had dysfunction. Two excellent patient–significant other booklets are available without charge from the American Cancer Society, written by Leslie Schorer, PhD, Section Head of Psychosexual Disorders, Dept. of Psychiatry and Urology, Cleveland Clinic Foundation: *Sexuality and Cancer: For the Woman Who Has Cancer and her Partner*; and *Sexuality and Cancer: For the Man Who Has Cancer and his Partner*.

SECTION B. NAUSEA AND VOMITING

Nausea and vomiting are common following chemotherapy, and pose a significant challenge to patients and to nurses caring for them. Nausea or vomiting can be *acute*, occurring soon after drug administration, such as with nitrogen mustard; *subacute*, occurring 6–12 hours later, as with cyclophosphamide; *delayed*, occurring 2–3 days later, as with cisplatin; and *anticipatory*, a conditioned response to past experience of nausea or vomiting after chemotherapy administration. It is estimated that 25–50% of patients with cancer delay one or more scheduled courses of therapy (Lazlo 1983) and that up to 10% of patients with

cancer refuse further chemotherapy, even curative treatment, because of the distress related to nausea and vomiting (Siegel and Longo 1981). Other potential complications of nausea and vomiting include esophageal tears (Mallory-Weiss syndrome), fractures, prolonged anorexia, malnutrition, metabolic abnormalities, and volume depletion (Craig and Powell 1987). Fortunately, progress has been made in the control of nausea and vomiting related to chemotherapy. Figure 4.11 illustrates the potential sequelae of nausea and vomiting in a nursing diagnostic framework.

Nausea refers to a vague, wavelike sensation and conscious need to vomit; *vomiting* refers to the actual forceful expulsion of gastric contents through the mouth, and *retching* is the rhythmic contraction of respiratory muscles causing up and down movement of gastric contents into the esophagus.

The vomiting or emetic center coordinates the reflex act of vomiting and is located in the lateral reticular formation of the medulla oblongata, close to the reflex centers controlling cardiovascular and respiratory function. Thus, shared efferent pathways bring about signs and symptoms of tachycardia; diaphoresis; weakness or dizziness during nausea; bradycardia and decreased blood pressure during vomiting; and increased rate and depth of respiration (Borison and McCarthy 1984). The vomiting center receives stimulation from five areas (Yasko 1985):

1. Intestinal tract through the vagus nerve (vagal visceral afferents), stimulated by delayed gastric emptying or gastrointestinal distention
2. Cortical pathway via hypothalamus (cerebral cortex and limbic system), stimulated by anxiety or increased intracranial pressure; the cortical pathway is probably responsible for anticipatory nausea and vomiting
3. Vestibular pathway via labyrinth system and vagus nerve, stimulated by rapid position changes; the pathway does not play a significant role in chemotherapy-induced emesis

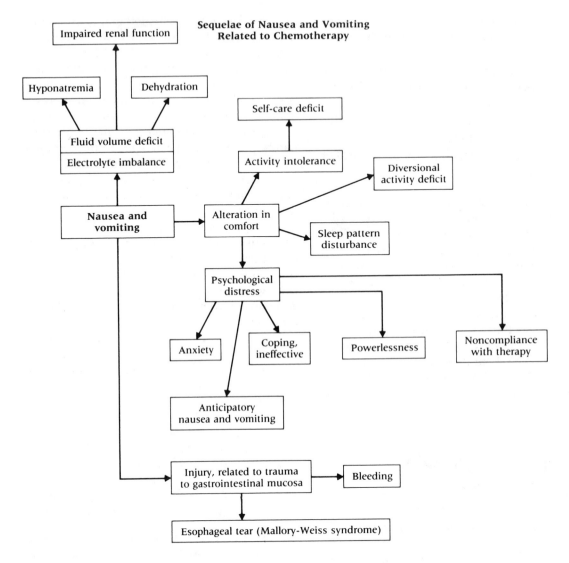

Figure 4.11   Potential patient problems related to nausea and vomiting

4. Peripheral pathways via sympathetic visceral afferents from the gastrointestinal tract, heart, and kidneys, stimulated by irritation or spasm
5. Chemoreceptor trigger zone (CTZ), stimulated by blood-borne toxins, drugs such as chemotherapy, and altered hormones of pregnancy

The chemoreceptor trigger zone (CTZ) contains receptors for histamine (H1 and H2), dopamine, acetylcholine, and opiates but the actual neurochemical physiology of chemotherapy-induced nausea and vomiting is not well known (Craig and Powell 1987). Blood-borne chemotherapy appears to stimulate the

CTZ, which then stimulates the vomiting center, probably via dopaminergic and serotonin pathways. The vomiting center has muscarinic (cholinergic) and histamine receptors, as do the vestibular and efferent vagal motor nuclei (Goodman 1987). Prostaglandins may also play a role in the stimulation of nausea and vomiting, and it is postulated that prostaglandin A2 may be released by trauma to the GI mucosa by chemotherapy (Ignoffo 1983). As shown in figure 4.12, there are multiple pathways of stimulation for nausea and vomiting; hence, the most effective antiemetic regimens include drugs that act on some or all of the different pathways. Although

it is quite likely that nausea and vomiting occurring after chemotherapy administration is related to the drugs given, it is important to exclude other potential causes. These include bowel obstruction or peritonitis, CNS metastasis, drugs such as narcotics, fluid and electrolyte imbalance, hepatic metastasis, infections (local or systemic), radiation therapy, and uremia.

Psychogenic factors can influence the occurrence of nausea and vomiting, and thus it is crucial to try to prevent this from occurring with the first treatment cycle. Anticipatory nausea and vomiting (ANV) refers to the learned conditioned response of nausea and vomiting when

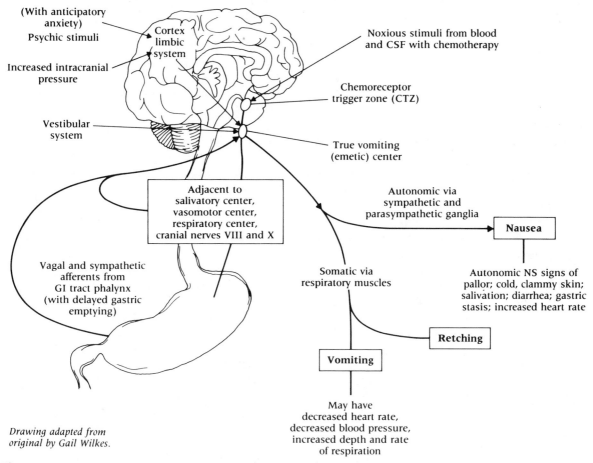

Drawing adapted from
original by Gail Wilkes.

Figure 4.12 Physiology of nausea and vomiting

triggered by the memory or reminder of chemotherapy administration, such as the smell of alcohol or the sight of the chemotherapy nurse. The vomiting center is stimulated by higher cortical areas (limbic system) resulting in pretreatment nausea or vomiting. ANV usually develops after the third or fourth cycle of therapy, and may affect as many as 33% of patients (Nicholas 1982). Studies have shown that behavioral techniques may be useful in decreasing the distress and degree of ANV. These techniques include hypnosis with guided imagery, systematic desensitization, and progressive muscle relaxation, where relaxation becomes the conditioned response. In addition, the drug lorazepam with its amnesiac quality, helps to decrease ANV. According to Morrow, patients at risk for developing ANV experience the triad of warm/hot sensation, severe nausea/vomiting, and diaphoresis following treatment (Morrow 1982). Yasko (1985) suggests increased risk in patients who experience a metallic taste after treatment, have anxiety or depression, and are less than fifty years old. Cotanch and Strum (1987) use five specific patient instructions together with behavioral techniques prior to chemotherapy administration. The patient is told that s/he will feel 1) restful sleep, 2) relinquishment of control, 3) swift passage of time, 4) thirst upon wakening but will fall back asleep again, and 5) satisfaction upon completion of therapy.

In contrast to ANV patients, who have great difficulty in tolerating treatment due to nausea and vomiting, it appears that patients with histories of alcohol abuse tend to have better results with antiemetics than other patients do (Hesketh et al. 1988).

The degree of nausea and vomiting, and duration of distress, is related to the drug, dose, frequency, and method of administration, where the risk is greater with IV administration than with oral dosing, and the risk is greater with shorter infusion than when the drug is administered over a longer time. Also affecting the degree and duration of emesis is the delayed excretion of the drug or drug metabolites, which may cause delayed nausea and vomiting. For example, it is possible to prevent nausea and vomiting during cisplatin administration, and then have the patient develop nausea and vomiting 24–48 hours after drug administration. This occurs in 30–60% of patients and lasts up to 7 days (Strum et al. 1985; Rhodes, Watson, and Johnson 1985). Thus, it is important to continue antiemetic protection post-cisplatin therapy to prevent emesis. While mild antiemetics are helpful in preventing emesis from low to moderate emetogenic drug combinations, aggressive, multidrug combinations are necessary for preventing emesis from highly emetogenic drugs such as high-dose cisplatin or DTIC (see table 4.15).

The nurse's prechemotherapy assessment should include hydration and electrolyte status, and these should be corrected prior to chemotherapy administration. Anxiety can be reduced by supportive and empathetic communication with the patient to explore concerns or provide distraction as appropriate, technical expertise of the nurse, and consistency of care providers between successive courses of therapy. Nursing care is directed toward preventing nausea and vomiting, decreasing anxiety, increasing comfort, and promoting self-care, as shown in the standardized nursing care plan at the end of this section.

ANTIEMETIC TREATMENT

In designing antiemetic treatment, antiemetics must be administered or have a duration of action for the period of expected nausea and vomiting from the specific chemotherapeutic agent. For example, peak nausea and vomiting from cyclophosphamide is 12 hours; therefore, antiemetic coverage should extend beyond this period. Drug administration schedules often begin the night before drug administration, especially if the patient has ANV. Antiemetic drugs should be given *prior* to chemotherapy so that receptors

Table 4.15   Emetic Potential of Chemotherapy Drugs

High (>80% Incidence)		Antiemetic Regimen
mechlorethamine (nitrogen mustard) dacarbazine (DTIC) cisplatin (platinol) Mitomycin C (BCNU, CCNU) high-dose cyclophosphamide high-dose methotrexate high-dose cytosine arabinoside		Aggressive combination antiemetics, metoclopramide or high-dose phenothiazine with dexamethasone nitrosoureas and lorazepam
Moderate (50%)		
doxorubicin (Adriamycin) daunorubicin (Daunomycin) cyclophosphamide (Cytoxan) ifosfamide dactinomycin (Actinomycin D) mitoxantrone (Novantrone) procarbazine etoposide hexamethylmelamine		Moderately aggressive therapy with IV phenothiazines (perphenazine, prochlorperazine)
Low (<25%)		
5-fluorouracil (5-FU) methotrexate bleomycin cytosine arabinoside (Ara-C) melphalan vincristine hydroxyurea etoposide	thiotepa thioguanine tamoxifen chlorambucil L-asparaginase vinblastine teniposide 6-mercaptopurine	oral phenothiazines

Source: Modified by permission of the publisher from Dorr and Fritz, *Cancer Chemotherapy Handbook*, pp. 103–104. Copyright 1980 by Elsevier Science Publishing Co., Inc.

in the CTZ can be effectively blocked, thus preventing the stimulation of nausea and vomiting:

oral antiemetics should be given 30–40 minutes before treatment;

when administered rectally, up to 60 minutes before;

by IM injection 20–30 minutes before;

and IV dosing should be given 10–20 minutes prior to treatment.

In this way the blockade is in place before the chemotherapy drug enters the bloodstream. In general, antiemetics should be administered prior to chemotherapy administration, and regularly after treatment for at least 24 hours for drugs that have moderate to high emetogenic potential (Yasko 1985).

The last ten years have seen many studies conducted in the search for more effective antiemetic regimens. Craig and Powell (1987) identify key elements to look for when reviewing antiemetic studies:

1. Is the study randomized and double-blind? Is it a parallel or cross-over study, which reduces bias; a cross-over design allows the patient to act as his or her own control.

2. Are there comparable, randomized patient populations in which it is the first treatment cycle for all patients, and patients are not taking any other medications that may have antiemetic potential? Are the patients receiving equally emetogenic chemotherapy drugs, and are they in the same treatment setting, i.e., inpatient or ambulatory setting?

3. Is there a clear definition of response? Is there a distinction between nausea and vomiting? Is patient preference evaluated? Is the number of vomiting episodes measured in a given period of time?

4. Is there an adequate sample to make a valid statistical statement?

As oncology nurses administering chemotherapy, it is essential to remain knowledgeable about current antiemetic research findings. Certain patients may not respond to standard antiemetic regimens, and it is important to be a patient advocate, discussing with the physician alternative antiemetic regimens that may be more effective.

PHARMACOLOGY OF ANTIEMETICS

The following seven groups of antiemetic drugs—phenothiazines, butyrophenones, substituted benzamides, benzodiazepines, glucocorticosteroids, cannabinoids, and antihistamines—are commonly used in antiemetic therapy for cancer chemotherapy side effects. This section presents information on selected drugs within each group.

Phenothiazines

Have been the mainstay of antiemetic therapy since the 1950s. Phenothiazines with a piperazine side-chain are more effective antiemetics (e.g., perphenazine, prochlorperazine) than those with an alkyl group (e.g., chlorpromazine).

Action: Blocks dopamine receptors in CTZ; also decreases vagal stimulation of vomiting center by peripheral afferents. Effective for low emetogenic drugs (e.g., methotrexate, 5-FU, low-dose cyclophosphamide) at usual doses, and more emetogenic chemotherapy agents at higher doses.

Efficacy: Prochlorperazine equally effective as droperidol and low-dose metoclopramide against cisplatin-containing chemotherapy, but less effective than cannabinoids, corticosteroids, and high-dose metoclopramide (Bakowski 1984). Carr et al. (1985) studied high-dose prochlorperazine

Drug	Dose/Schedule	Comments
Prochlorperazine (Compazine)	*PO:* 5, 10, 25 mg q 4–6 hr *Slow-release PO:* 10, 15, 30, 75 mg q 12 hr *PR:* 25 mg q 4–6 hr *IM/IV:* 5–40 mg (Carr et al. 1985) q 3–4 hr mix in 50 cc D$_5$W or NS and give over 20–30 mins	
perphenazine (Trilafon)	*PO:* 4 mg q 4–6 hr maximum 30 mg in 24 hours for inpatients, 15 mg for outpatients *IM/IV:* 5 mg IVB q 4–6 hr or then infusion at 1 mg/hr for 10 hrs (Smaglia 1984)	

and found increased effectiveness against cisplatin without increased toxicity when diphenhydramine is given. Prochlorperazine and perphenazine were found equally effective against cisplatin when equal doses were given (loading and continuous infusion) (Smaglia 1984).

Side Effects: Sedation, hypotension, and extrapyramidal side effects, especially dystonia. Rarely, can cause lowering of seizure thresholds, skin reactions, agranulocytosis, cholestatic jaundice, and increased prolactin levels.

Butyrophenones

Are potent neuroleptics. They are major tranquilizers used as antiemetics.

Action: Dopamine antagonists that suppress the CTZ and vomiting center; considered more potent than the phenothiazines. Also decreases stimulation of the vomiting center along vestibular pathway.

Efficacy: Droperidol appears to require higher doses to provide adequate protection against cisplatin-containing regimens. Citron et al. (1984) suggest a loading dose of 5–15 mg IVB then 5–7.5 mg IV every 2 hours for 6–8 hours (Wilson et al. 1981). Haloperidol IM or PO was shown to be equivalent to tetrahydrocannabinoid and superior to phenothiazines when

Drug	Dose/Schedule	Comments
droperidol (Inapsine)	*IM/IV:* 0.5–2.5 mg q 4–6 hr or drip but reports suggest large loading dose then intermittent IVB or continuous infusion for 6–10 hrs (Citron et al. 1984; Wilson et al. 1981)	Caution in patients with cardiac dysfunction on anticonvulsants
haloperidol (Haldol)	*PO:* 3–5 mg q 2 hr × 3–4 doses, beginning ½ hr before chemotherapy *IM:* 0.5–2 mg	oral well absorbed

tested against noncisplatin-containing regimens. IV haloperidol was not as effective as high-dose metoclopramide against cisplatin (Greenberg et al. 1984; Neidhart et al. 1981).

Side Effects: Sedation, restlessness, extrapyramidal reactions (less severe than with phenothiazines), and tardive dyskinesia may occur in older patients. Can induce respiratory depression when used with narcotic analgesics.

Substituted Benzamides

The only substituted benzamide with antiemetic potential is metoclopramide (Reglan), which is a procainamide derivative without cardiac effects.

Action: Acts both centrally and peripherally. Dopamine antagonist blocking CTZ; also stimulates upper GI tract motility thus increasing gastric emptying, and opposes retrograde peristalsis of retching (Goodman 1987).

Efficacy: Dose related, with 60% effectiveness against high-dose cisplatin, and increased to 66% with the addition of steroids, lorazepam (Strum et al. 1984). As a single agent, metoclopramide is superior to placebo, THC, dexamethasone, prochlorperazine, and haldol in controlling cisplatin-induced nausea and vomiting, and prevents *all* vomiting in 40% of patients (Gralla et al. 1984). Lower doses (1 mg/kg) appear equally effective to higher doses in patients receiving cisplatin $< 75mg/m^2$ (Raila et al. 1985). High-dose oral and continuous infusion administration appears equally effective to intermittent bolus administration (Craig and Powell 1987).

Side Effects: Sedation, akathisia (restlessness), other extrapyramidal side effects, especially in patients younger than 30 yrs where the incidence is 30% versus that of 1.8% in older adults (Allen et al. 1985). Diarrhea occurs in about 30% of patients and is well controlled by antidiarrheal medication, or may be prevented by the addition of dexamethasone to the regimen.

Drug	Dose/Schedule	Comments
metoclopramide hydrochloride (Reglan)	*IV:* 1–3 mg/kg IV 30 min before chemotherapy administration then repeat q 2 hrs for 2–4 doses *PO:* For delayed nausea and vomiting, 20–40 mg q 4 hr × 24 hours or 0.5 mg/kg qid × 4 days beginning 24 hrs after cisplatin together with dexamethasone 8 mg bid d 1–2, 4 mg bid d 3–4 (Kris and Gralla 1986)	Dosage of 2 mg/kg every 2 hrs for 3 to 5 doses is appropriate for high-dose CDDP (120 mg/m^2). PO route may result in increased number of stools.

Drug	Dose/Schedule	Comments
lorazepam (Ativan)	*IV:* 0.5–1.5 mg/m^2 to 4 mg total dose* IVP or in 50 cc D$_5$W or NS over 10 min, 30 mins prior to chemotherapy, q 4–6 hrs postchemotherapy *PO:* 1–3 mg 30 mins prior to chemotherapy, q 4–6 hrs postchemotherapy	Have someone accompany pt home if outpt Dosage should be titrated to induce arousable sleep state Should be mixed immediately prior to administration

*Dose reduce in elderly, debilitated patients; patients with severe hepatic dysfunction (Bilirubin >2 mg %); or serum albumin <2 mg %; and in patients with severe COPD where respiratory center depresssion is inadvisable.

Side Effects: Arousable sedation but may occasionally be profound; prolonged amnesia; hypotension; perceptual disturbances; and urinary incontinence.

Drug Interactions: CNS depression when given with alcohol, phenothiazines, barbiturates, MAO inhibitors, and other depressants. Increased sedation when combined with scopalamine.

Benzodiazepines

CNS depressants that decrease anxiety (anxiolytic), increase sedation, and cause anterograde amnesia so that if nausea or vomiting occur, they are not remembered.

Action: May work by blocking cortical pathways to the vomiting center, and thus may be useful in controlling anticipatory nausea and vomiting when begun the night before treatment. It is 90% absorbed from GI tract within 30 minutes of administration.

Efficacy: Lorazepam has been shown to be an effective addition to antiemetic regimens. A study by Gagen et al. (1984) comparing the effectiveness of metoclopramide to lorazepam and dexamethasone demonstrated that not only was the second combination more effective, but patients preferred the lorazepam combination 70% to 12% (Laszlo et al. 1985). However, lorazepam is most commonly used in combination with more active agents such as high-dose metoclopramide. Sublingual administration achieves peak and plasma levels similar to IV administration (Caille, Speneid, and Lacasse 1983).

Glucocorticosteroids

Glucocorticosteroids are usually used in conjunction with other antiemetic therapy.

Action: May inhibit prostaglandin release by stabilizing lysosomal membranes, thereby, theoretically, interrupting hypothalamic prostaglandin release and subsequent stimulation of nausea and vomiting (Goodman 1987).

Efficacy: Used in combination with other antiemetic agents, high doses of dexamethasone (oral or parenteral) have been effective in preventing nausea and vomiting in many patients (70–80% overall responses), especially in previously untreated patients (Markman et al. 1984). Also, the addition of high-dose dexamethasone in combination with high-dose metoclopramide significantly decreases the incidence of diarrhea from metoclopramide, as well as increasing the

Drug	Dose/Schedule	Comments
dexamethasone (Decadron)	*IV:* 10–20 mg begin ½ hr before chemotherapy, then q 4–6 hr *PO:* 4 mg q 4 × 4 doses beginning 1–8 hr before chemotherapy (Goodman 1987)	Use with caution in diabetics
Methylprednisolone (Solu-Medrol)	*IV:* 125–250 mg beginning ½ hr before chemotherapy, then q 4 × 3 more doses (Mason et al. 1982)	
Prednisone	*PO:* 25–50 mg 4 hr before chemotherapy and q 4 × 8 doses (Goodman 1987)	

Drug	Dose/Schedule	Comments
dronabinol (Marinol R)	*PO:* 5 mg/m^2–7.5 mg/m^2 1–3 hrs before chemotherapy then 2–4 hrs postchemotherapy for 4–6 doses per day	If ineffective, and no toxicity, can increase by 2.5 mg/m^2 increments to max 15 mg/m^2 dose (Sargeant and Fisher 1986)

effectiveness of the antiemetic action of metoclopramide in some studies (Gralla et al. 1987). As a single agent, corticosteroids are effective against low to moderate emetogenic agents.

Side Effects: During IVP administration, may have brief, intense perineal burning or pruritis which is prevented by infusion. Immediate vomiting has been reported and is self-limiting (Goodman 1987). Other side effects include lethargy, weakness, mood changes, hyperglycemia, leukocytosis secondary to demargination of WBC, and insomnia and agitation the evening following therapy. Side effects are usually mild as the drug is given for only short periods. High-dose steroids should be avoided in patients with a history of psychosis.

Cannabinoids

Synthetic preparations of marijuana have been proven effective in preventing or minimizing the nausea and vomiting that occurs as a side effect of chemotherapy.

Action: Active ingredient is delta-9-tetrahydrocannabinol (THC). Its mechanism of action is unclear but probably relates to central nervous system depression, and may involve disruption of higher cortical input, inhibition of prostaglandin synthesis, or may bind to opiate receptors in the brain to indirectly block the vomiting center.

Efficacy: More effective than placebo, in some cases equal or better than Prochlorperazine (Compazine R). However, not shown to be effective in patients receiving cisplatin (Gralla et al. 1984). Is an expensive drug, has high potential for abuse, and is indicated for patients who have failed standard antiemetics. Complete responses in 20–25%, partial responses in 40–55% against low emetogenic drugs (Sargeant and Fisher 1986).

Side Effects: Mood changes, disorientation, drowsiness, muddled thinking, dizziness; brief impairment of perception, coordination, and sensory functions. Rarely, dry mouth, increased appetite, general increase in central sympathomimetic activity with increased heart rate, and postural hypotension. Increased CNS toxicity in the elderly (up to 35%).

Antihistamines

Plays a major role in preventing extrapyramidal side effects of dopamine antagonists.

Action: Diphenhydramine (Benadryl) inhibits histamine, and has slight, if any, antiemetic activity by blocking the CTZ and decreasing vestibular stimulation.

Efficacy: Limited role in antiemesis but highly effective in the prevention of or resolution of extrapyramidal side effects.

Drug	Dose/Schedule	Comments
diphenhydramine (Benadryl)	*IV:* 50 mg before chemotherapy or 25 mg q 4 hr × 4 during metoclopramide or Trilafon (perphenazine) dosing, beginning prior to antiemetic *PO:* 25–50 mg q 4 *IM:* 25–50 mg q 4	Sedate to desired degree of sedation without compromising antiemetic activity

Side Effects: Drowsiness, dry mouth, dizziness.

EXTRAPYRAMIDAL SIDE EFFECTS: ASSESSMENT AND INTERVENTION

The most effective antiemetics to date seem to work by blocking or antagonizing dopamine receptors in the chemoreceptor trigger zone. All of these agents also have the potential to cause extrapyramidal side effects. Diphenhydramine (Benadryl) 50 mg IVP is rapidly effective in resolving acute dystonic reactions. If the symptoms are less acute, 50 mg IM usually brings relief within 15 minutes.

Symptoms of extrapyramidal reactions are:

tongue protrusion, neck dystonia (disordered muscle tone)

opisthotonus (spasm where the head and heels are bent backward and the body bowed forward)

trismus (spasm of chewing muscles so that mouth cannot open)

oligogyric crisis (movement of the eye around the anteroposterior axis, together with laryngeal and pharyngeal spasm can cause respiratory distress and ultimately anoxia)

limb dystonia (spasm of muscles of head, neck, back, which may resemble seizures)

akathesia (involuntary feeling of restlessness)

tremor

anxiety

insomnia

dizziness

Extrapyramidal side effects are so called because they result from excessive cholinergic activity in the extrapyramidal tract of the nervous system, caused by an unintentional blockade of the postsynaptic dopamine receptors by the antiemetic drug. Motor neurons which are responsible for movement lie in bundles located within tracts in the brain: those that pass through a pyramid-shaped area and that allow for direct cortical control, and initiation and patterning of skilled movement are called the *pyramidal tracts*. Those lying outside of this area are called the *extrapyramidal tracts*, and these are involved in motor activities such as the control and coordination of posture and locomotion. The extrapyramidal tracts inhibit muscle contractions that are "coordinated" by the cholinergic receptors in the pyramidal system. The pyramidal tracts are also able to inhibit cholinergic stimulation. The antiemetic drugs that work by blocking dopamine receptors (dopamine antagonists) also block postsynaptic dopamine receptors preventing completion of the nervous stimulation in the pyramidal tract. This imbalance leads to disinhibition of the extrapyramidal cholinergic receptors, with resulting *excessive* cholinergic activity as seen in the extrapyramidal side effects (Bickal 1987).

Dystonic reactions occur twice as commonly in young males, and in individuals younger than 35 years old (Gralla et al. 1987). Numerous studies have shown that adding diphenhydramine or lorazepam as part of combined antiemetics can prevent the development of this side effect in many cases. For example, diphenhydramine 50 mg can be given prior to initial metoclopramide dose. Lorazepam is especially effective in preventing akathesia (restlessness), as well as the other extrapyramidal symptoms (Kris et al. 1985).

In summary, prophylactic combination antiemetics should be given prior to all moderate and highly emetogenic chemotherapy agents.

Combinations containing metoclopramide, dexamethasone, and lorazepam, as developed by Gralla, offer the best antiemetic protection to date for highly emetogenic chemotherapy. Antiemetics should be continued for 4–7 days after cisplatin to prevent delayed nausea and vomiting. The use of metoclopramide plus dexamethasone orally has been shown in a study by Kris et al. (1989) to be superior to dexamethasone alone or placebo to prevent or control delayed nausea and vomiting. In providing antiemetic protection for moderately emetogenic chemotherapy, either metoclopramide or a phenothiazine, plus dexamethasone are effective, and should be continued for 24 hours postchemotherapy by either oral or IV route. For chemotherapeutic agents with low emetogenic potential, phenothiazine or dexamethasone alone, or no initial therapy, should be adequate.

It is critical to attempt to prevent nausea and vomiting at the first chemotherapy treatment, for only then can anticipatory nausea and vomiting be prevented. However, if ANV does occur, the use of intensive antiemetics, including lorazepam prior to therapy, and behavioral techniques may be helpful. If patients experience nausea and vomiting despite standard antiemetic therapy, patients may benefit from tetrahydrocannabinol (synthetic derivative Marinol) together with a phenothiazine to minimize central nervous system side effects (Craig and Powell 1987). Despite the best efforts using combination antiemetics, 30–40% of patients may experience nausea and vomiting related to chemotherapy, and it is important to continue the search for more effective antiemetic agents that do not possess distressing side effects.

Exciting new investigational work is being done on a serotonin-blocking drug which is believed to block 5-HT3 receptors in the chemoreceptor trigger zone (5-hydroxytryptamine or serotonin). However, because it does not involve dopamine antagonism, the side effects of dystonia do not occur. This selective serotonin antagonist (GR-C507/75) produces only mild toxicity (no extrapyramidal signs, mild increase in hepatic transaminase in 20% of patients, diarrhea in 12%, and mild sedation). Antiemetic effectiveness has been reported by various investigators, from 78–91% of patients having 0–2 emetic episodes while receiving cisplatin, and the drug is now being prospectively compared to standard antiemetics (Hesketh et al. 1988; Cunningham et al. 1987; Costall et al. 1987).

SECTION C. TOXICITY TO OTHER ORGAN SYSTEMS

INTRODUCTION

The following section addresses chemotherapy-related toxicities in other organ systems: systems that do not have a rapid cell proliferation rate, but which attract specific anticancer drugs. Consequently, damage may result from drug binding to tissue, such as doxorubicin and heart muscle myofibrils, when these cells have no affinity to other chemotheraputic agents. Toxicity may be found in certain organs responsible for drug elimination and excretion, such as the liver, kidneys, lungs, or sweat glands (Yasko 1983). The onset and degree of organ toxicity depends on the specific drug, dose received, and in many cases, the administration schedule (Yasko 1983).

Knowledge of drug-induced organ toxicity is critical to the oncology nurse administering chemotherapy. Certain tests must be performed prior to initial drug treatment, and periodically during treatment to identify early organ damage before symptoms become apparent. Although the ordering of these tests is the physician's responsibility, it is the nurse's responsibility to be certain the tests are performed and the results are within safe limits, prior to administering the drug. Also, prior to drug administration, the nurse assesses the patient for signs or symptoms of early organ toxicity.

Table 4.16 Standardized Nursing Care Plan for Patient Experiencing Nausea and Vomiting

Nursing Diagnosis	Expected Outcome	Nursing Interventions

I. Potential for altered nutrition, less than body requirements	I. A. Pt will maintain weight within 5% of baseline
	B. Pt will be without nausea and vomiting, and if it occurs it will be minimal
		I. A. Administer antiemetics prior to chemotherapy then regularly through expected duration of nausea and vomiting (depending on specific chemotherapeutic agent)
		  1. Evaluate past effectiveness of antiemetic regime
		  2. Evaluate need for beginning antiemetics 12–24 hrs after treatment
		  3. Attempt to prevent nausea and vomiting during first treatment cycle to prevent anticipatory nausea and vomiting
		B. Administer chemotherapy at night or late afternoon if possible
		C. Experiment with eating patterns: suggest patient avoid eating prior to, during, and immediately after initial treatment to assess tolerance. Discourage heavy, greasy, fatty, sweet, and spicy foods
		D. Encourage small, frequent, bland meals day of therapy (if tolerates eating day of therapy) and increase fluid intake to 3 quarts per day
		E. Encourage pt to suck hard candy during therapy
		F. Provide environment that is clean, quiet, subdued, without odors
		G. Encourage weekly weights; if pt unable to stabilize weight refer to dietician for intensive counseling, together with person responsible for doing the cooking
		H. Teach pt self-care measures
		  1. Self-administration of antiemetics, including indications, dose, schedule, and potential side effects
		  2. Dietary counseling encouraging bland, cool foods, cottage cheese, toast, if experiencing nausea and vomiting
		  3. Encourage favorite high-calorie, high-protein, small, frequent feedings as tolerated; encourage fluids to 3 quarts/day, including chicken soup, Gatorade, sherbet, gingerale
		  4. Give pt copy of *Eating Hints* (NCI free publication) with ideas such as whole milk plus 1–2 T powdered milk in eggnogs, snacks to increase protein, calorie intake

II. Potential for comfort alteration related to nausea and vomiting	II. A. Pt will verbalize decreased anxiety, and increased physical comfort	II. A. Encourage pt to verbalize feelings re prior treatments, if any, and significance of treatment to the patient B. Provide emotional support C. Consider anxiety-reducing drugs in antiemetic regime, such as lorazepam D. Minimize time pt is in waiting room, or chemotherapy room E. Provide distraction using VCR/TV, radio, as pt desires; for some pts, having a chaplain read the Psalms during therapy can be quite therapeutic F. Teach pt progressive muscle relaxation exercises and help pt to image peaceful past experiences; encourage fresh air G. Keep emesis basin within reach, provide cpp; cloth for face and hands if pt vomits H. Assist pt with mouth care after emesis I. Telephone pt, if treated as an outpt, the evening of, or day after, chemotherapy administration to assess tolerance and comfort
III. Potential powerlessness	III. A. Pt will have control over self-care activities	III. A. Pt and family teaching re potential side effects and self care measures. Offer pt and family *Chemotherapy and Use: A Self-Help Guide* (free NCI publication). B. Encourage pt to live as normal a life-style as possible, going out, and engaging in usual activities. Often, doing something "nice" for oneself *after* treatment helps to minimize the distress and increase control C. Involve pt and family in appropriate decisions in treatment as is possible

(continued)

Table 4.16 *(continued)*

Nursing Diagnosis	Expected Outcome	Nursing Interventions
IV. Potential for knowledge deficit of self-care measures	IV. A. Pt will verbally repeat self-care measures and schedule for carrying them out	IV. A. Instruct pt and family member in self-care measures 1. Self-administration of antiemetics postchemotherapy 2. Drink 3 quarts fluids per day, especially chicken soup, etc 3. Bland, cool, frequent, high-calorie, high-protein foods as tolerated 4. Call health care provider for persistent nausea and vomiting > 3 times/day, inability to keep fluids down B. Use a positive approach in teaching re the potential side effect of nausea and vomiting, stressing efforts to PREVENT nausea and vomiting from occurring C. If nausea and vomiting occur, reassure pt that there are other antiemetic regimens that can be used to control, and hopefully prevent it for the next cycle
V. Potential for injury related to nausea and vomiting (esophageal, tears, bleeding)	V. A. Pt will be free from injury B. Injury, if it occurs, will be detected early	V. A. Reinforce teaching to call clinic or health care provider if persistent nausea and vomiting occurs, as well as if pain, bleeding, or any other abnormality occurs B. If pt is taking steroids as part of chemotherapy or antiemetic regimen, teach pt to take pills with food

I. CARDIOTOXICITY OF ANTINEOPLASTIC DRUGS

Most well known of antineoplastic agents with cardiotoxicity potential are the anthracyclines, doxorubicin and daunomycin, and their analogues. These drugs are widely used in the treatment of breast and ovarian cancers, lymphomas and leukemias, and osteosarcomas. Often the patient with cancer is older, and may have pre-existing heart disease, so that a careful cardiovascular assessment must be performed prior to drug administration. Cardiotoxicity can be (1) *acute*, occurring soon after drug administration and manifested by EKG abnormalities (Tokaz and Von Hoff 1984); (2) *subacute*, fibrinous pericarditis with myocardial dysfunction, occurring during the first 4–5 weeks of therapy (Kaszyk, 1986); and (3) *cardiomyopathy*, usually occurring within months of treatment (Tokaz and Von Hoff 1984). The incidence of EKG abnormalities occurring during or soon after drug administration is estimated at 0%–41% (Ali et al. 1979). EKG abnormalities most often are benign, reversible, and do not prevent further drug administration: these include nonspecific ST-T wave changes, sinus tachycardia, and premature atrial and ventricular contractions (Tokaz and Von Hoff 1984). However, a decrease in QRS voltage may occur which often is irreversible, and may be associated with total dose of drug received (Cortes et al. 1975). Finally, there have been reports of sudden death and life-threatening arrythmias during or just after drug administration, so that caution is still important (Tokaz and Von Hoff 1984). It is not customary to use cardiac monitoring or serial EKGs during or after administration of anthracyclines.

The more serious, dose-limiting cardiomyopathy that may develop is related to cumulative drug dose, and high peak serum levels of bolus injection. Myofibril damage and degeneration is gradual, and if the patient becomes symptomatic while receiving treatment, maximum drug damage will not be seen for weeks to months after the last drug dose (Kaszyk 1986). However, most commonly, if patients do develop symptomatic cardiomyopathy, it occurs a week to 2½ months after the final dose of doxorubicin (Saltiel and McGuire 1983). When total dose of doxorubicin is controlled at < 550 mg/m^2, resultant cardiomyopathy is 1%–5% in comparison to 30% in patients receiving doxorubicin at cumulative dose > 550 mg/m^2 (Tokay and Von Hoff 1984). The pathophysiologic process centers around damage to the myofibril, the contractile element of the myocyte (Kaszyk 1986).

Within the myocyte, the sarcoplasmic reticulum swells, and then damage to the myofibril results in degeneration of the mitochondria (energy storehouse) and nucleus, and loss of contractility of the myofibril (Kaszyk 1986). Another biochemical change caused by doxorubicin that may increase myocyte damage is a decrease in cardiac glutathione peroxidase (the enzyme that converts toxic substances into harmless ones) resulting in damage to the heart cell membranes by destructive free radicals (Bristow 1982). It is suggested that there is preferential binding to heart cell mitochondria causing damage and possible alterations in calcium channel flow within the membrane (Kaszyk 1986). As more myofibrils are lost, the heart muscle has to work harder to compensate for the loss of pumping ability, and the heart enlarges (hypertrophy) and there is increased oxygen demand. The degree of damage can range from minor EKG changes to severe congestive heart failure (CHF), requiring digitalis and diuretics.

Early detection of cardiomyopathy is difficult without the use of invasive or noninvasive scans. The most precise measure of myocardial damage is endomyocardial biopsy, with quantification of damage using the Billingham scale of anthracycline damage (Bristow 1982). However, radionuclide angiography (gated blood pool scan) which measures left ventricular ejection fraction (pumping effectiveness) is noninvasive, and correlates well with cardiac damage and toxicity (Taylor, Applefeld, and Wiernik 1984).

Nursing assessment is aimed at identification of patients at risk for developing cardiomyopathy, examination for signs and symptoms of congestive heart failure, and knowledge of gated blood scan results.

Factors that appear to increase the *risk* of cardiomyopathy are as follows:

1. *Total cumulative drug dose:* A dose > 550 mg/m² increases risk, or doses > 400 mg/m² when concurrent chemotherapy is given with drugs such as cyclophosphamide, or if the patient has received prior mediastinal irradiation (Tokaz and Von Hoff 1984). Because not all patients develop the same cardiac damage at the same dose, risks and benefits must be weighed. Daunorubicin-related CHF is 1.5% at total dose of 600 mg/m² and 12% at 1 gm/m² (Von Hoff et al. 1977).

2. *Dosing schedule:* Apparent high peak serum drug levels, such as IV bolus drug administered every three weeks, increase risk over dosing schedules of low weekly dosing and continuous infusion (Legha et al. 1982).

3. *Age:* Young children and persons aged ≥ 50. The higher incidence with increasing age > 50 may be related to the increased incidence of preexisting myocardial damage (Tokaz and Von Hoff 1984).

4. *Preexisting myocardial damage:* abnormal EKG, hypertension

5. *Concurrent combination chemotherapy:* probable potentiation of risk with cyclophosphamide; possible risk with actinomycin D, mitomycin C, or dacarbazine (Tokaz and Von Hoff 1984)

6. *Prior radiation* (XRT) therapy to the mediastinum (Prior XRT potentiates myocardial damage induced by anthracyclines.)

Early signs and symptoms of CHF may be a nonspecific dry cough or tachycardia (Kaszyk 1986). As the cardiomyopathy progresses, the patient may be dyspneic at rest, and feel "winded." Physical exam may reveal an S_4 gallop heart rhythm on auscultation, distended neck veins, pedal edema, hepatomegaly, and cardiomegaly (Kaszyk 1984). Obviously at the first sign of CHF, doxorubicin would be discontinued pending further investigation. Recovery, if it occurs, is dependent on patient compensatory cardiac functions, and treatment is symptomatic with digoxin and diuretics.

Lastly, baseline and subsequent radionucleotide angiography or gated blood pool scans (GBPS) should be done to identify early changes in myocardial function. A GBPS will indicate left ventricular ejection fraction which shows the heart's pumping ability. Most chemotherapy protocols will determine frequency of testing, but in general, in addition to a baseline study prior to the first dose, GBPS is repeated after the patient has received 200 mg/m² of doxorubicin. If the ejection fraction drops significantly, then a then a GBPS is performed prior to each dose of the drug. In certain circumstances the drug is withheld, and a myocardial biopsy may be performed (Kaszyk 1986).

Other chemotherapeutic agents that may induce cardiac damage are shown in table 4.17.

Research is currently being conducted to develop new drugs with less risk of cardiotoxicity; to develop and utilize other drugs to block cardiotoxic damage; and to evaluate different administration schedules.

II. PULMONARY TOXICITY

Pulmonary toxicity is another dose-limiting potentially lethal toxicity of certain chemotherapeutic agents, generally manifested as pulmonary fibrosis. Most well known of the drugs that may cause toxicity are bleomycin, and the nitrosoureas (carmustine and busulfan). Others are listed in table 4.18.

Bleomycin is preferentially distributed to the skin and lungs, and thus, both these areas show

Table 4.17 Chemotherapeutic Agents Associated with Cardiac Toxicities

Drug	Dosage	Cardiac Toxicity	Occurrence	Comments
aminoglutethimide	250 mg po qid	hypotension, tachycardia	10%	Can occur at anytime during treatment.
amsacrine (AMSA)	100mg/m^2 IV qd × 3 or 75–150 mg/m^2 IV qd × 5	ventricular fibrillation cardiomyopathy	5%	Risk is increased by accumulative dose of greater than 900 mg/m^2 or greater than 200 mg/m^2 of AMSA in 48 hrs. Increased incidence with previous anthracycline exposure. Cardiac toxicity is enhanced by preexisting hypokalemia.
cyclophosphamide	120–270 mg/m^2 × 1–4 days	hemorrhagic myocardial necrosis	rare	Occurs with induced myelosuppression for bone marrow transplantation. Potentiates anthracycline-induced cardiomyopathy.
cisplatin	unknown	cardiac ischemia	rare	
cisplatin-based combination therapy	unknown	arterial occlusion events, MI, CVA	rare	Reports of myocardial infarction (MI), cerebrovascular accident (CVA) after treatment with cisplatin, velban, bleomycin, etoposide.
dactinomycin	0.25 mg/m^2 × 5 days	cardiomyopathy	rare	Seen with previous anthracycline exposure.
daunorubicin	400–550 mg/m^2 (lifetime dose)	transient EKG changes cardiomyopathy	0–41% 1.5%	Increased risk with concomitant cyclophosphamide or previous chest irradiation. Young children and the elderly are most susceptible.
doxorubicin	450–550 mg/m^2 (lifetime dose)	transient EKG changes cardiomyopathy	2.2% 1–5%	Same as for daunorubicin.
doxydoxorubicin (DXDX; synthetic Anthracycline)	25–30 mg/m^2	CHF (cumulative dose-related cardiotoxicity with 250 mg/m^2)	rare	Radionuclide ejected fraction performed after patient receives 150 mg/m^2 cumulative dose. Repeat at each dose of 250 mg/m^2.

(continued)

Table 4.17 (continued)

Drug	Dosage	Cardiac Toxicity	Occurrence	Comments
Estramustine	600 mg/m² po in 3 divided doses	Hypertension, angina, myocardial infarction, arrhythmias, pulmonary emboli	10%–15%	Increased risk with history of cardiovascular disease.
Estrogens	5 mg qd	CHF with ischemic heart disease, thromboembolic CVA	39%	Increased risk with history of cardiovascular disease.
Fluorouracil	12–15 mg/kg q wk	Angina 3–18 hrs after drug administered	rare	Not necessarily with preexisting cardiovascular disease. Can recur with subsequent doses. Cardiac enzymes are normal.
Mithramycin	25–50 mg/kg IV qod × 3–8 days	Cardiomyopathy	rare	Exacerbates subclinical anthracycline-induced cardiotoxicity.
Mitomycin	15 mg/m² q 6–8 wks	Cardiomyopathy	rare	Increased risk with previous chest irradiation or anthracycline exposure. Synergistic with anthracyclines.
Mitoxantrone (Novantrone)	a. 12–14 mg/m² q 3 wks; b. 100 mg/m² lifetime dose with prior exposure to anthracyclines; c. 160 mg/m² lifetime dose without prior exposure to anthracyclines	a. Transient EKG changes b. decreased ejection fraction c. CHF	a. 28% b. 44% c. 2.1%–12.5%	Increased risk of cardiomyopathy with previous anthracycline exposure, chest irradiation or cardiovascular disease. CHF has occurred in patients who have not received prior anthracycline therapy.
4′-epidoxorubicin (anthracycline analog)	75 mg/m² q 3 wks; 1100 mg/m² lifetime dose	transient EKG changes, ventricular extrasystole CHF	1%	Spectrum of activity is similar to doxorubicin. Incidence of CHF is 1% when doses equal to 1100 mg/m² are given.
vincristine and vinblastine	unknown	myocardial infarction	rare	Phenomena not well described.
etoposide (VP-16)	unknown	myocardial infarction	rare	May be worsened with prior mediastinal XRT and preexisting coronary artery disease.
diethylstilbestrol (DES)	5 mg q d	thromboembolic myocardial infarction	CVA, frequent	Risk decreased by decreasing dose to 1 mg qd.

Adapted with permission from Kaszyk 1986.

Table 4.18 Drugs that May Induce Pulmonary Toxicity

Drug	Risk Factors	Signs and Symptoms/Comments
Incidence: Frequent		
bleomycin	Age >70 Dose: At 400–500u constant low rate, at 500u rate increases but may occur at low doses High O_2 exposure, thoracic radiation, and renal dysfunction	Dry cough, dyspnea, tachypnea, fever, and rales which may progress to coarse rhonchi and occasional pleural friction rub Incidence: 5%–11%
carmustine (BCNU)	Preexisting lung disease, tobacco use, industrial exposure, possible synergism with cyclophosphamide and thoracic radiation Dose: >1000 mg/m², linear toxicity effect	Variable, none to dyspnea, dry cough, bibasilar crepitant rales Incidence: 20%–30% Mortality: 24%–80%
Incidence: Moderate		
busulfan	Thoracic radiation 500 mg may be threshhold dose for toxicity	Insidious onset; dyspnea, dry cough and fever progressive over weeks to months; bilateral basilar crepitant rales and tachypnea
methotrexate delayed	Daily and weekly schedules most likely to result in toxicity	Prodromal symptoms; headache and malaise, dyspnea, dry cough and fever for days to weeks, tachypnea, cyanosis, rales, skin eruptions—16%; eosinophilia—50%; steroid therapy may be helpful
Incidence: Moderate to Low		
mitomycin	High concentration of O_2	Progressive dyspnea, nonproductive cough, bibasilar rales; may occur with low doses, and after first dose; may be associated with renal toxicity
cyclophosphamide	None identified, but frequently reported in patients with Hodgkins and non-Hodgkins lymphoma possibly related to concurrent bleomycin	Dyspnea, fever, dry cough, tachypnea, scattered rales, rarely chest pain or pleural rub
Incidence: Low		
chlorambucil	None identified, duration of therapy 6 mos to >2 yrs; total dose >2 grams	Dyspnea, dry cough, fever developing over 1–2 months; bibasilar rales, anorexia, fatigue
cytosine arabinoside	None identified	Dyspnea and tachypnea develop during or posttherapy, associated with GI lesions; rare pulmonary edema
melphalan	None identified; total dose 80 mg to >3 gm duration of therapy 2 mos–83 mos	Rapid progressive dyspnea and fever over 2–10 days; tachypnea, rales common

(continued)

Table 4.18 (continued)

Drug	Risk Factors	Signs and Symptoms/Comments
Incidence: Rare		
procarbazine	None identified Potential risk for hypersensitivity-prone individuals	Fever, chills, eosinophilia, rash, cough, dyspnea, progressive pulmonary insufficiency; rapid recovery after discontinuation of drug
lomustine	Dose > 1100 mg/m^2 Questionable synergism with other pulmonary-toxic chemotherapy	Dypsnea, tachypnea, weight loss, anorexia
semustine	None identified	Exertional dyspnea, rales, and pleural friction rub
Zinostatin	None identified	Dry cough, hemoptysis, progressive pulmonary insufficiency
Chlorozotocin	None identified	Exertional dyspnea, rales, and fatigue
Spirogermanium	None identified Potential risk for pts previously treated with other chemotherapy or thoracic radiation	Progressive cough, dyspnea, fatigue and fever; onset of symptoms insidious
etoposide	Questionable synergism with methotrexate	Fever, dyspnea, cough, dry rales, cyanosis, tachypnea
vindesine and vinblastine	Seen in pts. treated simultaneously with mitomycin	Acute onset; dyspnea and cough, tachypnea, rales
teniposide	Previous treatment with XRT to spinal axis and BCNU	Dyspnea, cyanosis, tachypnea
mercaptopurine	None identified	Acute respiratory distress
methotrexate		Pulmonary edema, acute onset of dyspnea, tachypnea 6–12 hours after oral or intrathecal (IT) drug administration

Source: Modified from Wickham 1986. Reprinted with permission.

drug toxicity. In the lungs, there is a decrease in type I pneumocytes, and an increase and redistribution of type II pneumocytes into the alveolar spaces. There may be symptoms of pneumonitis. The alveolar septas become thickened, and decreased in number, and there is an increase in the amount of collagen secreted by the interstitial fibroblasts, with resulting generalized interstitial fibrosis of the lung (Ginsburg and Comis 1984). If damage continues, endstage interstitial fibrosis reveals obliteration of the alveoli and dilated airspaces, followed by a thickened, stiff interstitium (Seltzer, Goldstein, and Herman 1983). Pulmonary dysfunction is restrictive, with functionally decreased lung volume, increased work of breathing, and impaired gas exchange (Wickham 1986). The incidence of bleomycin-induced pulmonary toxicity is 5%–11% (Ginsburg and Comis 1984).

Nursing assessment features are 1) patients at risk for developing pulmonary toxicity, 2) signs and symptoms of dysfunction, and 3) evaluation of pulmonary function tests to identify early dysfunction.

Identified risk factors for bleomycin-induced pulmonary toxicity are the following:

1. *Age:* Risk increases with age, with risk 5% until age 70, then increasing to 15% after age 70 (Wickham 1986).

2. *Prior pulmonary or thoracic radiation:* Radiotherapy potentiates toxicity, and 35%–55% of patients develop severe bleomycin toxicity (over 50% of these patients die of this toxicity). *Concurrent* radiotherapy and low-dose bleomycin cannot be safely given simultaneously due to the high incidence of pneumonitis and respiratory failure (Einhorn et al. 1976; Ginsburg and Comis 1984).

3. *Total cumulative dose:* Increased risk when >400–500 units of bleomycin are administered. Overall, cumulative dose of <450 units had an incidence of 3%–5%, 450 units had 13% incidence, and 550 units had 17% incidence (10% mortality). However, this is *unpredictable*, and toxicity has occurred at lower cumulative doses (i.e., *50–60 units*) (Blum, Carter, and Agre 1973).

4. *High peak serum levels:* Higher IV bolus administration of bleomycin (25 ± 2u/wk) had greater decreases in pulmonary function than lower doses (16 ± 1.6u/wk) (Comis et al. 1979). *Continuous infusion* of bleomycin appears to decrease the risk of pulmonary toxicity (Carlson and Sikic 1983).

5. *Preexisting lung disease:* Not well studied, but requires careful administration; also, if patient smokes or has a smoking history risk may increase (Yasko 1983).

6. *Receiving combination chemotherapy* with another potentially pulmonary toxic drug, such as cyclophosphamide (Yasko 1983).

7. *Exposure to high oxygen concentrations after bleomycin treatment:* There is a synergistic effect of toxicity—therefore care must be taken to use $FiO_2 \ll 100\%$ during anesthesia for patients who have received bleomycin (Ginsberg and Comis 1984).

Early physical findings include dry hacking cough, fine bibasilar rales with dyspnea upon exertion, and decrease in DLCO (diffusing capacity). Chest X ray often has only minimal changes, but may show fine reticular bibasilar infiltrate (Ginsberg and Comis 1984).

Later signs are dyspnea at rest, tachypnea, fever, coarse rales, chest X ray changes with consolidation, significant decrease in DLCO, and hypoxemia.

Pulmonary function tests are routinely performed *prior* to initial dose of bleomycin to establish a baseline, and then are repeated serially during treatment. Diffusion capacity (DLCO) is the most sensitive indicator of injury (Wickham 1986). Bleomycin therapy should be discontinued if the DLCO falls to ≤40% of initial testing, if the FVC (forced vital capacity) falls to <25% of initial testing, or if symptoms or physical findings indicating bleomycin toxicity are found (Ginsberg and Comis 1984).

It appears that if pulmonary function is identified early, i.e., when physical findings are minimal, and the patient has normal resting arterial oxygenation (PO_2), progressive pulmonary failure does not occur. However, if signs and symptoms of severe dysfunction occur—dyspnea at rest, hypoxemia ($PO_2 < 55$ mm Hg), tachypnea, coarse rales, consolidation on chest X ray—then pulmonary injury is usually irreversible and progressive (Ginsberg and Comis 1984).

Acute hypersensitivity pulmonary toxicity may occur with a number of antineoplastic agents, including bleomycin, and is characterized by fever, diffuse infiltrates on chest X ray, and eosinophilia. The condition appears to respond to steroid therapy (Ginsberg and Comis 1984). It is important to distinguish between the agents; steroids are of questionable value in treating bleomycin toxicity. Doses of steroids may vary, and generally are 20–160 mg/day (Wickham 1986). Pulmonary toxicity related to other antineoplastic agents was shown in table 4.18.

The nursing goal is to identify early dysfunction and discontinue the drug to prevent progressive pulmonary toxicity.

III. HEPATOTOXICITY

The liver is an important site of cancer chemotherapy drug metabolism, yet it withstands significant damage from most of the drugs due to the slow growth of hepatocytes (Perry 1984). Drugs metabolized by the liver are alkylating agents (e.g., cyclophosphamide), nitrosoureas (e.g., BCNU, CCNU), plant alkaloids (e.g., vincristine), antimetabolites (e.g., 5-fluorouracil, cytosine arabinoside, methotrexate), antibiotics (e.g., doxorubicin), and miscellaneous drugs such as procarbazine. However, certain drugs are hepatotoxic, as shown in table 4.19.

Factors that increase the risk of hepatotoxicity when potentially hepatotoxic drugs are given are as follows (Goodman 1986):

1. previous or concurrent hepatic irradiation (vincristine and abdominal radiation)
2. concurrent administration of other hepatotoxic drugs (e.g., 6-mercaptopurine and doxorubicin; cyclophosphamide and methotrexate)
3. active hepatitis

Injury to the hepatocytes is first manifested by elevations of liver function tests (LFTs): the serum glutamic oxaloacetic transaminase (SGOT) and serum glutamic pyruvic transaminase (SGPT), bilirubin, lactic dehydrogenase (LDH), and alkaline phosphatase (Goodman 1986). Alterations in these liver function tests can be temporary and transient, or progress to hepatic cirrhosis when the drug (e.g., methotrexate, mercaptopurine) is used continuously on a long-term basis (Dorr and Fritz 1981). Certain drugs, such as L-asparaginase and mithramycin can cause acute injury to the liver, and require dose modifications. LFTs should be monitored when mithramycin is used in low doses for management of hypercalcemia. Other drugs produce more delayed or chronic injury as shown in table 3.17. A recent cause of hepatotoxicity is veno-occlusive disease of the liver, and as more bone marrow transplantations are performed, it is expected that this complication will increase. Veno-occlusive disease and subsequent hepatotoxicity have been reported after treatment with mitomycin C, carmustine, cytosine arabinoside, busulfan, and cyclophosphamide (Perry 1984).

Nursing management issues concern pre- and post-treatment analysis: 1) identifying the drugs that are potentially hepatotoxic, identifying patient risk factors such as preexisting liver disease or history of alcohol abuse, and monitoring the patient's baseline and pretreatment liver function values; and 2) assessment of the patient's hepatic function prior to subsequent drug administration. An abnormal liver test should be investigated to determine if it is drug related, and if the patient may require a liver biopsy.

Finally, because it is clear that many antineoplastic drugs are metabolized by the liver, if hepatic dysfunction occurs, certain drug dosages must be adjusted as shown in table 4.20. Otherwise, as the drug has a decreased rate of metabolic breakdown and excretion, and circulating serum levels of the drug would be higher than normal, increasing drug toxicity. The nurse should discuss dose modification with the physician prior to drug administration.

IV. NEPHROTOXICITY

Chemotherapy-induced renal damage can occur directly, via direct injury to renal cells by specific chemotherapeutic agents, e.g., cisplatin, methotrexate, or indirectly, by metabolic changes following treatment, e.g., hyperuricemic nephropathy related to rapid tumor cell lysis (Yasko 1984). Renal toxicity may be acute, chronic, or delayed. The usual signs are increased blood urea nitrogen (BUN), serum creatinine (Cr), and decreased renal clearance of creatinine. Risk factors are preexisting renal disease, volume depletion, and concommitant use of nephrotoxic drugs.

Table 4.19 Potential Hepatotoxicity of Chemotherapeutic Agents

Drug	Toxicity	Comments
amsacrine (investigational)	Mild increase in bilirubin in 20%–40% pts; rare hepatic failure	
Nitrosoureas (carmustine, lomustine)	Increased LFTs, normalize in 1 wk	Appears dose related, hold drug for prolonged elevations
streptozocin	Increased LFTs (in ~15% pts)	Occurs with usual doses, dose not usually require treatment
Antimetabolites methotrexate	Increased SGOT, LDH (short, freq doses) fibrosis, cirrhosis (long-term use)	Resolve within 1 mo after treatment stops. Avoid use in pts with Laennec's cirrhosis or preexisting liver disease.
6-Mercaptopurine	Increased bilirubin, SGOT, alkaline phosphatase. Cholestasis, necrosis	Usually not given to pts with preexisting liver disease, discontinue drug if increased LFTs occur— usually related to doses >2 mg/kg/day
cytosine arabinoside	Increased LFTs	
hydroxyurea	Rare increase in LFTs, hepatitis	
Antibiotics mithramycin	Acute necrosis, altered LFTs, clotting factors	Stop drug, or dose reduce
Bisantrene	Rare hepatitis	
Enzymes L-asparaginase	Fatty changes, with decreased albumin, clotting factor synthesis; impaired handling of lipids	Usually improves after treatment stopped, resolving over days to weeks
Miscellaneous dacarbazine	Transient increase in SGPT, SGOT, bilirubin (diffuse hepatocellular dysfunction); also reported veno-occlusive disease—rare.	Treatment not usually necessary
Alkylating Agents chlorambucil	Hepatitis, dysfunction	Stop drug
cisplatin	Steatosis & cholestasis	
busulfan	Cholestatic jaundice	

Sources: Perry 1984; Dorr and Fritz 1981; and Goodman 1986.

Specific drugs that are potential nephrotoxins are cisplatin, methotrexate, and the nitrosoureas as shown in table 4.21.

Cisplatin, a heavy metal with an alkylating action, can cause proximal and distal renal tubular necrosis (Schilsky 1984), and can decrease the ability of the renal tubules to resorb magnesium and calcium (Lydon 1986). Nephrotoxicity is a dose-limiting toxicity, is mild and reversible with low doses, but may become severe and permanent with high doses and multiple courses of therapy (Lydon 1986). Abnormalities include

Table 4.20 Suggested Dose Modification with Hepatic Dysfunction (% of Usual Dose to Administer if Any, on the Day of Treatment)

Drug	Bili < 1.5% and SGOT < 60 IU	Bili = 1.5–3.0 SGOT = 60–180	Bili = 3.1–5.0 or SGOT > 180	Bili > 5.0
5-Fluorouracil	100%	100%	100%	Omit
Cyclophosphamide	100%	100%	75%	Omit
Methotrexate	?%	? %	?75%	?Omit
Mitoxantrone	100%	75%	50%	0
Daunorubicin	100%	75%	50%	Omit
Doxorubicin	100%	50%	25%	Omit
Vinblastine	100%	50%	Omit	Omit
Vincristine	100%	50%	25%*	Omit
VP-16	100%	50%	25%*	Omit
VM-26	100%	50%	25%	Omit

Source: Modified from Perry 1984. Reprinted with permission.
*Fischer DS and Knobf MT (1989) *The Cancer Chemotherapy Handbook 3rd Edition.* Chicago: Year Book Medical Publishers, Inc., p. 193

increased BUN and creatinine, decreased creatinine clearance, hypomagnesemia, hypocalcemia, and proteinuria. On a cellular level, focal degeneration of basement membrane, hyaline droplets in renal tubules, and tubular necrosis can occur (Dentino et al. 1978). Newer platinum analogues, such as carboplatin, are not nephrotoxic, and may soon replace cisplatin use.

Renal toxicity is minimized by vigorous saline hydration of at least 100–150 cc/hr (as cisplatin reabsorption by the kidney is prevented by a platinum-chloride complex formation), to provide a urine output of at least 100 cc/hr. In some settings, mannitol is used to mobilize extracellular fluid into the vascular space and increase renal blood flow and filtration, or Lasix is used for similar purposes. Research has shown that mannitol and Lasix are equal in their protection (Ostrow et al. 1981), but it isn't clear that saline and diuretics are superior to saline hydration alone (Lydon 1986). Also, hypertonic saline and longer infusion time appear to decrease nephrotoxicity (Ozols et al. 1982). It appears that cisplatin is unstable in low chlorine concentrations, exchanging a chloride group for a hydroxyl or H_2O group, and the resulting molecule is felt to

be the nephrotoxic element (Lydon 1986). Hypertonic (3%) saline decreases the formation of these molecules and thus decreases cisplatin-induced nephrotoxicity (Ozols et al. 1982). Risk factors that increase toxicity are preexisting renal dysfunction, and administration of concurrent nephrotoxic antibiotics. Magnesium repletion is usually required, and can be given in the hydration fluid.

Methotrexate, an antimetabolite, is excreted via the kidneys, with 90% of conventional doses excreted unchanged in the urine (Schilsky 1984). It may cause injury by crystalizing or precipitating in the tubules and collecting ducts causing subsequent obstructive nephropathy (Abelson and Garnick 1982). Precipitation is increased in an acid environment. Damage is rare and reversible with short-term low-dose treatment, but the patient's BUN and Cr should be monitored prior to treatment. Incidence is high with high-dose methotrexate (1–15 gm/m^2) and can be permanent, but can be prevented by 1) vigorous hydration before, during, and after treatment (100 $ml/m^2/hr$) to produce a diuresis of at least 150 cc/hr; 2) alkalinization of the urine with sodium bicarbonate or diamox as this

Table 4.21 Relative Risks of Chemotherapeutic Agents: Nephrotoxicity

Drug	Pathophysiology	Laboratory Abnormalities	Nursing Interventions
I. High risk of immediate nephrotoxicity			
A. cisplatin	A. Proximal and distal renal tubule injury produces tubular necrosis, focal degeneration of basement membrane, hysline droplet deposits in renal tubules 1. *Mild*, reversible with low doses 2. *Severe*, permanent damage with high doses and multiple courses	A. ↑ BUN and creatinine, ↓ Creatinine clearance, azotemia, ↓ serum magnesium, ↓ serum calcium. Renal wasting with hypermagnesuria, hypercalciuria, proteinuria, enzymuria	A. 1. Saline hydration at least 100–150 mL/hr 2. Diuresis with mannitol or furosemide 3. Post-treatment hydration of at least 3 L/day 4. Prevent dehydration and vomiting

B. High-Dose methotrexate	B. Drug crystallizes or precipitates in renal tubules and collecting ducts; directly affects renal tubular cells; directly affects afferent vascular supply resulting in ↓ glomerular filtration rate (GFR)
	1. Rare and reversible with short-term low doses
	2. Occasional long-term, low-dose permanent dysfunction
	3. High incidence with high dose, usually reversible but with significant systemic drug toxicity
		B. ↑ BUN and creatinine, oliguria/anuria, azotemia, acidosis, hypokalemia, anemia, osteomalacia, hypophosphatemia, aminoaciduria	B. 1. Vigorous hydration to maintain high urine flow
			2. Alkalinize urine to pH ≥7.0
			3. Prevent dehydration, vomiting
			4. Prevent systemic drug toxicity
			  a. Leucovorin rescue *exactly* on time until methotrexate level $< 5 \times 10^{-8}$M (Shilsky 1984)
			  b. Effusions should be drained *prior* to drug administration
			  c. Eliminate concomitant administration of sulfonamides, salicylates, probenecid

(continued)

Table 4.21 (*continued*)

Drug	Pathophysiology	Laboratory Abnormalities	Nursing Interventions
I. C. streptozocin	I. C. 10–20% of intact, active drug is excreted by kidneys with primary injury on renal tubules and glomerulus, resulting in tubulointerstitial nephritis and tubular atrophy 1. Low doses produce transient, reversible damage 2. Continued therapy can lead to severe and permanent chronic renal failure 3. Dose-limiting factor	I. C. ↑ BUN and creatinine, ↓ creatinine clearance, hypophosphatemia, hypokalemia, hyperchloremia, proteinuria, glycosuria, aminoaciduria, phosphaturia	I. C. 1. Adequate hydration during and 24 hrs post treatment 2. Prevent vomiting, dehydration 3. Assess 24-hr urine creatinine clearance before treatment
D. High-Dose mithramycin	D. Direct damage to renal tubules causing distal and proximal tubule necrosis 1. Rare with low dose 2. High incidence with high dose, and may be permanent	D. ↑ BUN and serum creatinine, azotemia, proteinuria, hypophosphatemia, hypomagnesemia, hypokalemia, hypocalcemia	D. 1. Monitor renal function 2. No prevention strategies; however, high doses rarely administered

I. E. ifosfamide

I. E. Renal toxicity incidence ~6%, apparently related to tubular damage
1. Laboratory abnormalities usually transient
2. Bladder irritation, consisting of hemorrhagic cystitis, dysuria, and urinary frequency, occurs in 6%–92% of patients without uroprotection
3. Urotoxicity is dose-dependent

I. E. ↑ BUN and serum creatinine, ↓ urine creatinine clearance, rare proteinuria, acidosis
1. Microscopic hematuria

I. E. 1. Monitor kidney function (laboratory tests), vigorous hydration
2. Uroprotector must be administered with ifosfamide, i.e., mesna
   a. Assess urine for presence of RBC prior to subsequent dosing
   b. Manufacturer recommends urinalysis be assessed prior to each drug dose:
      1) if microscopic hematuria present (>10 RBC/high power field) dose should be held until complete resolution
      2) further drug administration (IFEX, Mead Johnson, 1/89) should be given with vigorous oral/parenteral hydration.

II. *High risk of nephrotoxicity from long-term use*

A. Nitrosoureas; BCNU, CCNU, MeCCNU

A. Postulated that drug binds irreversibly to amino acid residues → glomerular and tubular damage, decrease in kidney size
1. Uncommon with doses <1000 mg/m^2
2. In high dose chronic renal failure may occur

A. ↑ BUN and serum creatinine, ↓ glomerular filtration rate (GFR), azotemia, proteinuria

A. 1. No prevention strategies: suggest hydration during and post-drug administration (oral fluids to 3 L/day for 24 hrs)
2. Frequent long-term follow-up as renal failure may occur up to 5 years later

(continued)

Table 4.21 *(continued)*

Drug	Pathophysiology	Laboratory Abnormalities	Nursing Interventions
II. B. mitomycin C	II. B. Postulated drug interferes with DNA synthesis and induces immune complex deposits, damaging glomeruli and tubules 1. Cumulative toxicity 2. Mild and reversible, to fatal renal failure (i.e., if hemolytic uremic syndrome (HUS) develops) 3. Renal vasculitis may be increased with concurrent 5-fluorouracil administration	II. B. 1. ↑ BUN, azotemia, proteinuria 2. HUS: hypertension, hematuria, anemia, thrombocytopenia	II. B. 1. No prevention strategies 2. Suggest hydration during and 24 hrs post treatment 3. Assess renal function
III. *Moderate risk of nephrotoxicity*			
A. cyclo-phos-phamide	A. 1. Drug metabolites may injure collecting ducts, distal renal tubules, causing impaired water excretion and dilutional hyponatremia (SIADH) at high doses (>50 mg/kg) 2. Drug metabolites irritate stretched bladder capillaries causing hemorrhagic cystitis 3. Preventable 4. Dose-limiting	A. SIADH: Lab values of water intoxication: serum hyponatremia, ↑ urine osmolality, ↓ serum osmolality, ↓ urinary output	A. 1. Monitor electrolytes, treat SIADH if it occurs 2. Prevent by aggressive hydration (at least 3 L/day). 3. Encourage pt to void at least q 2–3 hrs. 4. Do not administer at noc.
B. Low-Dose metho-trexate	B. See pathophysiology as high-dose methotrexate. See Sec. I. B.	B. Hemorrhagic cystitis: urinary frequency, urgency, dysuria, hematuria	B. No nursing interventions

Drug	Description	Findings	Prevention
III. C. 5-azacytidine (Investigational)	III. C. Tubular damage and renal insufficiency possible when given in combination with other drugs	III. C. ↑ BUN and creatinine, azotemia, acidosis, hyperphosphatemia, hypomagnesemia, hypocalcemia, glycosuria, sodium wasting, aminoaciduria	III. C. No prevention strategies known. Assess renal function prior to each dose.
D. High-Dose 6-thioguanine	D. High dose (oral or IV) appears to induce reversible toxicity, possibly by inhibiting purine metabolism	D. ↑ BUN and creatinine, azotemia	D. No prevention strategies. Monitor renal function studies prior to each dose.
E. L-asparaginase	E. Prerenal azotemia	E. ↑ BUN	E. Use cautiously with nephrotoxic antibiotics. Monitor renal function studies.

IV. *Low-risk of nephroxicity*
- A. Anthracyclines (doxorubicin in high doses, daunorubicin)
- B. Low-Dose Mithramycin
- C. Tenoposide (VM-26)
- D. 5-Fluorouracil
- E. Vincristine (SIADH, ↓ serum Na^{++}, inappropriate urinary sodium wasting)
- F. 6-Mercaptopurine (hematuria, requires dose reduction)
- G. Carboplatin (rare tubular damage)
- H. Hydroxyurea (mild, reversible, requires dosage reduction)

Modified from Lydon 1986.

decreases drug precipitation in the renal tubule; 3) close monitoring of serum methotrexate levels; and 4) administration of calcium leukovarin rescue doses exactly on time (Lydon 1986). Risk factors increasing nephrotoxicity include pre-existing renal dysfunction; pleural and other effusions in which the drug can be sequestered and released slowly into the systemic circulation; dehydration or volume depletion; concomitant use of salicyclates, sulfonamides, and probenecid which displace drugs from albumin; and increased circulating serum levels of methotrexate.

In the event of renal dysfunction resulting from high-dose methotrexate (HDMTX) therapy, renal excretion of the drug is decreased and systemic serum levels of the drug are elevated. This causes more severe systemic toxicity, such as mucositis and bone marrow depression. Therefore, nursing care of patients receiving HDMTX therapy is quite precise, and demands scrupulous attention to details to prevent nephrotoxicity.

In caring for patients receiving nephrotoxic drugs, assessment *must* include renal function, electrolyte balance, and degree of hydration (Goodman 1986). Drug administration may have to wait until these are corrected.

Assessment of renal function is essential prior to administration of any drug that is excreted by the kidneys. If there is compromised renal function, then the drug dose is often reduced or discontinued until renal function improves. These drugs include bleomycin, cisplatin, cyclophosphamide, methotrexate, mithramycin, and the nitrosoureas.

The *nitrosoureas* include streptozocin. Streptozocin may cause tubulointerstitial nephritis and tubular atrophy, resulting in 1) electrolyte imbalance (hypophosphatemia, hypokalemia, hyperchloremia), and 2) renal dysfunction (elevated BUN and creatinine, decreased creatinine clearance, with urinary wasting of protein, glucose, phosphorus, and amino acids) (Lydon 1986). Injury to the renal tubules and glomerulus is transient and reversible with low doses but

with continued therapy, often causes chronic interstitial nephritis with progressive renal failure which continues after treatment is stopped (Perry 1984). Hydration during and 24 hours post therapy is important, as well as pretreatment BUN, creatinine, and 24 hour creatinine determination. The other nitrosoureas (BCNU, CCNU, and MeCCNU) cause glomerular and renal tubule damage at cumulative doses above 1000 mg/m^2. Hydration is important, but renal failure can develop up to five years after treatment is completed, and long-term renal follow-up is essential.

Indirect injury to the kidneys can occur when there is rapid tumor lysis. Patients with large bulky chemosensitive tumors or rapidly proliferating tumors, such as acute leukemia, Burkitt's lymphoma, and diffuse histiocytic lymphomas are at risk to develop hyperuricemic nephropathy and renal failure. With the destruction (lysis) of large numbers of malignant cells, there is a release of excessive amounts of nucleic acids which are converted to uric acid. In an acid environment, uric acid is less soluble, and the high concentration of uric acid to be excreted may lead to precipitation of uric acid crystals in the distal nephron, especially the collecting ducts where urine concentration is maximal (Fields, Josse, and Bergsagel 1982). Signs and symptoms are characteristic of acute renal failure with oliguria or anuria, hyperuricemia (>8 mg/dl), and often uric acid crystals in the urine. Without intervention, this progresses to uremia. Rapid reversal of renal failure usually occurs with the administration of allopurinol but may require hemodialysis (Schilsky 1984). Early recovery is manifested by the onset of diuresis (Fields, Josse, and Bergsagel 1982).

The most important intervention is the *prevention* of acute hyperuricemic nephropathy, using the following treatment (Schilsky 1984):

1. *Intravenous hydration* to produce a urinary output of at least 100 cc/hr (requires >3 L/24 hrs) to increase renal tubular filtration

2. *Urinary alkalinization* to increase urine pH ≥ 7.0, thus increasing uric acid solubility (requires adding NaH_2O_3 50–100 mg to each liter of IV fluid, or administration of acetazolamide 250–500 mg/day (if not contraindicated)

3. *Allopurinol* administration to decrease the formation of uric acid (requires 500 mg/m² for 2–3 days then reduced to 200 mg/m²/day). Allopurinal inhibits xanthine oxidase, an enzyme that is essential to the degradation of nucleic acid (purines) to uric acid.

Hyperuricemic nephropathy may occur as a separate entity, or if accompanied by the rapid release of intracellular ions is called *tumor lysis syndrome* (TLS). This syndrome is considered a metabolic emergency. Patients at risk for both TLS and hyperuricemic nephropathy are those with large, rapidly proliferating tumors (i.e., lymphomas with LDH >1500, leukemias, and small cell lung cancer). Also at risk are patients with preexisting renal dysfunction with creatinine ≥ 1.6 mg/dl and uric acid ≥ 8 mg/dl (Moore 1985).

Symptoms are characteristic of the metabolic abnormalities, and include:

weakness

confusion

irritability

numbness, tingling

muscle cramping

Preventative treatment should begin 12–24 hours prior to chemotherapy administration in high risk patients as previously discussed (Schilsky 1984): 1) vigorous hydration, 2) urinary alkalinization, 3) administration of allopurinol. During the first 24–48 hours of therapy, serum electrolytes, calcium, phosphorus, and creatinine should be assessed every 6–8 hours (Schilsky 1984). In addition, the nurse should strictly monitor 1) intake and output, total balance, and daily weights to identify fluid overload, retention or inadequate renal flow; 2) vital signs, to assess circulatory tolerance of hydration, and the development of arrythmias; and 3) urine for pH ≥ 7.0 and assess for the presence of uric acid crystals. The risk period of rapid tumor cell lysis lasts 5–7 days after chemotherapy administration, and usually the above measures are adequate to prevent TLS. However, if severe metabolic derangements occur, hemodialysis may be necessary. See table 4.22 for nursing interventions.

V. NEUROTOXICITY

Neurotoxicity may occur following specific drug treatment, but, as neurologic signs and symptoms usually occur at some time during the course of malignancy, it is important to distinguish those related to drug toxicity (Kaplan and Wiernik 1984). Injury can be to the central nervous system with resulting acute or chronic encephalopathies, or to peripheral nerves producing neuropathies related to demyelination and axonal degeneration (Goodman 1986; Holden and Felde 1987). Toxicity may occur soon after drug administration, or up to years after treatment (Yasko 1983). The potential neurotoxicities that may occur are summarized in table 4.23. Table 4.24 describes the specific drug-related neurotoxicity.

Central Nervous System (CNS) Toxicity

Chemotherapy may be toxic to the central nervous system through a number of different mechanisms. The following section describes specific drugs, their associated neurological toxicities, and nursing implications.

Following intrathecal administration of drugs such as methotrexate or cytosine arabinoside to treat or prevent CNS metastasis, there may be signs of arachnoiditis or meningeal irritation. These signs include stiff neck, headache, nausea

Table 4.22 Nursing Protocol for the Management of Tumor Lysis Syndrome

Problem	Intervention
Fluid balance	Administer IV hydration. Monitor weight, intake and output, response to diurectics. Observe for signs of fluid overload, especially patients with potential or preexisting cardiac damage.
Electrolyte balance	Monitor electrolytes q day or q 6–12 hrs as indicated. Correct imbalances as prescribed. Observe for signs of hyperkalemia: weakness, flaccid paralysis, ECG changes, cardiac arrest.
Potential renal failure	Monitor Ca^{++}, PO_4^+, uric acid, BUN, and creatinine daily for the 5–7-day period of cytolysis. Maintain hydration, especially if preexisting renal insufficiency (creatinine > 1.6 mg/dL, uric acid ≥ 8 mg/dL). Administer allopurinol 300–800 mg PO q day. Monitor urine pH: maintain ≥ 7 by administering IV $NaHCO_3$ as prescribed. Report decreased urine output, lethargy. Prepare to manage patient on temporary hemodialysis.
Potential effects of drug therapy	Observe for side effects from allopurinol: skin rashes, GI disturbances, fever (rarely), vasculitis, and blood dyscrasias. Decrease doses of 6-MP and azathioprine if given concurrently with allopurinol.
Potential cardiac irritability	Monitor lab values for increased K^+ and decreased Ca^{++}. Check pulse rate and rhythm frequently. Report irregularity. Observe for ECG changes, cardiac arrest.
Potential neuromuscular irritability	Monitor serum Ca^{++} level. Observe for symptoms of hypocalcemia: tetany, positive Chvostek's and Trousseau's signs.

Source: Moore 1985. Reprinted with permission.
Ca^{++}, ionized calcium; K^+, ionized potassium; 6-MP, 6-mercaptopurine; $NaHCO_3$, sodium bicarbonate; Po_4^+, phosphate ion(s).

and vomiting, fever, and lethargy, and begin 2–4 hours after drug administration, and last 12–72 hours (Kaplan and Wiernik 1984). The incidence of arachnoiditis is significantly reduced by 1) the use of *preservative-free* drug and diluent (if the nurse assists the physician in intrathecal drug administration, it is imperative to ensure that this is used) and 2) delivery of small doses of drug over several days, perhaps via an Ommaya reservoir, rather than large, intermittent doses (Kaplan and Wiernik 1984).

Both methotrexate and cytosine arabinoside in high doses effectively cross the blood-brain barrier, and it is therefore critical that these drugs

be reconstituted with a preservative-free diluent, again to prevent arachnoiditis.

Chronic encephalopathies may occur with intraventricular or intrathecal methotrexate administration, and can be subacute and transient, or chronic. Radiation increases the risk of CNS damage when given in combination with intrathecal methotrexate, or if radiotherapy to the CNS is given prior to methotrexate (Kaplan and Wiernik 1984). One syndrome is necrotizing leukoencephalopathy which is characterized by demyelination, multifocal white matter necrosis, and damage to the nerve axons (Kaplan and Wiernik 1984). Signs and symptoms include

Table 4.23 Possible Neurologic Syndromes Caused by Antineoplastic Agents

Acute Encephalopathies	Chronic Encephalopathies
Intrathecal methotrexate (MTX)—XRT	Necrotizing leukoencephalopathy
Radiotherapy (XRT) ± intrathecal (IT) MTX	Radiotherapy—IT MTX
High-dose MTX ("Stroke-like")	IT or IV MTX
Asparaginase (early and late)	IT cytosine arabinoside (Ara-C)
Hexamethylmelamine	Mineralizing microangiopathy
5-Fluorouracil (with allopurinol)	XRT ± IT MTX
Procarbazine	Cerebral atrophy
BCNU (intracarotid)	IT MTX ± XRT
Cisplatin (intracarotid)	IT Ara-C ± XRT
Cyclophosphamide	Pontine myelinolysis
5-Azacytidine	XRT ± IT MTX
High-dose cytosine arabinoside (Ara-C)	

Arachnoiditis/Myelopathy	Acute Cerebellar Syndromes/Ataxia
Encephalomyelopathy	5-Fluorouracil
IT or intraventricular	Procarbazine
MTX or high-dose MTX	Hexamethylmelamine
IT Ara-C	?BCNU
IT thiotepa	

Neuropathies		
Peripheral	**Cranial**	**Ototoxicity**
Axonal degeneration	Vinca alkaloids	Cisplatin
Vinca alkaloids	Cisplatin	Misonidazole
Misonidazole	5-Fluorouracil	
Demyelination		
Cisplatin		
Sensory		
Vinca alkaloids		
Cisplatin		
Procarbazine		
Misonidazole		
Sensorimotor		
Vinca alkaloids		
Hexamethylmelamine		
5-Azacytidine		
Uncertain		
Hexamethylmelamine		
Procarbazine		
5-Azacytadine		
VP-16		

Source: Modified from Kaplan and Wiernik 1984. Reprinted with permission.

confusion, drooling, somnolence or irritability, ataxia, tremors, dementia, spasticity, quadraparesis, and slurred speech.

Cytosine arabinoside in high doses (greater than 3 grams/m^2 times 4–8 doses for treatment of adult acute myelocytic leukemias) has resulted in dose-limiting acute encephalopathies characterized by somnolence, altered personality, difficulty carrying out calculations, headaches or seizures. This was seen frequently with cerebellar dysfunction and the severity was parallel. Age over 50 was an increased risk factor (Herzig et al. 1987).

An acute cerebellar syndrome may occur after high-dose bolus injection of 5-fluorouracil, believed related to high peak plasma levels of the drug (Goodman 1986). Signs include dysmetria

Table 4.24 Neurotoxicity of Anticancer Agents

Drug	Incidence	Signs/Symptoms	Crosses BBB	Onset/ Resolution	Dose Relation
Vinca alkaloids					
vincristine	common, dose-limiting	paresthesias, constipation, loss of deep tendon reflexes (DTR), weakness, SIADH	−	1–2 weeks to 1–3 months	High dose (>2 mg/dose) and high cumulative doses
vinblastine	rarely dose-limiting	same as vincristine	−	same as vincristine	same as vincristine
Alkalyting agents					
Nitrogen mustard (mechlorethamine hydrochloride)	rare (intra-arterial, toxic IV doses)	tinnitus, coma, seizures, death	+ high dose	immediate to rapidly progressive	toxic in high IV doses, normal intra-arterial doses
Chlorambucil	rare	hypersensitivity, coma, seizures	+ high dose	immediate with rapid recovery	accidental overdose
Nitrosoureas					
Lomustine (CCNU)	rare	confusion, lethargy, ataxia	+ +	delayed (days to weeks)	usual doses
Semustine (MeCCNU)	very rare	acute metabolic encephalopathy	+ +	2 days → 2 weeks	
Carmustine (BCNU)	very rare	optic neuroretinitis	+ +	onset 8 days → slow resolution	unknown
Antimetabolites					
5-Fluorouracil	very rare (<1%)	ataxia, cerebellar dysfunction	+	immediate to 1 week with slow recovery	variable
Methotrexate	common with intrathecal dose but preventable using *preservative-free* diluent	stiff neck, headache, meningismus, rare seizures	low dose − high dose + (IV)	2–4 onset 12–72 hr duration	large intrathecal (IT) doses or prolonged therapy
Cytarabinoside (Ara-C)	rare IT	meningismus, headache, vomiting	low dose − high dose + +	immediate to 1 hr, lasting 12 hrs–2 days	↑ with larger doses
5-Azacytidine	rare	some cases of myalgia leading to somnolence and coma	+	during week-long infusions	dose dependent

(continued)

Table 4.24 (*continued*)

Drug	Incidence	Signs/Symptoms	Crosses BBB	Onset/ Resolution	Dose Relation
Others					
L-Asparaginase	common, 30%–60% incidence; may be dose limiting	somnolence, lethargy, personality changes	–	within the first day to 1–3 days after drug cessation	none
Procarbazine	infrequent (po), dose-limiting when given IV	optic neuroretinitis, somnolence, CNS depression, manic psychosis, peripheral neuropathies	+ +	• onset in 8 days with slow resolution when oral dosing • onset immediate with rapid recovery with IV dosing	unknown in high doses
Cisplatin	becoming more common	uni- or bilateral ototoxicity, peripheral neuropathy	unknown	rapid onset unknown recovery	dose-related
Mitotane	40% of pts	lethargy, sedation, vertigo	+ +	rapid onset with slow resolution	may be related to cumulative dose

Source: Modified from Dorr and Fritz (1980). Reprinted by permission of the publisher from Dorr RT, Fritz WL, *Cancer Chemotherapy Handbook*, pp. 120–122. Copyright 1980 by Elsevier Science Publishing Co., Inc.

(difficulty controlling muscle movement), ataxia of trunk or extremities, unsteady gait, slurred speech, nystagmus, dizziness, and oculomotor disturbances (Kaplan and Wiernik 1984). The syndrome is reversible within 1–6 weeks of drug discontinuance. This toxicity has not been seen with continuous infusion therapy (120 hours) despite the fact that higher doses are administered. Hexamethylmelamine may cause CNS symptoms with continuous high-dose oral administration, characterized by depression, hallucinations, somnolence or insomnia, dysphagia, questionable seizures, prominent ataxia, and tremors (Kaplan and Wiernik 1984).

Procarbazine is a weak monoamine oxidase inhibitor which rapidly crosses the blood-brain barrier, and may cause altered levels of consciousness and rarely, ataxia, which is reversible (Kaplan and Wiernik 1984). It is important to remember that procarbazine potentiates the effects of phenothiazines, barbiturates, and narcotics, so that concurrent administration of these medications should be done with caution.

The Syndrome of Inappropriate Antidiuretic Hormone (SIADH) occurs rarely, following administration of the vinca alkaloids (vincristine, vinblastine) or cyclophosphamide. Kaplan and Wiernik describe the hyponatremia related to the vinca alkaloids as moderate to severe, developing within 10 days of drug administration, and resolving in 1–2 weeks. It is believed that there is a direct drug effect on the hypothalamus, neurohypophyseal tract, or posterior pituitary (Stuart et al. 1975). It is possible that rare mental changes, confusion, delirium, and seizures reported after vincristine administration may be due to SIADH-induced hyponatremia (Kaplan and Wiernik 1984). Cyclophosphamide-induced SIADH appears related to a transient decrease in free-water clearance and urine volume as active metabolites of the drug are excreted in the urine, and there is a consequent fall in serum sodium concentration 4–12 hours after drug infusion, lasting up to 20 hours (DeFronzo et al. 1973). It is possible that slower infusion of cyclophosphamide may minimize neurotoxic reactions (Kaplan and Wiernik 1984).

Neuropathies

The drugs most commonly associated with neuropathies are the vinca alkaloids and cisplatin, and they will be discussed in detail. Of the three vinca alkaloids, vincristine has the greatest potential to cause neurotoxicity because it has been shown to be rapidly taken up by unsheathed nerves and is extensively tissue bound leading to prolonged exposure of neural tissue (Nelson, Dyke, and Root 1980). However, vindesine and vinblastine may cause similar toxicity. An early sign of vincristine neurotoxicity is the loss of the Achilles tendon reflex, and with continued treatment, the other deep tendon reflexes may be lost even though the patient is asymptomatic (Sandler, Tobin, and Henderson 1969). The most common symptom is parasthesia of the hands or feet, occurring in up to 57% of patients, which may progress to muscle pain, weakness, gait disturbance, and sensory impairment with continued drug dosing (Kaplan and Wiernik 1984). However, neurotoxic drugs are not usually discontinued unless there is loss of deep tendon reflexes. Loss of dorsiflexion reflexes of the foot leads to distressing foot drop or a slapping gait, and then may continue to severe muscle weakness (Weiss, Walker, Wiernik 1974). The sensory and motor impairment is symmetrical and appears to be dose related, although patients with lymphoma appear to develop neuropathies earlier in the treatment course (Kaplan and Wiernik 1984). If treatment is stopped when loss of reflexes or parasthesia are first identified, then recovery occurs in 1–3 months; in contrast, if vincristine is continued, loss of deep tendon reflexes may be permanent (Kaplan and Wiernik 1984).

Cisplatin is a heavy metal and appears to act as an alkylating agent. Neuropathy is an increasingly more common side effect as higher doses of cisplatin are administered, and the impact on the patient can be devastating. The neuropathy is generally dose dependent, but there is much variability in symptoms. Patients first experience numbness and tingling of the extremities, and may have decreased vibratory sensation and decreased deep tendon reflexes. This progresses to impaired position sense, and in some, to sensory ataxia (Mollman et al. 1988). Because cisplatin-induced nephropathy is easily preventable, neuropathy is now becoming the dose-limiting factor. In an effort to try to decrease the neurotoxicity of cisplatin, Mollman and colleagues (1988) used the radioprotective agent WR-2721 and showed a significantly lower incidence of neuropathy in a study of 69 patients receiving cisplatin-containing chemotherapy regimens. They also found the highest incidence of severe peripheral neuropathy at cisplatin doses of 40 mg/m^2 on 5 consecutive days repeated monthly, while in another report by Legha and Dimery (1985), the median cumulative dose of cisplatin was 775 mg/m^2 in patients developing neurotoxicity.

Damage to cranial nerves can occur in up to 10% of patients receiving vincristine, and damage is usually reversible when treatment is interrupted (Kaplan and Wiernik 1984). The signs of damage to cranial nerves are as follows:

recurrent laryngeal nerve→vocal cord paresis or paralysis

oculomotor nerve→bilateral ptosis, diplopia

rare optic neuropathy→transient cortical blindness

trigeminal nerve→severe jaw pain after 1st dose

Holden and Felde (1987) describe five categories of sensory-perceptual losses. The first, *auditory*, includes the ototoxicity experienced by many patients receiving high-dose cisplatin. It is estimated that reversible tinnitus occurs in about 9% of patients receiving doses up to 60 mg/m^2; symptomatic hearing loss occurs in about 6%; and audiogram abnormalities (high frequency pure-tone hearing loss) that occur in at least 24% may not be reversible (Kaplan and

Wiernik 1984). As higher doses of cisplatin are administered, these percentages will increase. Audiograms should be performed prior to cisplatin therapy, and repeated if the patient develops impaired speech perception; at that time a decision based on potential risks and benefits would be made about continuing therapy (Kaplan and Wiernik 1984).

The second loss is *visual loss*, and patients may experience blurred vision and impaired color vision (color saturation and discrimination along the blue-yellow axis) (Wilding et al. 1985). In Holden and Felde's survey (1987), the loss of precise color vision was most distressing to patients. Other changes, although rare, are similar to heavy metal poisoning such as papilledema and retrobulbar neuritis (see table 4.25). Patient problems include mistaken colors, potential for injury, and decreased appreciation for food and environment related to loss of color discrimination.

Taste changes occur, but may be related to other factors, and often involve hypersensitivity to red meat.

Tactile changes are distressing, and develop as bilateral, symmetrical paresthesias and dysethe-sias in a stocking-and-glove distribution (Kaplan and Wiernik 1984), from fingertips to wrist, and toes to knees. Vibration sense is often disturbed, as well as fine motor movement. Patient problems include potential for injury related to insensitivity to temperature.

Proprioceptive losses can be devastating due to the loss of ability to determine the position of body parts without visual cues. Patients may have gait disturbances and difficulty with hand writing (Kaplan and Wiernik 1984). Patient problems may include alterations in role and self-esteem if proprioceptive and sensory changes require changes in occupation, and altered ability to perform activities of daily living.

Lastly, autonomic neuropathy is very common, especially constipation and colicky abdominal pain. This occurs in 33%–46% of patients, and may precede the onset of parasthesias or diminished deep tendon reflexes (Kaplan and Wiernik 1984). Nurses should make certain that patients receiving vinca alkaloids are receiving a bowel regime containing stool softeners and laxatives as needed to *prevent* constipation, as this can lead to adynamic ileus and severe morbidity.

Table 4.25 Ocular Toxicity

Drug	Direct Effect
busulfan	cataracts
chlorambucil	rare diplopia, papilledema, retinal hemorrhage
cisplatin	rare papilledema, blurry vision, retrobulbar neuritis
cytosine arabinoside (high dose)	increased lacrimation, conjunctivitis as drug is excreted in tears
corticosteroids	cataracts
cyclophosphamide	rare blurred vision
doxorubicin	rare conjunctivitis
5-fluorouracil	increased lacrimation, blurred vision photophobia (drug excreted in tears)
methotrexate	rare ocular irritation (some drug found in tears)
nitrosoureas	rare optic neuroretinitis, loss of depth perception, blurred vision, retinopathy
procarbazine	rare retinal hemorrhage, nystagmus, diplopia, photophobia
tamoxifen (high dose)	decreased visual acuity, retinopathy, corneal opacities
vinca alkaloids	ptosis, diplopia, nerve palsies, photophobia, optic neuropathy

Source: Modified from Brager and Yasko 1984. Adapted from Vizel 1982.

Table 4.26 Standardized Nursing Care Plan for the Patient Experiencing Neuropathy

Nursing Diagnosis	Expected Outcome	Nursing Interventions

I. Potential for injury related to ↓ sensitivity to temperature, gait disturbance, ↓ proprioception	I. A. Pt will be without injury
	 B. Pt will report changes in tactile and proprioceptive function
	 C. Pt will develop safe measures to compensate for losses
		I. A. Assess integrity of *tactile* and *proprioceptive* functions
		    1. Sensory perception to light touch, pinprick, vibration, temperature; vision, color vision
		    2. Pt's ability to tolerate light touch, cool water, presence of numbness and tingling, presence of painful sensations
		    3. Proprioception testing of station, gait, deep tendon reflexes, muscle weakness or atrophy, and balance
		    4. Pt's ability to sense placement of body parts, ability to write, evidence of muscle weakness
		 B. Discuss alterations in sensation, proprioception, and impact on ability to do activities of daily living (ADLs)
		 C. Discuss alternative strategies to prevent injury
		    1. Instruct pt in safety measures and use of visual cues
		    2. Encourage pt to take time to complete activities, focus attention to task
		    3. Use potholder when cooking
		    4. Use gloves when washing dishes, gardening
		    5. Inspect skin for cuts, abrasions, burns daily, especially arms, legs, toes, fingers
		 D. Refer as appropriate for occupational or physical therapy, diagnostic testing using EMG
		 E. If pt presents with S/S of peripheral neuropathy, hold chemotherapy and discuss with physician

II. Potential for impaired self-care related to tactile and proprioception dysfunction	II. A. Pt will identify activities of self-care that are difficult
	B. Pt will identify strategies to meet needs
		II. A. Assess pt's ability to perform ADLs such as eating, hygiene, dressing, walking, and handwriting
		B. Discuss and develop strategies to meet self-care needs
		  1. Referral to occupational therapy for splint, etc.
		  2. Involve family members in care planning
		  3. Community resource referral as appropriate (homemaker, home health aide, visiting nurse)

III. Potential for alteration in comfort related to painful parasthesias	III. A. Pt will have decreased pain	III. A. Assess comfort level and presence of severe tingling or prickling sensation, cramping or burning B. Assess intensity, quality, and frequency of discomfort C. Identify precipitating factors, such as warm or cold stimulation, and develop realistic plan to avoid precipitating factors D. Consider adjunctive analgesics with neurologic action for dysaesthetic pain: amitriptyline HCl (Elavil), phenytoin sodium (Dilantin) E. Consider nonpharmacologic intervention: teach pt guided imagery, progressive muscle relaxation, massage, etc.
IV. Impaired mobility related to decreased proprioception, muscle dysfunction	IV. A. Pt will ambulate safely	IV. A. Assess pt's level of activity, muscle strength, and mobility level prior to chemotherapy, then prior to each treatment, and at each visit once therapy is completed B. Encourage pt to use visual cues to determine position of body parts C. Teach measures to prevent injury D. Refer for physical, occupational therapy, and assistive devices as needed

(continued)

Table 4.26 *(continued)*

Nursing Diagnosis	Expected Outcome	Nursing Interventions
V. Potential for sexual dysfunction related to altered tactile sensation, muscle weakness, changes in role	V. A. Pt and significant other (SO) will identify alterations in sexual expression B. Pt and SO will identify alternative methods of sexual expression	V. A. Discuss with pt the impact of treatment-related dysfunction on sexuality, social role, and self-esteem B. Discuss appropriate alternative means of sexual expression C. Refer for specific sexual counseling if diminished ability to have erection D. Observe for changes in needs related to affection and emotional support
VI. Potential for role change with changes and alterations in self-esteem and self-concept related to sensory/perceptual dysfunction, changes in social function, changes in ability to perform occupational role	VI. A. Pt and family will demonstrate positive coping strategies	VI. A. Assess impact of sensory/perceptual dysfunction on social and work roles: ability to meet role expectations of self and family B. Discuss modifications in job and role, as appropriate and available C. Refer pt to OT/PT to see if appliances available to foster rehabilitation (braces, etc.) D. Encourage independence and provide positive reinforcement for accomplishments E. Support pt as s/he grieves loss(es); assess need for support groups or counseling F. Support pt and family by providing information to help explain these behavioral responses to treatment-related dysfunction

VII. Potential for alteration in nutrition: less than body requirements related to taste distortions, anorexia, hypersensitivity to foods	VII. A. Pt will eat balanced diet from 4 food groups B. Pt attains ideal body weight following completion of treatment	VII. A. Assess dietary preferences, changes in food tolerances B. Teach pt to select high-calorie, high-protein foods C. Suggest dietary modifications based on taste changes; e.g., Crazy Jane Salt and spices if foods are tasteless D. Perform periodic weights prior to each treatment cycle E. Evaluate pt's ability to do fine motor movements to feed self, cook F. Referral to nutritionist or dietician as needed G. Monitor laboratory values, especially magnesium, calcium on cisplatin therapy
VIII. Potential for constipation related to autonomic neuropathy (vinca alkaloids)	VIII. A. Pt will move bowels at least every other day	VIII. A. Assess normal elimination pattern B. Encourage pt to drink at least 3 liters of fluid/day C. Encourage daily exercise D. Teach pt to include bulky, high-fiber foods in diet E. Teach pt to self-administer stool softeners and laxatives as needed

IX. Knowledge deficit related to self-care measures related to neuropathic changes	IX. A. Pt identifies risk of development of neuropathy
	B. Pt identifies signs and symptoms to report to health care provider
		IX. A. Teach pt re potential side effect(s) of neuropathy
		1. Constipation
		2. Numbness/tingling in hands/feet
		3. Motor weakness
		  a. Gait changes (e.g., foot drop)
		  b. Loss of fine-motor movement (buttoning shirt, picking up dime)
		4. Inability of males to have erection
		5. Difficulty urinating
		B. Teach pt to report the occurrence of signs and symptoms of neuropathies

Sources: Ogrinc 1985; Holden and Felde 1987; Brager and Yasko 1984; Kaplan and Wiernik 1984.

BIBLIOGRAPHY

Potential Toxicities

Levine ME (1978) Cancer chemotherapy—a nursing model. *Nursing Clinic of North America* 13(2): 271–280

Perry MC and Yarbro JW (1984) Complications of chemotherapy: an overview, in Perry MC, and Yarbro JW (eds), *Toxicity of Chemotherapy*. Orlando, Fla: Grune & Stratton

Bone Marrow Depression

Antman KD, Griffin JD, Elias A, et al (1988) Effect of recombinant human granulocyte-macrophage colony stimulating factor on chemotherapy-induced myelosuppression. *NEJM* 319(10): 593–598

Bergsagel DE (1971) Assessment of massive dose chemotherapy of malignant disease. *Can Med Assoc J* 104: 31–36

Blesch KS (1988) The normal physiological changes of aging and their impact on the response to cancer treatment. *Seminars in Oncology Nursing* 4(3): 178–188 (August)

Bodey GP (1984) Current status of prophylaxis of infection with protected environments. *The American Journal of Medicine* 76: 678–684

Bodey GP, Buckley M, Sathe YS, et al (1966) Quantitative relationship between circulating leukocytes and infections in patients with acute leukemia. *Ann Int Med* 64(2): 328–340

Brager BL, Yasko JM (1984) *Care of the Client Receiving Chemotherapy*. Reston, Va.: Reston Publishing Company, 96, 106, 178, 180

Brandt B (1984) A nursing protocol for the client with neutropenia. *Oncology Nursing Forum* 11(2): 24–28

Carlson AC (1985) Infection prophylaxis in the patient with cancer. *Oncology Nursing Forum* 12(3): 60

Dorr RT, Fritz W (1980) *Cancer Chemotherapy Handbook*. New York, Elsevier Press, 102

Fox LS (1981) Granulocytopenia in the adult cancer patient. *Cancer Nursing* (December): 24

Golden W (1971) Routine protective isolation: worth the trouble in neutropenic patients. *JAMA* 242(19): 2045

McConnell EA (1986) Leukocyte studies: what the counts can tell you. *Nursing 86* (March): 42–43

Neuseff W, Maki D (1981) A study of the value of simple protective isolation in patients with granulocytopenia. *NEJM* 304(8): 448–453

Pizzo PA (1983) *Management of Fever and Infection in Patients with Cancer*. New York, Della Corte Publications, 2, 3

Pizzo PA, Schimpff SC (1983) Strategies for the prevention of infection in the immunosuppressed cancer patient. *Cancer Treatment Reports* (Mar): 223–234

Rodriquez V, Ketchel SJ (1981) Acute infections in patients with malignant disease, chapter 11 in Yarbro JW, Bornstein RS (eds): *Oncologic Emergencies*. New York, Grune and Stratton

Schimpff SC, Young VM, Green WH, et al (1972) Origin of infection in acute ANLL: significance of hospital acquisition of pathogens. *Ann Int Med* 77: 707–714

Spross JA (1985) Protective mechanisms: bone marrow, chapter 9 in Johnson BL, Gross J (eds): *Handbook of Oncology Nursing*. New York, John Wiley and Sons, 250–251

Wroblewski SS, Wroblewski SH (1981) Caring for the patient with chemotherapy-induced thrombocytopenia. *American Journal of Nursing* 81(4): 746

Stomatitis

Adrian RM, Hood AF, Skarin AT (1980) Mucocutaneous reactions to antineoplastic agents. *Cancer J Clin* 30: 142–157

Beck S (1979) Impact of a systemic oral care protocol on stomatitis after chemotherapy. *Cancer Nursing* 2: 186 (June)

Beck S, Yasko JM (1984) *Guidelines for Oral Care*. Cary, Illinois, Sage Products

Bersani G, Carl W (1983) Oral care for cancer patients. *American Journal of Nursing* 83: 533

Brager BL, Yasko JM (1984) *Care of the Client Receiving Chemotherapy*. Reston, Va.: Reston Publishing Co.

Capizzi RL, DeConti RC, Marsh JC, et al (1970) Methotrexate therapy of head and neck cancer: improvement in therapeutic index by the use of leukovorin rescue. *Cancer Research* 30: 1783

Daeffler RJ (1985) Protective mechanisms: mucous membranes, in Johnson BL, Gross J (eds): *Handbook of Oncology Nursing*. New York, John Wiley and Sons, 253–274

Dreizen S, Boday G, and Rodriques V (1975) Oral complications of cancer chemotherapy. *Postgraduate Medicine* 58: 76

Dudjak LA (1987) Mouth care for mucositis due to radiation therapy. *Cancer Nursing* 10(3): 131-140

Engleking C (1988) Managing stomatitis: a nursing process approach, in *Supportive Care for the Patient with Cancer*. Richmond, Va.: AH Robins Co, 20-28

Fardal O, Turnbull RS (1986) A review of the literature on use of chlorhexidine in dentistry. *JADA* 112: 863-869 (June)

Ferraro JM, Mattern JQA (1984) Sucralfate suspension for stomatitis. *Drug Intell Clin Pharmacol* 18: 153

Ferretti GA, Ash RC, Brown AT, et al (1987) Chlorhexidine for prophylaxis against oral infections and associated complications in patients receiving bone marrow transplants. *JADA* 114: 461-467 (April)

Ferretti GA, Hanse IA, Whittenburg K, et al (1987) Therapeutic use of chlorhexidine in bone marrow transplant patients: case studies. *Oral Surgery*, 63(6): 683-687 (June)

Ferretti, GA, Raybould T, Whittenberg A, et al (1987) Effect of chlorhexidine mouthrinse on mucogisis in patients receiving intensive chemotherapy. *J. Dental Research* 66 (Special Issue): 342

Frattore L, Larson RA, Mostofi RS (1986) Dental management of cancer patients receiving chemotherapy. *Illinois Medical Journal* 169: 223-227

Goodman MS, Stoner C (1985) Mucous membrane integrity, impairment of stomatitis, chapter 37, in McNally JC, Stair JC, Somerville ET: *Guidelines for Cancer Nursing Practice*. Orlando, Grune and Stratton, 178-182

Lavalle C, Proctor D (1978) *Clinical Pathology of the Oral Mucosa*. Hagerstown, Md.: Harper and Row

Lockhart P, Sonis S (1979) Relationship of oral complications to peripheral blood leukocyte and platelet counts in patients receiving cancer chemotherapy. *Oral Surgery* 48: 21-28

McGaw WT and Belch A (1985) Oral complications of acute leukemia: prophylactic impact of a chlorhexidine mouth rinse regimen. *Oral Surgery, Oral Medicine, Oral Pathology* 60 (3): 275-280 (Sept)

McNally JC, Stair J, Somerville ET (eds.) (1985) *Guidelines for Cancer Nursing Practice*. Orlando, Grune and Stratton

Peterson DE (1984) Toxicity of chemotherapy: oral lesions, chapter 6, in Perry MC, Yarbro JW (eds): *Toxicity of Chemotherapy*. Orlando, Grune and Stratton, 155-180

Poland JM (1987) Comparing Moie-stir to lemon glycerine swabs. *American Journal of Nursing* 87: 87

Siena S, et al (1988) Amelioration of severe mucositis by misoprostol following total body irradiation and high dose melphalan with autologous bone marrow transplantation. *Gastroenterology International* 1 (Suppl): 1044

Sonis ST, Sonis AL, Lieberman A (1978) Oral complications in patients receiving treatment for malignancies other than head and neck. *Journal of the American Dental Assoc* 97: 468-472

Wilkes GM (1986) Sucralfate suspension for mucositis. *Oncology Nursing Forum* 13(1): 71-72

Yasko, JM (1983) *Guidelines for Cancer Care: Symptom Management*. Reston, Va., Reston Publishing Co

Zinner SH, Belcher AE, Murphy C (1988) *Assessing the risk of herpes in immunocompromised patients*. Research Triangle Park, N.C., Burroughs Wellcome

Esophagitis and Diarrhea

Brager BL, Yasko JM (1984) *Care of the Client Receiving Chemotherapy*. Reston, Va, Reston Publishing Co, 247-255

Culhane B (1983) Diarrhea, in Yasko J (ed): *Guidelines for Cancer Care: Symptom Management*. Reston, Va: Reston Publishing Co

Daeffler RJ (1985) Mucous membranes, in Johnson BL, Gross J (eds): *Handbook of Oncology Nursing*. New York, John Wiley and Sons, 253-274

Davis M (1985) Bowel elimination, alterations in: diarrhea, chapter 49, in McNally JC, Stair JC, Somerville ET (eds): *Guidelines for Cancer Nursing Practice*. Orlando, Grune and Stratton, 239-242

Dorr RT, Fritz WL (1980) *Cancer Chemotherapy Handbook*. New York, Elsevier Press

Frattore L, Larson RA, Mostofi RS (1986) Dental management of cancer patients receiving chemotherapy. *Illinois Medical Journal* 169: 223-227

Kris MG, Gralla RJ, Clark RA, et al (1988) Control of chemotherapy-induced diarrhea with the synthetic enkephalin BW 942C: a randomized trial with placebo in patients receiving cisplatin. *Journal of Clinical Oncology* 6(4): 663-669 (April)

Nunnally C, Donoghue M (1986) Nursing management of gastrointestinal dysfunction, in Yasko JM, *Nursing Management of Symptoms Associated with Chemotherapy*. Columbus, Ohio, Adria Laboratories

Nunnally C, Donoghue M, and Yasko JM (1983) Esophagitis, in Yasko JM (ed): *Guidelines for Cancer Care: Symptom Management*. Reston, Va: Reston Publishing Co.

Perry MC, Yarbro JW (1984) *Toxicity of Chemotherapy*. New York, Grune and Stratton

Ropka ME (1985) Nutrition, chapter 8, in Johnson BL, Gross J (eds): *Handbook of Oncology Nursing*. New York, J Wiley and Sons, 205

Alopecia

Baxley KO, Erdman LK, Henry EB, et al (1984) Alopecia: effect on cancer patients' body image. *Cancer Nursing* 7(6): 499–502

Brager BL, Yasko JM (1984) *Care of the Client Receiving Chemotherapy*. Reston, Va, Reston Publishing Co, 247–255

Chernecky CC, Yasko JM (1986) Alopecia, in Yasko JM (ed): *Nursing Management of Symptoms Associated with Chemotherapy*. Columbus, Ohio, Adria Labs

Cline BW (1984) Prevention of chemox-induced alopecia: a review of the literature. *Cancer Nursing* 7(3): 221–228

Dean JC, Griffith KS, Cetus TC, et al (1983) Scalp hypothermia: a comparison of ice packs and the kold kap in the prevention of doxorubicin-induced alopecia. *J Clin Oncology* 1(1): 33–37

Dorr RT, Fritz WL (1980) *Cancer Chemotherapy Handbook*. New York, Elsevier, 107–109

Dunagin WG (1984) Dermatologic toxicity, in Perry MC, Yarbro JW (eds): *Toxicity of Chemox*. Orlando, Greene and Stratton

Keller JF, Blausey LA (1988) Nursing issues and management in chemotherapy-induced alopecia. *ONF* 15(5): 603–607

Lindsey AM (1985) Building the knowledge base for practice: alopecia, self-breast exam and other human responses, part 2. *ONF* 12(2): 27–34

Parker R (1987) The effectiveness of scalp hypothermia in preventing cyclophosphamide-induced alopecia. 14(6): 49–55 (Nov/Dec)

Perez JE, Macchiavelli M, Leone BA, et al (1986) High dose alpha-tocopherol as a preventative of doxorubicin-induced alopecia. *Cancer Treatment Reports* 70(10): 1213–1214

Gonadal Dysfunction

Block E (1952) Quantitative morphological investigations of the follicular system in women, variations at different ages. *Acta Anat* 14: 108–123

Bonfante V, Santoro A, Bajetta E, et al (1985) Hodgkin's disease: an overview and ABVD studies in Milan, in Sikic BI, Rozencweig M, Carter SK (eds): *Bleomycin Chemotherapy*. New York, Academic Press

Brager BL, Yasko J (1984) *Care of the Client Receiving Chemotherapy*. Reston, Va, Reston Publishing Co

Chapman RM (1984) Effect of cytotoxic therapy on sexuality and gonadal function, chapter 13, in Perry MC, Yarbro JW (eds): *Toxicity of Chemotherapy*. Orlando, Grune and Stratton, 343–365

Chapman RM, Sutcliffe SB, Malpas JS (1979) Cytoxic-induced ovarian failure in females with Hodgkin's disease: I. Hormone function. *JAMA* 242: 1877–1881

Drasga RE, Einhorn LH, Williams SD, et al (1983) Fertility after chemotherapy for testicular cancer. *Journal of Clinical Oncology* 1: 179–183

Fisher SG (1983) The psychosexual effects of cancer and cancer treatment. *Oncology Nursing Forum* 10(2): 63–68

Glasgow M, Halfin V, Althausen A (1987) Sexual response and cancer. *CA—A Cancer Journal for Clinicians* 37(6): 322–333 (Nov-Dec)

Howard–Ruben, J (1985) Sexual dysfunction related to disease process and treatment, chapter 56, in McNally JC, Stair JC, Somerville ET, (eds): *Guidelines for Cancer Nursing Practice*. Orlando, Greene and Stratton, 268–277

Kaempfer S (1981) The effect of cancer chemotherapy on reproduction—a review of the literature. *ONF* 8: 11–18

Kaempfer SH, Wiley FM, Hoffman DJ, et al (1985) Fertility considerations and procreative alternatives in cancer care. *Seminars of Oncology Nursing* 1(1): 25–34 (Feb)

Kreuser ED, Hetzel WD, Heit W, et al (1988) Reproductive and endocrine gonadal function in adults following multidrug chemotherapy for acute lymphoblastic or undifferentiated leukemia. *Journal of Clinical Oncology* 6(4): 588–596 (April)

Perry MC, Yarbro JW (1984) *Toxicity of Chemotherapy*. New York, Grune and Stratton

Santoro A, Viviani S, Zucoli R, et al (1983) Comparable results and toxicity of MOPP vs ABVD combined with radiotherapy in PS IIB, III(A&B) HD. *Proc Amer Soc Clin Oncol.*

Sherins RJ, DeVita VT (1973) Effects of drug treatment of lymphoma on male reproductive capacity. *Ann Int Med* 79: 216–220

Smith DB (1989) Sexual rehabilitation of the cancer patient. *Cancer Nursing* 12(1): 10–15

Tarpy CC (1985) Birth control considerations during chemotherapy. *Oncology Nursing Forum* 12(2): 75–78

Viviani S, Santoro A, Ragni G, et al (1985) Gonadal toxicity after combination chemotherapy for Hodgkin's disease. Comparative results of MOPP vs. ABVD. *European Journal of Cancer Clinical Oncology* 21: 601–605

Yarbro CH, Perry MC (1985) The effect of cancer therapy on gonadal function. *Seminars in Oncology Nursing* 1(1): 3–8

Yasko JM (1984) Sexual and reproductive dysfunction, in Yasko JM (ed): *Guidelines for Cancer Care: Symptom Management*. Reston, Va, Reston Publishing Co, 269–290

Nausea and Vomiting

Allen TC, Gralla R, Reilly L, et al (1985) Metoclopramide: dose-related toxicity and preliminary antiemetic studies in children receiving cancer chemotherapy. *Journal of Clin Oncology* 3: 1136–1141

Bakowski M (1984) Advances in antiemetic therapy. *Cancer Treat Rev* 11: 237–256

Bickal T (1987) A protocol for the diagnosis and treatment of extrapyramidal symptoms of neuroleptic drugs. *Nurs Prac* 12(1): 25–38

Borison H, McCarthy L (1984) Neuropharmacology of chemotherapy-induced emesis. *Drugs* 25 (Suppl 1): 8–17

Caille G, Speneid J, Lacasse J (1983) Pharmacokinetics of two lorazepam formations, oral and sublingual, after multiple doses. *Biopharm Drug Dispos* 4: 31–42

Carr B, Blayney D, Leong L, et al (1985) A prospective, double-blind dose-response study of prochlorperazine therapy for cisplatin-induced emesis. *Proc ASCO* 4: 268

Citron M, Johnson–Early A, Boyer M, et al (1984) Droperidol: optimal dose and time of initiation. *Proc ASCO* 3: 106

Costall B, Domeney AM, Gunning ST, et al (1987) GR 38032F: A potent and novel inhibitor of cisplatin-induced emesis in the ferret. *Br J Pharmacol* 90: 90

Cotanch PM, Strum S (1987) Progressive muscle relaxation as antiemtic therapy for cancer patients. *Oncology Nursing Forum* 14(1): 33–37

Craig JB, Powell BL (1987) Review: the management of nausea and vomiting in clinical oncology. *Am Journal of Medical Sciences* 293(1): 34–41 (Jan)

Cunningham D, Pople A, Ford HT, et al (1987) Prevention of emesis in patients receiving cytotoxic drugs by GR38032F, a selective 5-HT3 receptor antagonist. *Lancet*(27 Jun): 1461–1462

Dorr RT, Fritz W (1980) *Cancer Chemotherapy Handbook*. New York, Elsevier Press, 103–104

Fiore JJ, Gralla RJ (1984) Pharmacologic treatment of chemotherapy-induced nausea and vomiting. *Cancer Investigation* 2(5): 351–361

Gagen M, Gochnour D, Young D, et al (1984) A randomized trial of metoclopramide and a combination of dexamethasone and lorazepam for prevention of chemotherapy-induced vomiting. *Journal of Clinical Oncology* 2: 696–701

Goodman M (1987) Management of nausea and vomiting induced by outpatient cisplatin therapy. *Seminars in Oncology Nursing* 3(1) (Suppl 1): 23–35

Gralla RJ, Tyson L, Bordin L, et al (1984) Antiemetic therapy: a review of recent studies and a report of a random assignment trial comparing metoclopramide with delta-9-tetrahydrocannabinol. *Cancer Treat Rep* 68(1): 163–172

Gralla RJ, Tyson LB, Kris MG, et al (1987) The management of chemotherapy-induced nausea and vomiting. *Med Clin North America* 71(2): 294–297

Greenberg S, Gala K, Lampenfeld M, et al (1984) Comparison of the antiemetic effect of high-dose metoclopramide and high-dose IV haloperidol. *J Clin Oncology* 21: 782–783

Hesketh PJ, Murphy WK, Khojasten A, et al (1988) GR-C507175 (GR38032F): A novel compound effective in the treatment of cisplatin induced nausea and vomiting. *Proc ASCO* 7: 280

Hesketh PJ, Murphy WK, Lester EP, et al (1988) GR38032F (GR-C507/75): A novel compound effective in the prevention of acute cisplatin-induced emesis. *Proc ASCO* 7: 280

Ignoffo RJ (1983) Conversations with the pharmacist. *Highlights on Antineoplastic Drugs* (Aug): 3

Kris MG, et al (1985) Consecutive dose-finding trials adding lorazepam to the combination of metoclopramide plus dexamethasone: improving subjective effectiveness over the combination of diphenhydramine plus metoclopramide plus dexamethasone. *Can Treat Rep* 69: 1257–1262

Kris M, Gralla R (1986) Antiemetic trials to control delayed vomiting following high-dose cisplatin. *Proc ASCO* 5: 1005

Kris MG, Gralla RJ, Tyson LB, et al (1989) Controlling delayed vomiting: double-blind, randomized trial comparing placebo, dexamethasone alone, and metoclopramide plus dexamethasone in patients receiving cisplatin. *Journal of Clinical Oncology* 7(1): 108–114

Laszlo J (1983) Nausea and vomiting as major complications of cancer chemotherapy. *Drugs* 25 (Suppl 1): 1–7

Laszlo J, Clark RA, Harrison DC, et al (1985) Lorazepam in cancer patients treated with cisplatin: a drug having antiemetic, amnesic and anxiolytic effects. *J Clin Oncology* 3: 864–869

Markman M, Scheidler V, Ettinger DS, et al (1984) Antiemetic efficacy of dexamethasone. *NEJM* 311: 549–552

Mason BA, Dambra J, Grossman B (1982) Effective control of cisplatin-induced nausea using HD steroids and droperidol. *Cancer Treatment Reports* 66(2): 243–245

Morrow GA (1982) Clinical characteristics associated with the development of anticipatory nausea and vomiting in cancer patients undergoing chemotherapy treatment. *J Clin Oncology* 2(10): 1170

Neidhart J, Gagen M, Wilson H, et al (1981) Comparative trial of antiemetic effects of THC and haloperidol. *J Clin Pharmacology* 21: 385–390

Nicholas D (1982) The prevalence of anticipatory nausea and emesis in cancer chemotherapy patients. *J Behav Med* 5(3): 461–63

Raila F, Tonato M, Basusto C, et al (1985) Antiemetic activity of two different high doses of metoclopramide in cisplatin-treated cancer patients. *Cancer Treatment Rep* 69: 1353–1357

Rhodes VA, Watson PM, Johnson MH (1985) Patterns of nausea and vomiting in chemotherapy patients: a preliminary study. *Oncology Nursing Forum* 12(3): 42–48

Roxane Laboratories (1986) Marinol (dronabinol) Manufacturer's Information Sheet. Roxane Laboratories

Sargeant KS, Fisher JM (1986) Delta-9-tetrahydrocannabinol as antiemetic. *Drug Intell and Clin Pharm* 20: 271–272

Siegel LJ, Longo DL (1981) The control of chemotherapy-induced emesis. *Ann Int Med* 95: 352–359

Smaglia RA (1984) Antiemetic effect of perphenazine versus prochlorperazine intravenously before cisplatin therapy. *Am J Hosp Pharm* 41: 560 (Mar)

Strum S, McDerned HM, Abrahano-Umali R, et al (1985) Management of platinum-induced delayed onset nausea and vomiting: preliminary results with two drug regimens. *Proc Am Soc Clin Oncol* 4: 263

Strum SB, McDermed JE, Pileggi J, et al (1984) Intravenous metoclopramide: prevention of chemotherapy-induced nausea and vomiting. *Cancer* 53(6): 1432–1439

Wilson JM, Weltz M, Solimando D, et al (1981) Continuous infusion droperidol: Antiemetic therapy for cis-Platinum toxicity. *Proc ASCO* 22: 421

Yasko JM (1985) Holistic management of nausea and vomiting caused by chemotherapy. *Topics in Clinical Nursing* (April): 26–29

Cardiac Toxicity

Ali MK, Soto A, Maroongronge D, et al (1979) Electrocardiographic changes after Adriamycin chemotherapy. *Cancer* 43: 465–471

Bristow MR (1982) Toxic cardiomyopathy due to doxorubicin. *Hospital Practices* (Dec) 102–111

Cortes EP, Lutman G, Wanka J, et al (1975) Adriamycin cardiotoxicity: a clinicopathologic correlation. *Cancer Chemotherapy Report*, Part 3, 6(2): 215–225

Doll DC, List AF, Greco A, et al (1986) Acute vascular ischemic events after cisplatin-based combination chemotherapy for germ-cell tumors of the testes. *Annals of Internal Medicine* 105: 48–51

Doll DC, Ringenberg QS, Yarbro JW (1986) Vascular toxicity associated with antineoplastic agents. *Journal of Clinical Oncology* 4(9): 1450–1417 (Sept)

Druck MN, Gulenchyn KY, Evans WK, et al (1984) Radionucleotide angiography and endomyocardial biopsy in the assessment of doxorubicin cardiotoxicity. *Cancer* 53(8): 1667–1674

Kaszyk LK (1986) Cardiac toxicity associated with cancer therapy. *Oncology Nursing Forum* 13(4): 81–88

Legha S, Benjamin RS, MacKay B, et al (1982). Reduction of doxorubicin cardiotoxicity by prolonged continuous intravenous infusion. *AIM* 96: 133–139

Minow RA, Benjamin RS, Gottlieb JA (1975) Adriamycin cardiomyopathy—an overview with determination of risk factors. *Cancer Chemotherapy Reports* 6: 195–201

Saltiel E, McGuire W (1983) Doxorubicin cardiomyopathy. *West J Med* 139(3): 332–341

Taylor AL, Applefeld MM, Wiernik PH (1984) Acute anthracycline cardiotoxicity: comparative morphologic study of 3 analogues. *Cancer* 53(8): 1660–1666

Tokaz LK, Von Hoff DD (1984) The toxicity of anticancer agents, in Perry MC, Yarbro JW (eds): *Toxicity of Chemotherapy*. Orlando, Greene and Stratton 199–226

Tomitotti M, Riundi R, Pulici S, et al (1984) Ischemic cardiomyopathy from CIS-diammine Dichloroplatinum (CDDP). *Tumori* 70: 235–236

Von Hoff D, Rozencweig M, Layard M, et al (1977). Daunomycin-induced cardiotoxicity in children and adults: a review of 110 cases. *American Journal of Medicine* 62: 200–208

Yasko JM (1983) *Guidelines for Cancer Care: Symptom Management*. Reston, Va, Reston Publishing Co

Pulmonary Toxicity

Blum RH, Carter SK, Agre K (1973) A clinical review of bleomycin—a new antineoplastic agent. *Cancer* 31(4): 903–914

Carlson RW, Sikic BI (1983) Continuous infusion or bolus injection in cancer chemotherapy. *Annals of Internal Medicine* 99(6): 823–833

Comis RL, Kuppinger MS, Ginsberg SG, et al (1979) Role of single-breath carbon monoxide diffusion capacity in monitoring the pulmonary efforts of bleomycin in germ cell tumor patients. *Cancer Research* 39(12): 5078–5080

Einhorn L, Krause M, Hornbach N, et al (1976) Enhanced pulmonary toxicity with bleomycin and radiotherapy in oat cell lung cancer. *Cancer* 37(5): 2414–2416

Ginsberg SJ, Comis RL (1984) The pulmonary toxicity of antineoplastic agents, in Perry MC, Yarbro JW (eds): *Toxicity of Chemotherapy*. New York, Greene and Stratton, 227–268

Goodman MS (1987) *Cancer: Chemotherapy and Care*. Evansville, IN, Bristol-Myers USP&NG 33–34

Holoyl PY, Luna MA, Mackay B, et al (1978) Bleomycin hypersensitivity pneumonitis. *AIM* 88: 47–49

Iacovino JR, Leitner J, Abbas A, et al (1976) Fatal pulmonary reaction from low doses of bleomycin. *JAMA* 235(12): 1253–1255

Seltzer SE, Goldstein JD, Herman PG (1983) Iatrogenic thoracic complications induced by drugs, in Herman P: *Iatrogenic Complications*. New York, Springer-Verlag, 1–8

Wickham R (1986) Pulmonary toxicity secondary to cancer treatment. *ONF* 13(5): 69–76 (Sept/Oct)

Yasko JM (1983) *Guidelines for Cancer Care: Symptom Management*. Reston, Va, Reston Publishing Co

Hepatotoxicity

Dorr RT, Fritz WL (1981) *Cancer Chemotherapy Handbook*. New York, Elsevier Press, 130–133

Fischer DS, Knobf MT (1989) *The cancer chemotherapy handbook* (ed 3). Chicago, Year Book Medical Publishers

Goodman, MS (1987) *Cancer: Chemotherapy and Care*. Evansville, IN, Bristol-Myers USP&NG, 32–33

Menard DB, Gisselbrecht C, Marty M, et al (1980) Antineoplastic agents and the liver. *Gastroenterology* 78: 142–164

Perry MC (1984) Hepatotoxicity, in Perry MC, Yarbro JW (eds): *Toxicity of Chemotherapy*. Orlando: Grune and Stratton, 297–312

Woods WG, Denner LP, Nesbit ME, et al (1980) Fatal veno-occlusive disease of the liver following high-dose chemotherapy, irradiation, and bone marrow transplantation. *American Journal of Medicine* 68: 285–290

Zafrani ES, Pinaudeau Y, Dhumeaux D (1983) Drug-induced vascular lesions of the liver. *Arch Internal Medicine* 143: 495–502

Nephrotoxicity

Abelson HT, Garnick MD (1982) Renal failure induced by cancer chemotherapy, in Rieselbach RE, Garnick, MB (eds): *Cancer and the Kidney*. Philadelphia, Lea and Febriger

Cohen D (1983) Metabolic complications of induction therapy for leukemia and lymphoma. *Cancer Nursing* 6: 307

Dentino M, Luft FC, Yum MN, et al (1978) Long-term effect of Cis-diammine-dichloroplatinum (CDDP) on renal function and structure in man. *Cancer* 41(4): 1224–1281

Fields ALA, Josse RG, Bergsagel DE (1982) Metabolic emergencies, in DeVita VT, Hellman S, Rosenberg SA (eds): *Cancer: Principles and Practice of Oncology*. Philadelphia, JB Lippincott Co

Garnick M, Mayer R (1978) Acute renal failure associated with neoplastic disease and its treatment. *Seminars in Oncology* 5(2): 155

Goodman MS (1987) *Cancer: Chemotherapy and Care*. Evansville, IN, Bristol-Myers USP&NG

Lydon, J (1986) Nephrotoxicity of cancer treatment. *ONF* 13(2): 68–77

Moore J (1985) Metabolic emergencies: tumor lysis syndrome, in Johnson BL, Gross J (eds): *Handbook of Oncology Nursing*. New York, John Wiley and Sons, 470–476

Ostrow S, Egorin MJ, Hahn D, et al (1981) High-dose cisplatin therapy using mannitol vs. furosemide diuresis: comparative pharmacokinetics and toxicities. *Cancer Treatment Reports* 65(1–2): 73–78

Ozols RF, Javadpour N, Messerschmidt GL, et al (1982) Poor prognosis non-seminomatous testicular cancer: an effective high-dose *cis*-Platinum regimen without increased renal toxicity. *Proc Am Soc Clin Oncol* 1: 113

Perry MC, Yarbro JW (1984) *Toxicity of Chemotherapy*. New York, Grune and Stratton

Schilsky RL (1984) Renal and metabolic toxicities of cancer treatment, in Perry MC, Yarbro JW (eds): *Toxicity of Chemotherapy*. Orlando, Greene and Stratton, 317–333

Weiss RB, Poster DS (1982) The renal toxicity of cancer chemotherapy agents. *Cancer Treatment Rev* 9(1): 37–56

Yasko JM (1983) *Guidelines for Cancer Care: Symptom Management*. Reston, Va, Reston Publishing Co

Neurotoxicity

Brager BL, Yasko JM (1984) *Care of the Client Receiving Chemotherapy*. Reston, Va, Reston Publishing Co

DeFronzo RA, Braine H, Colvin OM, et al (1973) Water intoxification in man after cyclophosphamide therapy. *Annals of Internal Medicine* 78: 861–869

Dorr RT, Fritz WL (1980) *Cancer Chemotherapy Handbook*. New York, Elsevier Press, 120–122

Goodman MS (1986) *Cancer: Chemotherapy and Care*. New York, Bristol Myers Oncology

Herzig RH, Herzig GP, Wolff SN, et al (1987) Central nervous system effects of high-dose cytosine arabinoside. *Seminars in Oncology* 14(2) (Suppl 1): 21–24 (June)

Holden S, Felde G (1987) Nursing care of patients experiencing cisplatin-related peripheral neuropathies. *Oncology Nursing Forum* 14(1): 13–19

Kaplan RS, Wiernik PH (1984) Neurotoxicity of antitumor agents, in Perry MC, Yarbro JW (eds): *Toxicity of Chemotherapy*. Orlando, Grune and Stratton, 365–431

Legha SS, Dimery IW (1985) High-dose cisplatin administration without hypertonic saline: observation of disabling neurotoxicity. *J Clin Oncol* 3: 1373–1378

Maciewicz R, Bouckoms A, Martin J (1985) Drug therapy of neuropathic pain. *The Journal of Pain* 1(1): 39–49

Mollman JE, Glover DJ, Hogan M, et al (1988) Cisplatin neuropathy: risk factors, prognosis, and protection by WR-2721. *Cancer* 56(8): 1934–1939

Nelson RL, Dyke RW, Root MA (1980) Comparative pharmacokinetics of vindesine, vincristine, and vinblastine in patients with cancer. *Cancer Treat Rev* 7(Suppl): 17–24

Ogrinc M (1985) Sensory/perceptual alterations related to peripheral neuropathy, chapter 39 in McNally JC, Stair JC, Somerville ET (eds): *Guidelines for Cancer Nursing Practice*. Orlando, Grune and Stratton, 185–188

Sandler SG, Tobin W, Henderson ES (1969) Vincristine-induced neuropathy: a clinical study of fifteen leukemic patients. *Neurology* (Minn) 19: 367–374

Schaefer SD, Post JD, Close LG, et al (1985) Ototoxicity of low- and moderate-dose cisplatin. *Cancer* 56(8): 1934–1939

Seifert P, Baker LH, Reed ML, et al (1975) Comparison of continuously infused 5-fluorouracil with bolus injection in treatment of patients with colorectal adenocarcinoma. *Cancer* 36: 123–128

Stuart MJ, Cuaso C, Miller M, et al (1975) Syndrome of recurrent increased secretion of antidiuretic hormone following multiple doses of vincristine. *Blood* 45: 315–320

Weiss HD, Walker MD, Wiernik PH (1974) Neurotoxicity of commonly used anticancer agents. *NEMJ* 291: 75–81

Wilding G, Caruso R, Lawrence T, et al (1985) Retinal toxicity after high-dose cisplatin therapy. *J Clin Oncol* 3(12): 1683–1689

Vizel M, Oster M (1982) Ocular side effects of cancer chemothrapy. *Cancer* 49: 1999–2002

Yasko JM (1983) *Guidelines for Cancer Care: Symptom Management*. Reston, Va, Reston Publishing Co

5

CHEMOTHERAPEUTIC AGENTS: STANDARDIZED NURSING CARE PLANS TO MINIMIZE TOXICITY

CONTENTS

Acridinyl anisidide (AMSA, M-AMSA) 141
Adrenocorticoids 145
Aminoglutethimide 149
Androgens 153
5-Azacytidine 156
Aziridinylbenzaquinone (AZQ) 159
Bleomycin sulfate 163
Busulfan 169
Carboplatin (Paraplatin) 171
Carmustine 175
Chlorambucil 179
Cisplatin 183
Cyclophosphamide 188
Cytarabine, cytosine arabinoside 193
Dacarbazine 197
Dactinomycin 203
Daunorubicin hydrochloride 208
Doxorubicin hydrochloride 213

Estramustine phosphate 218
Estrogens 223
Etoposide 227
Floxuridine 233
5-Fluorouracil 238
Flutamide (Eulexin) 242
Hexamethylmelamine 244
Hydroxyurea 247
Idarubicin 251
Ifosfamide 256
L-asparaginase 261
Leucovorin calcium 266
Leuprolide acetate 268
Lomustine (CCNU, CeeNU) 270
Mechlorethamine hydrochloride 273
Melphalan 280
6-Mercaptopurine 285
Mesna 288
Methotrexate 290

Methyl-CCNU (semustine, MeCCNU) 295
Mitoguazone dihydrochloride (methyl-GAG) 299
Mitomycin 305
Mitotane 310
Mitoxantrone (Novantrone) 313
Pentostatin 318
Plicamycin 322
Procarbazine hydrochlorozide 326
Progestational agents 330
Streptozocin 332
Tamoxifen citrate 337
6-Thioguanine 340
Thiotepa 343
Trimetrexate 346
Vinblastine (Velban) 349
Vincristine 355
Vindesine 360
VM-26 (teniposide) 365

INTRODUCTION

Nursing process is the basis for nursing practice. It is solely the purview of nursing's domain. Nursing diagnosis is an integral part of the nursing process. This chapter integrates nursing process with chemotherapy administration. The content of both the drug information forms and the mini-care plans is meant to be information that the nurse needs to know at the time of administration in order to give the medication safely. The information is not meant to replace any hospital formulary or manufacturer information. The writers and publisher of this book have made every effort to ensure that the dosage regimens set forth in the text are accurate and in accord with current labeling at the time of publication. However, in view of the constant flow of information resulting from ongoing research and clinical experience, as well as changes in government regulations, nurses are urged to check the package insert of each drug they plan to administer to be certain that changes have not been made in its indications or contraindications or in the recommended dosage for each use. This is particularly important when a drug is new or infrequently employed.

The following information is a synthesis of many sources reviewed by the authors. In-depth drug information can be gathered from the sources at the back of the chapter and from the numerous books that are available solely on cancer chemotherapy. The drug care plans are meant to be shorthand for the larger side effect care plans that are in chapters 4 and 6.

The nursing diagnoses used in this chapter are analogous to the NANDA-approved nursing diagnoses. These diagnoses occur when a patient receives the specific chemotherapeutic agent. At times these diagnoses seem repetitive as do the nursing interventions, but the reader will notice that the defining characteristics are always individualized to the specific drug. The nursing interventions should be individualized to the specific patient being cared for, using the plan as a basis for care.

Patient education is an integral part of all nursing care. The authors have included aspects of patient education under specific nursing interventions, rather than separating patient education into a specific nursing diagnosis of its own.

All authors have contributed to the writing of the care plans; thus writing styles of the plans vary due to the individual style of each author. The authors encourage the reader to create an individualized plan of care to meet the needs of each patient.

DRUG

Acridinyl anisidide (AMSA, M-AMSA)

Class: Investigational agent

MECHANISM OF ACTIONS

Cell cycle phase specific—S phase. The primary mechanism of action is not yet clearly understood. It is believed that AMSA binds with DNA by intercalating between base pairs and thus prohibiting RNA synthesis.

METABOLISM

Broken down into metabolites in the liver and excreted in the bile and urine. The initial halflife of AMSA is 12 minutes; the halflife of the metabolites is 2.5 hours.

DOSAGE/RANGE

Drug is undergoing clinical trials. Consult individual protocol for specific dosages.

DRUG PREPARATION

AMSA is available as 2 sterile liquids. One ampule with an orange-red solution of AMSA; a second with the dilutant L-lactic acid.

The solution, once mixed, is chemically stable for 48 hours. It should be discarded after 8 hours because of lack of bacteriostatic preservatives.

AMSA is not stable in sodium-chloride-containing solutions. Precipitates form. Only 5% dextrose solutions should be used.

DRUG ADMINISTRATION

Dilute the AMSA solution further in D_5W and infuse over 1 hour, unless contraindicated.

SPECIAL CONSIDERATIONS

Drug is a vesicant.

Drug is investigational.

No anaphylaxis reported.

Do not dilute AMSA with chloride-containing solutions.

Impaired liver function may require dose modifications.

Skin discoloration (yellow to orange) has been reported in 10% of patients.

Drug is orange-red when reconstituted.

Acridinyl Anisidide

I. *Altered nutrition, less than body requirements related to*

Nursing Diagnosis	Defining Characteristics	Expected Outcomes	Nursing Interventions
A. Nausea and vomiting	I. A. The frequency and severity of the nausea or vomiting is dose dependent. Only occurs in ~10% of patients and lasts only a few hours	I. A. Pt will be without nausea and vomiting. Nausea and vomiting, if it occurs, will be minimal	I. A. 1. Premedicate with antiemetics and continue prophyllactically × 24 h to prevent nausea and vomiting, at least first treatment 2. Encourage small frequent feedings of cool, bland foods and liquids
B. Stomatitis	B. Mild to moderate	B. Oral mucous membranes will remain intact without infection	B. 1. Teach pt oral assessment 2. Encourage pt to report early stomatitis 3. Teach pt oral hygiene 4. See sec. on stomatitis, chap. 4
C. Diarrhea	C. Infrequent and mild	C. Pt will have minimal diarrhea	C. 1. Encourage pt to report onset of diarrhea 2. Administer or teach pt to self-administer antidiarrheal medications 3. See sec. on diarrhea, chap. 4
D. Hepatic dysfunction	D. Hepatitis is rare but may occur. Also disturbances in liver function studies, especially elevated serum alkaline phosphatase and serum bilirubin	D. Hepatic dysfunction will be identified early	D. 1. Monitor LFTs, i.e., alkaline phosphatase and bilirubin, periodically during treatment 2. Monitor pt for any elevations 3. Dose modifications may be necessary if LFT elevation occurs

II. *Infection and bleeding related to bone marrow depression*	II. A. Hematologic toxicity is the dose-limiting toxicity B. Leukopenia nadir 7–14 days with recovery by day 25 C. Relatively platelet-sparing with only mild thrombocytopenia except in patient with history of radiation to major marrow-producing sites D. Mild anemia	II. A. Pts will be without s/s of infection or bleeding B. Early s/s of infection or bleeding will be identified	II. A. Monitor CBC, platelet count prior to drug administration as well as s/s of infection and bleeding B. Instruct pt in self-assessment of s/s of infection and bleeding C. Dose reduction necessary if compromised bone marrow function D. Refer to sec. on bone marrow depression, chap. 4
III. *Alteration in cardiac output, related to high-dose AMSA*	III. A. Pts have developed ventricular fibrillation when the serum potassium level was low B. CHF has been reported in patient with prior history of antitumor antibiotics, e.g., doxorubicin or daunorubicin C. Cardiac arrest has been reported during amsacrine infusions	III. A. Early s/s of CHF and cardiac irregularities will be identified	III. A. Assess patient for s/s of CHF and quality/regularity of heartbeat B. Monitor I & Os C. Discuss gated blood pool scans with MD D. Instruct pt to report dyspnea, shortness of breath, palpitations, swelling in extremities E. Monitor for cardiac irregularities associated with low serum potassium levels

(continued)

Acridinyl Anisidide (*continued*)

Nursing Diagnosis	Defining Characteristics	Expected Outcomes	Nursing Interventions
IV. *Impaired skin integrity related to phlebitis*	IV. A. Pain may occur if drug is not properly diluted B. Skin discoloration (yellow-orange) has been reported in 10% of patients	IV. A. AMSA will be diluted according to manufacturer's recommendations B. Pt will verbalize any pain related to chemotherapy administration	IV. A. Follow manufacturer's recommendations for drug preparation B. Assess pt for s/s of immediate or late pain/phlebitis C. Teach pt s/s of phlebitis and to report any symptoms early D. Discuss with patient potential skin discoloration and strategies to minimize distress
V. *Potential for injury related to* A. *Hypersensitivity reactions*	V. A. Range from transient skin rashes to anaphylactic reactions in ~ 0.4% of patients	V. A. Early s/s of hypersensitivity will be identified	V. A. 1. Teach pt the potential of a hypersensitivity reaction and to report any unusual symptoms 2. Obtain baseline vital signs and note pt's mental status 3. Assess pt for s/s of a reaction: localized flare reaction—anaphylaxis. See sec. on reactions, chap. 6 4. Administer therapy in case of reaction according to MD orders
B. *Neurological reactions*	B. At very high doses of AMSA, transient paresthesias, hearing loss, and seizure activity have been reported	B. Early s/s of paresthesias and seizure activity will be identified	B. 1. Teach pt the potential of neurologic reactions and to report any unusual symptoms 2. Obtain baseline neurologic mental and hearing functions 3. Assess pt for any unusual neurosymptoms and report changes to MD

Note: ~ means approximately

DRUG

Adrenocorticoids (Cortisone, Hydrocortisone, Dexamethasone, Methylprednisone, Methyl-prednisolone, Prednisone, Prednisolone)

Class: Hormones

MECHANISM OF ACTION

Cause lysis of lymphoid cells, which led to their use against lymphatic leukemia, myeloma, malignant lymphoma. May also recruit malignant cells out of G_0 phase, making them vulnerable to damage caused by cell cycle phase-specific agents.

METABOLISM

Metabolized by the liver, excreted in urine. Prednisone is activated by the liver in its active form, prednisolone.

DOSAGE/RANGE

Varies according to which preparation is used. Dexamethasone is 25 times the potency of hydrocortisone.

Sample doses:

Cortisone	25 mg
Hydrocortisone	20 mg
Prednisone, prednisolone	5 mg
Methylprednisone, Methylprednisolone	4 mg
Dexamethasone	0.75 mg

DRUG PREPARATION

None

DRUG ADMINISTRATION

Oral

SPECIAL CONSIDERATIONS

Chronic steroid use is associated with numerous side effects. Intermittent therapy is safer and in some conditions just as effective as daily therapy.

Adrenocorticoids

Nursing Diagnosis	Defining Characteristics	Expected Outcomes	Nursing Interventions
I. *Altered nutrition: less than body requirements related to*			
A. Gastric irritation	I. A. 1. Steroids can cause increase in secretion of hydrochloric acid & decreased secretion of protective gastric mucus 2. May exacerbate existing gastric ulcer	I. A. Gastric irritation will be avoided/minimized	I. A. 1. Administer drug with meals or antacid. Instruct pt in optimal schedule for drug administration 2. Instruct pt to report evidence of gastric distress immediately
B. Decreased carbohydrate metabolism; hyperglycemia	B. Steroids use insulin antagonists and may cause gluconeogenesis	B. Blood sugar will remain within normal limits	B. 1. Obtain baseline glucose levels; monitor blood sugar periodically throughout therapy 2. Teach pt to recognize s/s of hyperglycemia (polyuria, polydipsia, polyphagia) and to report these to doctor or nurse 3. Dipstick urine for glucose
II. *Potential for injury related to*			
A. Sodium and water retention	II. A. Occurs occasionally	II. A. Fluid and electrolyte balance will be maintained	II. A. 1. Identify patients at risk for complications associated with fluid/sodium retention (pts with preexisting cardiac, renal, hepatic dysfunction) 2. Inform pts of potential for sodium/water retention, of s/s to watch for, and to report to MD 3. Assess pt daily (if inpatient) for s/s of fluid/electrolyte imbalance

II. B. Hypokalemia/ hypocalcemia	II. B. 1. Causes increased excretion of potassium, calcium 2. Osteoporosis may occur with long-term therapy	II. B. Potassium, calcium levels will remain within normal limits	II. B. 1. Teach pt to report s/s of hypocalcemia (leg cramps, tingling in fingertips, muscle twitching) 2. Instruct pt to report s/s hypokalemia (anorexia, muscle twitching, tetany, polyuria, polydipsia) 3. Monitor eletrolytes on a regular basis; report abnormal values 4. Encourage high-potassium, high-calcium diet. If indicated, discuss supplements 5. Instruct pt in safety measures to avoid injury
C. Steroid-induced immunosuppression	C. 1. Increases susceptibility to infections, tuberculosis 2. May mask or aggravate infection 3. May prolong or delay healing of injuries	C. Pt will remain free of infection	C. 1. Instruct pt to report slow healing of wounds and signs of infection (inflammation, redness, soreness, etc) or colds 2. Instruct pt in hygene regimens: mouth, perineal, foot care
III. *Potential sensory/ perceptual alterations*	III. A. Cataracts or glaucoma may develop with prolonged steroid use B. Increased risk of ocular infections resulting from viruses or fungi	III. A. Pt's vision will remain at baseline levels	III. A. Opthalmascopic exams recommended every 2–3 months B. Instruct pt to report s/s eye infection (discharge, vision changes), or decreased vision

(continued)

Adrenocorticoids *(continued)*

Nursing Diagnosis	Defining Characteristics	Expected Outcomes	Nursing Interventions
IV. *Potential for body image disturbance*	IV. A. Cushingoid state may occur with prolonged use B. Every other day therapy can reduce Cushingoid changes C. May include acne, moonface, striae, purpura, hirsutism	IV. A. Pt will verbalize feelings about altered body image and identify strategies for coping with changes	IV. A. Discuss possible body changes with pt and emphasize that they will resolve when therapy is discontinued B. Assess pt for Cushingoid features C. Offer emotional support D. Administer drug in early morning with breakfast
V. *Potential alteration in behavior*	V. A. Commonly causes behavioral changes which include emotional lability, insomnia, mood swings, psychosis, increased appetite	V. A. Pt will avoid significant changes in behavior B. Behavioral changes, should they occur, will be tolerable to pt	V. A. Inform pt and family that behavioral change may occur, and that they will resolve when therapy is discontinued B. Encourage pt to report troublesome behavioral changes to physician
VI. *Potential for immobility*	VI. A. Loss of muscle mass may occur with chronic use and may be serious enough to impair walking B. Muscle cramping can occur with discontinuation of treatment	VI. A. Pt will maintain baseline mobility	VI. A. Inform pt that muscle weakness may occur with therapy and that muscle cramping may occur on discontinuation of therapy B. Encourage pts to report weakness, cramping. Weakness may necessitate discontinuation of therapy as recovery is not always complete

DRUG

Aminoglutethimide (Cytadren, Elipten)

Class: Adrenal Steroid Inhibitor

MECHANISM OF ACTION

Causes "chemical adrenalectomy." Blocks adrenal production of steroids, reducing levels of glucocorticoids, mineralcorticoids, and estrogens. Also inhibits peripheral aromatization of androgens to estrogens.

METABOLISM

Well-absorbed orally. Hydroxylated in liver, undergoes enterohepatic circulation. Most of drug is excreted in urine.

DOSAGE/RANGE

750–2000 mg orally daily in divided doses

40 mg hydrocortisone daily given to replace glucocorticoid deficiencies

DRUG PREPARATION

None

DRUG ADMINISTRATION

Oral

SPECIAL CONSIDERATIONS

Skin rash may develop within 5–7 days, lasting 8 days, often with malaise and fever (100°–102°F). If not resolved in 7–14 days, drug should be discontinued.

Adjuvant corticosteroids need to be administered.

Aminoglutethimide

Nursing Diagnosis	Defining Characteristics	Expected Outcomes	Nursing Interventions
I. Impairment of skin integrity related to rash	I. A. Seen within one week of treatment and disappears in 5–8 days B. If rash does not disappear within expected time, drug may be discontinued C. May be accompanied by malaise and low-grade fever D. Symptoms may include: erythema, pruritis, and unexplained dermatitis	I. Pt will verbalize feelings regarding changes in skin and identify s/s of potential alterations	I. A. Assess skin for any cutaneous changes including location and description B. Instruct pt in self-care measures, including 1. Avoid abrasive products, clothing 2. Avoid tight-fitting clothing 3. Avoid scratching involved areas
II. Sensory/perceptual alteration related to chemotherapy	II. A. Second-most common reaction is often lethargy B. Other s/s include: somnolence, visual blurring, vertigo, ataxia and nystagmus C. Symptoms may be general and transient	II. Sensory-perceptual neurological disturbances will be identified early	II. A. Obtain baseline neurologic/motor function prior to administering chemotherapy B. Teach pt self-assessment techniques and risks of disturbances C. Encourage patient to report any disturbances early D. Further dose reductions may be necessary
III. Infection related to myelosuppression	III. A. Leukopenia is rare	III. A. Pt will be without infection B. Early s/s of infection will be identified	III. A. Monitor CBC including WBC, differential prior to drug administration B. Drug dosage may be reduced or held for lower than normal blood values C. See sec. on bone marrow depression, chap. 4

IV. Altered nutrition, less than body requirements related to

A. Nausea and vomiting		
B. Anorexia		
IV. A. Nausea and vomiting usually mild	IV. A. Pt will be without nausea or vomiting. Nausea or vomiting, if it occurs, will be minimal	IV. A. 1. Premedicate with antiemetics and continue prophylactically × 24 hrs to prevent nausea and vomiting at least for first treatment 2. Encourage small frequent feedings of cool bland foods and liquids
B. Mild	B. Patient will maintain baseline weight ± 5%	B. 1. Encourage small, frequent feedings of favorite foods, especially high-calorie, high-protein (HCHP) foods 2. Encourage use of spices 3. Weekly weights 4. Nutritional consult as needed

V. Alteration in fluid/electrolyte balance

V. A. Possible with high dose aminoglutethamide	V. A. Fluid and electrolyte balance will be maintained	V. A. Monitor pt for weight gain, edema with daily weights
B. Symptoms of hyponatremia include: headache, nausea/vomiting, muscle weakness, lethargy		B. Monitor I/O
C. Symptoms of hyperkalemia include: abdominal cramping, muscle weakness, tingling, cardiac irregularities, mental status changes		C. Check electrolytes daily, monitor for clinical s/s of imbalance

(continued)

Aminoglutethimide (continued)

Nursing Diagnosis	Defining Characteristics	Expected Outcomes	Nursing Interventions
VI. Potential for endocrine dysfunction related to adrenal insufficiency	VI. A. Causes reversible chemical adrenalectomy (adrenal insufficiency) by blocking synthesis of all steroid hormones B. Additional s/s of cortisol insufficiency C. Hyponatremia, postural hypotension (aldosterone), possible hypothyroidism D. Possible ovarian malfunction resulting in virilization	VI. A. Pt will verbalize feelings regarding sexual dysfunction and body image changes due to hormonal alterations B. Side effects from corticosteroid replacement therapy will be identified early	VI. A. Educate pt (significant other) in self-administration of hormone replacement therapy, i.e., preferred time of administration, potential side effects, tapering schedule B. Encourage pt to report any untoward effects especially while on steroid replacement C. Monitor electrolytes especially Na^+, K^+, Ca^{++} D. Encourage diet high in carbohydrates and protein E. Q weekly weights F. Assess for s/s of infection G. Monitor I and O H. Assess pt for behavioral changes I. Assess pt for Addisonian/adrenal crisis J. As appropriate, explore with pt, significant other, reproductive and sexuality patterns and impact chemotherapy may have. See sec. on gonadal dysfunction, chap. 4

DRUG

Androgens: testosterone propionate (Neo-hombreol, Oreton), fluoxymesterone (Halotestin, Ora-Testryl), testolactone (Teslac)

Class: Hormones

MECHANISM OF ACTION

Has stimulatory effect on red blood cells that results in an increased hematocrit. Other mechanism of action unknown.

METABOLISM

Metabolized by the liver; excreted in the urine and feces.

DOSAGE/RANGE

Testosterone propionate	50–100 mg IM 3 times weekly
Fluoxymesterone	10–30 mg orally daily (3–4 divided doses)
Testolactone	100 mg IM 3 times weekly or 250 mg orally 4 times daily

DRUG PREPARATION

Drug comes in ready-to-use vials or tablets.

DRUG ADMINISTRATION

Before IM administration, shake vial vigorously and give injection immediately to avoid solution settling.

SPECIAL CONSIDERATIONS

Fluoxymesterone may increase sensitivity to oral anticoagulants. Should be administered in divided doses because of its short action.

Androgens

Nursing Diagnosis	Defining Characteristics	Expected Outcomes	Nursing Interventions
I. Altered nutrition: less than body requirements related to nausea and vomiting	I. A. Uncommon, but may occur	I. A. Pt will be without nausea and vomiting	I. A. 1. Inform pt that nausea and vomiting can occur; encourage pt to report nausea or vomiting 2. Encourage small, frequent feedings of cool, bland foods and liquids 3. Refer to sec. on nausea and vomiting, chap. 4.
II. Potential for injury related to			
A. Sodium and water retention	II. A. Occur occasionally, and may imply need for dose reduction or diuretic therapy	II. A. Fluid and electrolyte balance will be maintained	II. A. 1. Identify pts at risk for complications associated with fluid/sodium retention: cardiac history, renal or hepatic disease, low serum protein 2. Inform pt of potential for sodium/water retention, of s/s to watch for, and to report to MD 3. Assess pt daily (if inpatient) for s/s of fluid/electrolyte imbalance
B. Hypercalcemia	B. 1. Uncommon in everyone except those patients with bony metastases 2. Risk is highest during induction therapy	B. 1. Serum calcium will remain within normal limits 2. Hypercalcemia will be identified and treated early	B. 1. Identify pts at risk and monitor serum calcium closely during the first few weeks of therapy: hypercalcemia is an indication to discontinue treatment 2. Teach pts s/s of hypercalcemia (drowsiness, increased thirst, constipation, increased urine output). Instruct pt to notify MD if s/s occur
C. Obstructive jaundice	C. Has occurred with methyltesterone, fluoxymesterone, and oxymethalone	C. LFTs will remain within normal limits	C. 1. Teach pt to report GI distress, diarrhea, onset of jaundice 2. Monitor LFTs

III. Sexual dysfunction related to masculinization	III.	III.	III.
	A. Occurs commonly in women; increased risk when therapy duration exceeds 3 months. Prolonged use may cause irreversible masculinization	A. Pt will report onset of changes in sexual characteristics	A. Instruct pt to report onset of symptoms, indicating changes in sexual characteristics, functioning; those symptoms may necessitate terminating therapy
	B. Symptoms include increased libido, deepening of voice, excessive body hair growth, especially noticeable on face, acne, clitoral hypertrophy	B. Pt and significant others will verbalize understanding of changes in sexuality that may occur	B. As appropriate, explore with pt and significant other issues of reproductive and sexuality patterns, and impact that therapy may have on them
	C. In men drug may cause priapism (sustained and often painful erections) and reduced ejaculatory volume	C. Pt and significant other will identify strategies to cope with sexual dysfunction	C. Discuss strategies to preserve sexual and reproductive health
			D. See sec. on gonadal dysfunction, chap. 4

DRUG

5-Azacytidine (Azacytidine, 5AZ)

Class: Investigational

MECHANISM OF ACTION

Acts by interfering with nucleic acid metabolism by acting as a false metabolite when incorporated into DNA and RNA; cell cycle phase-specific for S phase.

METABOLISM

90% of the total administered dose is excreted in the urine during the first 24 hours. Drug half-life depends on the route of administration: SQ—3.5 hours and IV—4.2 hours.

DOSAGE/RANGE

100–400 mg/m^2 daily, weekly, biweekly or continuous infusion schedule. Consult individual clinical trials protocol for specific dose.

DRUG PREPARATION

This drug is supplied by the National Cancer Institute. The powder is reconstituted with sterile water for injection. DO NOT RECONSTITUTE with 5% Dextrose.

DRUG ADMINISTRATION

SQ administration may be painful and may result in a brownish discoloration at the injection site.

IV bolus or continuous infusion.

This drug is rapidly metabolized and once reconstituted it decomposes quickly. The infusion bottles need to be changed every 3–4 hours due to drug decomposition. Stable in Lactated Ringers solution for 4 hours.

SPECIAL CONSIDERATIONS

Patients develop side effects as a result of nephrotoxicity, hepatotoxicity, and CNS involvement

Thromboembolic phenomena may occur

5-Azacytidine

Nursing Diagnosis	Defining Characteristics	Expected Outcomes	Nursing Interventions
I. *Altered nutrition; less than body requirements related to*			
A. Nausea and vomiting	I. A. 1. Dose-related with a frequency of about 75% 2. Usually occurs 1–3 hours after administration 3. Symptoms are worse the first 2 days of infusion and lessen as infusion progresses	I. A. 1. Pt will be without nausea and vomiting 2. Nausea and vomiting, should they occur, will be minimal	I. A. 1. Premedicate with antiemetics and continue propyllactically × 24 h to prevent nausea and vomiting 2. Encourage small, frequent feedings of cool, bland foods and liquids 3. If vomiting occurs, assess for s/s of fluid/electrolyte imbalance: monitor I/O, daily weights, lab results 4. Refer to sec. on nausea and vomiting, chap. 4
B. Diarrhea	B. Develops in about 50% of pts	B. Pt will have minimal diarrhea	B. 1. Encourage pt to report onset of diarrhea 2. Administer or teach administration of anti-diarrheal medications 3. Check all stools for blood 4. If diarrhea is protracted, ensure adequate hydration, monitor I/O and electrolytes and teach perineal hygiene regimen 5. See sec. on diarrhea, chap. 4
C. Stomatitis	C. Rare	C. Oral mucous membranes will remain intact and without infection	C. 1. Teach pt oral assessment and mouth care regimen 2. Encourage pt to report early stomatitis 3. Provide pain relief measures, if indicated 4. See sec. on stomatitis, chap. 4
D. Hepatotoxicity	D. 1. Develops in a small percentage of pts 2. Marked by abnormal LFTs	D. Hepatic dysfunction will be identified early	D. 1. Monitor SGOT, SGPT, LDH alkaline phosphatase and bilirubin periodically during treatment 2. Notify MD about any changes

(continued)

5-Azacytidine (continued)

Nursing Diagnosis	Defining Characteristics	Expected Outcomes	Nursing Interventions
II. Infection and bleeding related to bone marrow depression	II. A. Leukopenia, thrombocytopenia, anemia all occur B. Leukopenia nadir days 14–17; lasts 2 weeks, recovery in 14 days	II. A. Pt will be without s/s of infection or bleeding B. S/s of infection or bleeding will be identified early	II. A. Monitor CBC, platelet count prior to drug administration, as well as s/s of infection or bleeding B. Instruct pt in self-assessment of s/s infection or bleeding C. Refer to sec. on bone marrow depression, chap. 4
III. Sensory/perceptual alterations	III. A. Neurologic syndrome has been observed, characterized by lethargy, myalgia, and coma B. Most likely to occur on the 2nd or 3rd day of therapy	III. A. Neurotoxicity will be identified early B. Pt safety will be assured	III. A. Teach patient s/s of neurotoxicity: encourage pt to report s/s early B. Assess for neurotoxicity; notify MD if it occurs C. Institute safety precautions when warranted—explain precautions to pt
IV. Impairment of skin integrity	IV. A. Pruritic, follicular skin rash occurs in about 2% of pts B. Usually transient, does not require dose reduction	IV. Skin integrity will be maintained	IV. A. Assess and teach pt to assess skin for rash, other dermatologic changes B. Administer antihistamines/ antipruritic medication as ordered
V. Alteration in comfort	V. A. Fever can occur within 1–2 hrs after infusion (rare), up to 24 hrs later B. Hypotension (rare) C. Fever and hypotension have been associated with rapid IV infusion	V. A. Fever will be recognized early and treated B. Pt will maintain adequate blood pressure	V. A. Monitor temp frequently after drug given B. Report fever to MD C. Administer antipyretic medications and measures as ordered D. Monitor BP during and after infusion; report changes to MD

DRUG

Aziridinylbenzaquinone (AZQ)

Class: Investigational

MECHANISM OF ACTION

Structure suggests alkylating activity and is also a class of drug that crosslinks DNA. Lipid-soluble synthesized drug designed to penetrate CNS.

METABOLISM

Excreted by the kidney. Extra precautions should be taken with patients with impaired renal function.

DOSAGE/RANGE

20–28 mg/m^2/day

DRUG PREPARATION

AZQ should be mixed in 0.9% Sodium Chloride or Lactated Ringers. AZQ is less stable in a 5% Dextrose solution.

DRUG ADMINISTRATION

Intravenous infusion. Administer immediately after reconstitution as there is 25% loss of potency after 3 hours.

SPECIAL CONSIDERATIONS

Dosages may vary with individual protocols, so protocol should be checked for specific dosage ranges.

Can cause anaphylactic reactions.

Aziridinylbenzaquinone (AZQ)

Nursing Diagnosis	Defining Characteristics	Expected Outcomes	Nursing Interventions
I. *Infection bleeding, and anemia related to bone marrow depression*	I. A. 33% of pts experience leukopenia/thrombocytopenia B. Dose-limiting toxicity C. Leukopenia nadir 2–3 weeks after treatment, lasting 1–3 weeks D. Thrombocytopenia is rarer with a nadir comparable to leukopenia E. Anemia occasionally occurs	I. A. Pt will be without s/s of infection, anemia, or bleeding B. Early s/s of infection, anemia, or bleeding will be identified	I. A. Monitor CBC, platelet count prior to drug administration as well as s/s of infection, bleeding, anemia B. Instruct pt in self-assessment of s/s of infection, bleeding, anemia C. Dose reduction often necessary with compromised bone marrow function
II. *Altered nutrition, less than body requirements related to* A. Nausea and vomiting	II. A. 1. Occurs in 75% of pts and may be severe 2. Nausea and vomiting start within 1–3 hours after injection; abates in 3–4 hrs. Usually by 10 days after injection nausea and vomiting have completely subsided	II. A. 1. Pt will be without nausea/vomiting 2. Nausea/vomiting, if it occurs, will be minimal 3. Pt will maintain baseline weight $\pm 5\%$	II. A. 1. Premedicate with antiemetics 24–48 hours before treatment and continue prophylactically to prevent nausea/vomiting, especially for first treatment 2. Encourage small, frequent feedings of cool, bland foods 3. Refer to sec. on nausea and vomiting, chap. 4
B. Stomatitis	B. Noted occasionally	B. Oral mucous membranes will remain intact without infection	B. 1. Teach pt oral assessment 2. Encourage pt to report early stomatitis 3. Teach pt oral hygiene 4. See sec. on stomatitis, chap. 4

II. C. Diarrhea

II. C. 1. Occurs in 50% of pts and may be severe
2. Starts 2–3 days after treatment and subsides spontaneously

II. C. Patient will have minimal diarrhea

II. C. 1. Encourage pt to report onset of diarrhea
2. Administer or teach pt to self-administer antidiarrheal medications
3. See sec. on diarrhea, chap. 4

D. Hepatic dysfunction

D. 1. Rare but may be serious
2. S/s may include changes in liver function tests to hepatic coma
3. AZQ contra-indicated in pts with hepatic metastasis or with elevated albumin levels

D. Hepatic dysfunction will be identified early

D. 1. Monitor SGOT, SGPT, LDH, alkaline phosphatase, and bilirubin periodically during treatment
2. Notify MD of any elevations

III. *Potential for injury, hypersensitivity reactions*

III. A. Rare
B. Transient fevers lasting 24 h after treatment
C. Hypotension

III. Early s/s of hypersensitivity will be identified

III. A. Teach pt about the potential of a hypersensitivity reaction and to report any unusual symptoms
B. Obtain baseline vital signs and note pts mental status
C. Assess pt for s/s of a reaction. See sec. on reactions, chap. 6
D. Administer therapy for reactions according to MD orders

IV. *Impaired skin integrity, related to dermatitis*

IV. A. Rare
B. Transient pruritic rash

IV. Pt will identify any changes in the skin

IV. A. Assess pt for changes in skin
B. Discuss with pt impact of changes and strategies to minimize distress
C. Topical medications as ordered

(continued)

Aziridinylbenzaquinone (AZQ) (continued)

Nursing Diagnosis	Defining Characteristics	Expected Outcomes	Nursing Interventions
V. *Potential for injury related to neuromuscular complications*	V. A. Rare B. Onset of symptoms likely within 2–3 days of treatment C. Symptoms range from lethargy, muscle pain, tenderness, weakness, to confusion or somnolence	V. Pt will identify s/s of neuromuscular changes early	V. A. Teach pt about the potential for injury due to neuromuscular changes and to report any unusual symptoms B. Teach pt self-assessment techniques C. Obtain baseline physical, muscular, and mental status D. Assess pt for s/s of any complications E. Administer therapy as ordered

DRUG

Bleomycin sulfate (Blenoxane)

> **Class:** antitumor antibiotic—isolated from fungus *Streptomyces verticullus*. Possesses both antitumor and antimicrobial actions.

MECHANISM OF ACTION

Primary action of bleomycin is to induce single-strand and double-strand breaks in DNA. DNA synthesis is inhibited. The action of drug is not exerted against RNA.

METABOLISM

Excreted via the renal system. About 70% is excreted unchanged in urine. 30–60 minutes after IV infusion, urine levels are 10 times the serum level.

DOSAGE/RANGE

5–20 U/m^2 once a week

10–20 U/m^2 twice a week

(frequency and schedule may vary according to protocol and age)

DRUG PREPARATION

Dilute powder in Normal Saline or sterile water.

DRUG ADMINISTRATION

IV, IM, or SC doses may be administered. Some clinical trials protocol may utilize 24-hour infusions. There is a risk for anaphylaxis and hypotension with some diseases and with higher doses of drug. It may be recommended that a test dose be given before the first dose to detect hypersensitivity.

SPECIAL CONSIDERATIONS

Because of pulmonary toxicities with increasing dose, PFTs and CXR should be obtained before each course or as outlined by protocol.

Incidence of anaphylaxis increases over the age of 70.

May cause chemical fevers up to 103°–105°F (60%). May need to administer premedications such as acetaminophen, antihistamines, or in some cases steroids.

Watch for signs/symptoms of hypotension and anaphylaxis. Test dose needed.

May cause irritation at site of injection (is considered an irritant, not a vesicant).

Maximum cumulative lifetime dose: 400 U

Decreases the oral bioavailability of digoxin when given together.

Decreases the pharmacologic effects of phenytoin when given in combination.

Bleomycin sulfate

Nursing Diagnosis	Defining Characteristics	Expected Outcomes	Nursing Interventions
I. Potential alteration in comfort			
A. Fever and chills	I. A. 1. Fever and chills occur in 60% of pts 4–10 hours after drug dose, persisting up to 24 hours 2. Severity of reaction decreases with successive doses	I. A. Pt will remain comfortable during therapy	I. A. 1. Assess pt for these symptoms during the hour following treatment 2. Discuss with MD premedication with acetaminophen, antihistamines, or steroids 3. Evaluate the effectiveness of the symptomatic relief that is prescribed 4. Monitor the quantity of cumulative dose
B. Pain at tumor site	B. Pain at tumor site due to chemotherapy-induced cellular damage	B. Pt will be supported during therapy	B. 1. Offer emotional support to patient 2. Reinforce information on the action and side effects of bleomycin 3. Discuss with MD medicating with acetaminophen
II. Potential for impaired skin integrity			
A. Alopecia	II. A. Usually occurs late, 3–4 weeks after dose	II. A. Pt will verbalize feelings re hair loss and identify strategies to cope with changes in body image	II. A. 1. Discuss with pt impact of hair loss 2. Suggest wig as appropriate prior to actual hair loss 3. Explore with pt response to actual hair loss and plan strategies to minimize distress, i.e., wig, scarf, cap 4. Refer to sec. on alopecia, chap. 4
B. Skin changes	B. Skin changes occur in 50% of pts (e.g., striae, pruritis, skin peeling—fingertips, hyperpigmentation, and hyperkeratosis)	B. 1. Skin discomfort will be minimized and skin will remain intact 2. Pt will verbalize feelings re: skin changes	B. 1. Skin changes are not an indication to stop the drug 2. Discuss with MD symptomatic management 3. Reinforce pt teaching on the action and side effects of bleomycin 4. Offer emotional support

II. C. Skin eruptions	II. C. Macular rash (hands and elbows) urticaria and vesiculations are the type of eruptions most likely to be seen	II. C. 1. Skin discomfort will be minimized and skin will remain intact 2. Pt will verbalize feelings re: skin changes	II. C. 1. Skin erruptions are not an indication to stop the drug 2. Discuss with MD symptomatic management 3. Reinforce pt teaching on the action and side effects of bleomycin 4. Offer emotional support
D. Nail changes	D. Nail changes and possible nail loss can occur	D. Pt will verbalize feelings about nail changes and identify strategies to cope with loss	D. 1. Nail changes are not an indication to stop the drug 2. Discuss with MD symptomatic management 3. Reinforce pt teaching on the action and side effects of bleomycin 4. Offer emotional support
III. Potential alteration in nutrition			
A. Nausea and vomiting	III. A. Nausea and vomiting are rare	III. A. Pt will be without nausea and vomiting; if it occurs, it will be minimal	III. A. 1. Premedicate with antiemetic if needed, and continue prophyllactically to prevent nausea and vomiting 2. Encourage small, frequent feedings of favorite foods, especially high-calorie, high-protein foods 3. Refer to sec. on nausea and vomiting, chap. 4
B. Anorexia and weight loss	B. Anorexia and weight loss may occur and may be prolonged	B. Pt will maintain baseline weight ± 5%	B. 1. Encourage small frequent feedings of favorite foods, especially high-calorie, high-protein foods 2. Encourage use of spices 3. Weekly weights
C. Stomatitis	C. Stomatitis may decrease ability and desire to eat	C. Oral mucous membranes will remain intact and without infection	C. 1. Teach pt oral assessment 2. Encourage pt to report early stomatitis 3. Teach pt oral hygiene 4. See sec. on stomatitis, chap. 4

(continued)

Bleomycin sulfate (*continued*)

Nursing Diagnosis	Defining Characteristics	Expected Outcomes	Nursing Interventions
IV. *Potential for impaired gas exchange related to pulmonary toxicity*	IV. A. Incidence 8%–10% Pneumonitis (rales, dyspnea, infiltrate) may progress to irreversible pulmonary fibrosis. PFTs decrease before X ray changes B. High risk: 1. Age > 70 years old 2. Dose > 150 U (maximum lifetime dose is 400) 3. XRT to chest (prior to chemotherapy or concomitantly)	IV. A. Early s/s or pulmonary toxicity will be identified	IV. A. Discuss with MD the need for pulmonary function tests and CXR prior to beginning therapy B. Assess lung sounds prior to drug administration C. Instruct pt to report cough, dyspnea, shortness of breath D. See sec. on pulmonary toxicity, chap. 4
V. Potential for sexual dysfunction	V. A. Drug is mutagenic and probably teratogenic	V. A. Pt and significant other will understand needs for contraception B. Pt and significant other will identify strategies to cope with sexual dysfunction	V. A. 1. As appropriate, explore with pt and significant other issues of reproductive and sexuality pattern and impact chemotherapy may have on them. 2. Discuss strategies to preserve sexual and reproductive health (i.e., sperm banking, contraception) 3. See sec. on gonadal dysfunction, chap. 4

VI. Potential for injury related to anaphylaxis	VI. A. 1% of lymphoma pts experience anaphylaxis	VI. A. Early s/s of hypersensitivity will be identified	VI. A. Review standing orders for management of pt in anaphylaxis and identify location of anaphylaxis kit containing epinephrine 1:1000, hydrocortisone sodium succinate (Solucortef), diphenhydramine HCL (Benadryl), Aminophylline, and others
	B. S/s include tachycardia, wheezing, hypotension, facial edema		B. Prior to drug administration, obtain baseline vital signs and record mental status
			C. Observe for following s/s during infusion, usually occurring within first 15 minutes of start of infusion:
			1. *Subjective* generalized itching nausea chest tightness crampy abdominal pain difficulty speaking anxiety agitation sense of impending doom uneasiness desire to urinate or defecate dizziness chills
			2. *Objective* flushed appearance (angioedema of face, neck, eyelids, hands, feet) localized or generalized urticaria respiratory distress ± wheezing hypotension cyanosis

(continued)

Bleomycin sulfate (*continued*)

Nursing Diagnosis	Defining Characteristics	Expected Outcomes	Nursing Interventions
			VI. D. If reaction occurs, stop infusion and notify MD
			E. Place pt in supine position to promote perfusion of visceral organs
			F. Monitor vital signs until stable
			G. Provide emotional reassurance to pt and family
			H. Maintain patent airway, and have CPR equipment ready if needed
			I. Document incident
			J. Discuss with MD desensitization versus drug discontinuance for further dosing
			K. See sec. on reactions, chap. 6

DRUG

Busulfan (Myleran)

Class: Alkylating agent

MECHANISM OF ACTION

Forms carbonium ions through the release of a methane sulfonate group. This results in the alkylating of DNA. Acts primarily on granulocyte precursors in the bone marrow and is cell cycle phase nonspecific.

METABOLISM

Well absorbed orally; almost all metabolites are excreted in the urine. Has a very short half-life.

DOSAGE/RANGE

2–10 mg/day PO for 2–3 weeks initially then maintenance dose of 2–6 mg/m^2 PO qd or 0.05 mg/kg PO qd. Dose titrated to WBC counts.

DRUG PREPARATION

None

DRUG ADMINISTRATION

Available in 2-mg scored tablets given PO.

SPECIAL CONSIDERATIONS

If WBC is high, pt is at risk for hyperuricemia. Allopurinol and hydration may be indicated.

Follow weekly CBC and platelet count initially, then monthly. Dose is decreased to maintenance when leukocyte count falls below 50,000 mm^3.

Hyperpigmentation of skin creases may occur due to increased melanin production.

If given according to accepted guidelines, patient should have minimal side effects.

Busulfan

Nursing Diagnosis	Defining Characteristics	Expected Outcomes	Nursing Interventions
I. *Potential for infection*			
A. Myelosuppression	I. A. Nadir 11–30 days with recovery occurring over 24–54 days	I. A. Pt will have normal recovery of bone marrow function	I. A. Monitor WBC weekly initially, then at least monthly
B. Delayed, refractory pancytopenia	B. Delayed, refractory pancytopenia has occurred	B. Pt will be without infection, bleeding	B. Monitor WBC closely; Drug dose adjustment or discontinuance is based on the WBC
II. *Potential for impaired gas exchange related to interstitial pulmonary fibrosis (rare)*	II. A. Rare complication. May occur within a year of beginning therapy but usually occurs after long-term theapy	II. A. Pt will be without pulmonary dysfunction	II. A. Carefully assess pulmonary function of pts receiving long-term therapy
	B. Symptoms may be delayed and usually occur after 4 years: anorexia, cough, dyspnea, fever	B. Pulmonary dysfunction will be identified early	
	C. Usually fatal due to rapid diffuse fibrosis; high-dose corticosteroids may be helpful		
III. *Potential for sexual dysfunction*	III. A. Testicular atrophy, impotence, and amenorrhea may occur	III. A. Pt will understand potential dysfunction and that sterility may occur	III. A. Prechemo assessment of sexual patterns and function; institute pt and significant other teaching
	B. Successful pregnancies have been described after and during treatment with busulfan	B. Pt and significant other will discuss potential impact of sterility on their lives	B. Facilitate discussion between patient and partner re: reproductive issues. Provide information, support counseling, and referral as needed
	C. Men may experience gynecomastia	C. Pt will understand importance of birth control if appropriate	C. As appropriate discuss birth control measures
	D. Drug is potentially teratogenic		

DRUG

Carboplatin (Paraplatin)

Class: Alkylating agent (heavy metal complex)

MECHANISM OF ACTION

A second-generation platinum analog. The cytotoxicity is identical to that of the parent, *Cis*-platinum. Cell cycle phase nonspecific.

Reacts with nucleophilic sites on DNA, causing predominantly intrastrand and interstrand cross-links rather than DNA–protein cross-links. These cross-links are similar to those formed with *Cis*-platinum but are formed later.

METABOLISM

At 24 hours post administration, approximately 70% of carboplatin is excreted in the urine. The mean half-life is roughly 100 minutes.

DOSAGE/RANGE

Drug is undergoing clinical trials, consult individual protocol for specific dosages. As single agent, dose may be 400–500 mg/m^2 q 4 weeks, less for patients with bone marrow reserve or in combination chemotherapy.

FDA approved for ovarian cancer.

DRUG PREPARATION

Available as a white powder in amber vial

Reconstitute with sterile water for injection, D$_5$W, or NSS

Dilute further in D$_5$W or Normal Saline

The solution is chemically stable for 24 hours; discard solution after 8 hours because of the lack of bacteriostatic preservative

DRUG ADMINISTRATION

Administered by IV bolus over 30 minutes to 1 hour

May also be given as a continuous infusion over 24 hours

SPECIAL CONSIDERATIONS

Does not have the renal toxicity seen with *Cis*-platinum

Mix in 5% Dextrose or Normal Saline

Monitor urine creatinine clearance

Carboplatin (Paraplatin)

Nursing Diagnosis	Defining Characteristics	Expected Outcomes	Nursing Interventions
I. *Potential for infection and bleeding related to bone marrow depression*	I. A. Myelosuppression is major dose-limiting toxicity B. Thrombocytopenia nadir 14–21 days with recovery by day 28 C. Leukopenia nadir usually follows thrombocytopenia by 1 week but may take 5–6 weeks to recover D. Mild anemia frequently observed	I. A. 1. Pt will be without s/s of infection or bleeding B. S/s of infection or bleeding will be identified early	I. A. Monitor CBC, platelet count prior to drug administration, as well as s/s of infection or bleeding B. Instruct pt in self-assessment of s/s of infection or bleeding C. Dose reduction often necessary (35%–50%) if compromised bone marrow function D. Refer to sec. on bone marrow depression, chap. 4
II. *Altered nutrition; less than body requirements related to* A. Nausea and vomiting	II. A. 1. Nausea and vomiting begin 6+ hours after dose and usually lasts for <24 hours 2. 80% of pts experience some nausea or vomiting but often mild to moderate in severity	II. A. 1. Pt will be without nausea and vomiting 2. Nausea and vomiting, should they occur, will be minimal	II. A. 1. Premedicate with antiemetics and continue prophylactically × 24 hrs to prevent nausea and vomiting 2. Encourage small, frequent feedings of cool, bland foods and liquids 3. If vomiting occurs, assess for s/s of fluid/electrolyte imbalance; monitor I/O, daily weights, lab results 4. Refer to sec. on nausea and vomiting, chap. 4
B. Anorexia	B. Somewhat common but usually lasts for less than 1 day	B. Patient will maintain baseline weight ± 5%	B. 1. Encourage small, frequent feedings of favorite foods, especially high-calorie, high-protein foods 2. Encourage use of spices 3. Weekly weights 4. Nutritional consulting as needed

Nursing Diagnosis	Defining Characteristics	Expected Outcomes	Nursing Interventions
II. C. Stomatitis	II. C. Occurs in ~10% of pts but usually mild	II. C. 1. Oral mucous membranes will remain intact without infection	II. C. 1. Teach pt oral assessment and oral hygiene regimen 2. Encourage pt to report early stomatitis 3. See sec. on stomatitis, chap. 4
D. Diarrhea	D. Occurs in ~10% of pts but usually mild	D. 1. Pt will have minimal diarrhea	D. 1. Encourage pt to report onset of diarrhea 2. Administer or teach pt to self administer antidiarrheal medications 3. See sec. on diarrhea, chap. 4
E. Hepatic dysfunction	E. Mild to moderate reversible disturbances in liver function studies, especially alkaline phosphatase and SGOT, rarely SGPT and bilirubin	E. Hepatitic dysfunction will be identified early	E. 1. Monitor LFTs, i.e., alkaline phosphatase, SGOT, SGPT, and bilirubin, periodically during treatment 2. Monitor pt for any elevations in LFTs 3. Dose modifications may be necessary if elevation occurs
III. *Altered urinary elimination related to nephrotoxicity*	III. A. Does not have the renal toxicity seen with *Cis*-platinum B. Minimal diuresis and hydration needed. If occurs, usually mild	III. A. Pt will be without renal dysfunction B. Early s/s of renal dysfunction will be identified	III. A. Monitor BUN and creatinine prior to initiating drug dose, as drug excreted by the kidneys B. Check parameters of BUN and creatinine established in protocol as myelotoxicity is directly related to the renal function status C. Dose modifications may be made for renal impairment based on urine creatinine clearance

(continued)

Carboplatin (Paraplatin) (*continued*)

Nursing Diagnosis	Defining Characteristics	Expected Outcomes	Nursing Interventions
IV. *Potential for sensory/ perceptual alterations due to high-dose carboplatin*	IV. A. Neurotoxicity and ototoxicity rare; similar to those seen with *Cis*-platinum (but not as severe) B. Neurotoxicity: peripheral neuropathies, reversible confusion and dementia C. Ototoxicity: transient	IV. A. Neuropathies and ototoxicities will be identified early	IV. A. If pt is to receive high-dose carboplatin, obtain baseline neurological and auditory test B. Assess pt for changes during treatment course C. Teach pt the potential for neurologic toxicity problems and to report any changes
V. *Potential for sexual dysfunction*	V. A. Drug is mutagenic and probably teratogenic	V. A. Patient and significant other will understand needs for contraception B. Pt and significant other will identify strategies to cope with sexual dysfunction	V. A. As appropriate, explore with pt and significant other issues of reproductive and sexuality pattern and impact chemotherapy will have B. Discuss strategies to preserve sexual and reproductive health (i.e., sperm banking, contraception) C. See sec. on gonadal dysfunction, chap. 4
VI. *Potential for injury related to hypersensitivity reactions*	VI. A. Anaphylaxis or anaphylactic-like reactions have been reported (reactions similar to parent drug *Cis*-platin) 1. Tachycardia 2. Wheezing 3. Hypotension 4. Facial edema B. Occurs within a few minutes of initiating the drug and usually responds to steroid, epinephrine, or antihistamines	VI. A. Early s/s of hypersensitivity will be identified	VI. A. Teach pt about the potential of a hypersensitivity reaction and ask pt to report any unusual s/s B. Assess baseline vs. mental status C. Adverse reaction kit with epinephrine in room D. IF REACTION OCCURS, administer treatment per MD orders E. Document anaphylactic incident F. Discuss with MD precautionary measures to be taken before next drug dose is given OR drug discontinuance

DRUG

Carmustine (BiCNU, BCNU)

Class: Nitrosoureas

MECHANISM OF ACTION

A nitrosourea that alkylates DNA by causing cross-links and strand breaks. Also carbamoylates cellular proteins of nucleic acid synthesis. Alkylates DNA in the same manner as classic mustard agents. Is cell cycle phase nonspecific.

METABOLISM

Rapidly distributed and metabolized with a plasma half-life of one hour. 70% of IV dose is excreted in urine within 96 hours. Significant concentrations of drug remain in CSF for 9 hours due to lipid solubility of drug.

DOSAGE/RANGE

75–100 mg/m^2 IV/day × 2 days
or
200–225 mg/m^2 every 6 weeks
or
40 mg/m^2 day on 5 successive days

DRUG PREPARATION

Add sterile alcohol (provided with drug) to vial, then add sterile water for injection

May be further diluted with 100–250 ml D$_5$W or NS

DRUG ADMINISTRATION

Discard solution 2 hours after mixing

Administer via volutrol over 45–120 minutes as tolerated by patient

SPECIAL CONSIDERATIONS

Wear gloves during mixing to prevent skin discoloration.

Drug is an irritant—avoid extravasation.

Pain at the injection site or along the vein is common—treat by applying ice pack above the injection site and decreasing the infusion flow rate.

Patient may act inebriated related to the alcohol diluent and may experience flushing.

Increased myelosuppression when given with cimetidine.

Can decrease the pharmacologic effects of phenytoin.

Carmustine

Nursing Diagnosis	Defining Characteristics	Expected Outcomes	Nursing Interventions
I. Potential for infection related to myelosuppression	I. A. Nadir: 3–5 weeks after dose, and persists 1–3 weeks longer B. Myelosuppression is cumulative and may be delayed	I. A. Pt will be without infection B. Early s/s of infection will be identified	I. A. Monitor CBC, including WBC differential, prior to drug administration B. Drug dosage may be reduced or held for lower than normal blood values C. See sec. on bone marrow depression, chap. 4
II. Alteration in comfort related to drug administration			
A. Pain along vein	II. A. 1. Drug diluent is absolute alcohol 2. Drug is an irritant and can cause pain along a vein 3. True thrombophlebitis is rare 4. Venospasms commonly occur during rapid infusion	II. A. Pt will be without pain or will have minimal discomfort during infusion	II. A. 1. Administer drug in 100–250 ml D₅W or NS over 45–120 min 2. Use ice pack above injection site, decrease infusion rate, further dilute drug if pain occurs
B. Flushing of skin or burning of eyes	B. Occurs with rapid drug infusion	B. Pt will be without flushing or burning of eyes	B. Administer drug slowly; if symptoms occur, slow rate of infusion
III. Alterated nutrition; less than body requirements related to drug administration			
A. Nausea and vomiting	III. A. Severe nausea and vomiting may occur 2 hrs after administration and last 4–6 hrs	III. A. 1. Pt will be without nausea and vomiting 2. Nausea and vomiting, if it occurs, will be minimal	III. A. 1. Premedicate with antiemetics and continue prophylactically × 24 hrs to prevent nausea and vomiting, at least for first treatment 2. Encourage small frequent feedings of cool, bland foods and liquids

Nursing Diagnosis	Characteristics	Goals	Interventions
III. B. Liver dysfunction (rare) related to subacute hepatitis	III. B. Abnormal SGOT, alkaline phosphatase, serum bilirubin have occurred; also painless jaundice and hepatic coma, usually reversible	III. B. Laboratory abnormalities will be identified early	III. B. 1. Monitor LFTs (SGOT, SGPT, LDH, alkaline phosphatase, bilirubin) during treatment 2. Notify MD of elevations
IV. Altered urinary elimination related to nephrotoxicity	IV. A. Increased BUN occurs in ~ 10% of treated pts, usually reversible	IV. A. Pt will be without renal dysfunction B. Early s/s of renal dysfunction will be identified	IV. A. Monitor BUN and creatinine prior to initiating drug dose, as drug is excreted by the kidneys B. Check parameters of BUN and creatinine established in protocol, as myelotoxicity is directly related to the renal function C. Dose modifications may be made for renal impairment
V. Potential for impaired gas exchange related to pulmonary fibrosis	V. A. Presents as insidious cough and dyspnea, or sudden onset of respiratory failure B. CXR shows interstitial infiltrates C. Pulmonary function tests show hypoxia with diffusion and restrictive defects D. Risk may increase with concurrent cyclophosphamide E. Risk increases as dose exceeds 1 g/m^2 F. Incidence 20%–30% with mortality of 24%–80%	V. A. Early dysfunction will be identified	V. A. Assess pts at risk: 1. Cumulative dose 1 g/m^2 2. Preexisting lung disease 3. Concurrent cyclophosphamide and thoracic irradiation 4. Assess breath sounds and presence of dyspnea 5. Monitor pulmonary function studies periodically for evidence of pulmonary dysfunction

(continued)

Carmustine (*continued*)

Nursing Diagnosis	Defining Characteristics	Expected Outcomes	Nursing Interventions
VI. *Potential for sexual dysfunction*	VI. A. Drug is teratogenic	VI. A. Pt and significant other will understand needs for contraception	VI. A. 1. As appropriate, explore with pt and significant other issues of reproductive and sexuality pattern and impact chemotherapy may have 2. Discuss strategies to preserve sexual and reproductive health (i.e., sperm banking, contraception) 3. See sec. on gonadal dysfunction, chap. 4

DRUG

Chlorambucil (Leukeran)

Class: Alkylating agent

MECHANISM OF ACTION

Alkylates DNA by causing strand breaks and cross-links in the DNA. Is a derivative of a nitrogen mustard.

METABOLISM

Pharmacokinetics are poorly understood. Is well absorbed orally, with a plasma half-life of 1.5 hours. Degradation is slow; appears to be eliminated by metabolic transformation with 60% of drug excreted in urine in 24 hours.

DOSAGE/RANGE

0.1–0.2 mg/kg/day (equals 4–8 mg/m^2/day) to initiate treatment
or
14 mg/m^2/day × 5 days with a repeat every 21–28 days depending upon platelet count and WBC.

DRUG PREPARATION

(oral) 2 mg tabs

DRUG ADMINISTRATION

Simultaneous administration of barbiturates may increase toxicity of chlorambucil due to hepatic drug activation.

SPECIAL CONSIDERATIONS

None

Chlorambucil

Nursing Diagnosis	Defining Characteristics	Expected Outcomes	Nursing Interventions
I. *Potential for infection related to myelosuppression*	I. A. WBC decreases for 10 days after last dose B. Neutropenia, thrombocytopenia occur with prolonged use and may be irreversible occasionally C. Secondary malignancies have been reported (acute myelogenous leukemia) D. Increased toxicity may occur with prior barbiturate use	I. A. Pt will be without infection B. Early s/s of infection will be identified	I. A. Monitor CBC including WBC differential prior to drug administration B. Drug dosage may be reduced or held for lower than normal blood values C. See sec. on bone marrow depression, chap. 4
II. *Potential for sexual dysfunction*	II. A. Drug is mutagenic, teratogenic and suppresses gonadal function with consequent sterility (permanent or temporary) B. Amenorrhea C. Oligospermia	II. A. Pt and significant other will understand needs for contraception	II. A. As appropriate, explore with pt and significant other issues of reproductive and sexuality pattern and impact chemotherapy will have B. Discuss strategies to preserve sexual and reproductive health (i.e., sperm banking, contraception) C. See sec. on gonadal dysfunction, chap. 4

III. *Potential alteration in nutrition related to*

A. Nausea and vomiting	III. A. 1. Nausea and vomiting are rare	III. A. 1. Pt will be without nausea and vomiting 2. If it occurs, it will be minimal	III. A. 1. Premedicate with antiemetic if ordered, and continue prophylactically to prevent nausea and vomiting 2. Encourage small, frequent feedings of favorite foods, especially high-calorie, high-protein foods 3. Administer oral dose on an empty stomach 4. Refer to sec. on nausea and vomiting, chap. 4
B. Anorexia and weight loss	B. 1. Anorexia and weight loss may occur and be prolonged	B. 1. Pt will maintain baseline weight ±5%	B. 1. Encourage small frequent feedings of favorite foods, especially high-calorie, high-protein foods 2. Encourage use of spices 3. Weekly weights
C. Hepatic dysfunction	C. 1. Hepatitis is rare but may occur (also disturbances in liver function)	C. 1. Hepatitic dysfunction will be identified early	C. 1. Monitor LFTs, i.e., alkaline phosphatase and bilirubin, periodically during treatment 2. Monitor pt for any elevations 3. Dose modifications may be necessary if elevation occurs
IV. *Potential for impaired skin integriy*	IV. A. Dermatitis and urticaria may occur (rarely) B. Cross hypersensitivity may exist between Alkeran and cholorambucil (skin rash)	IV. A. Skin will remain intact B. Early skin impairment will be identified	IV. A. 1. Assess skin for integrity 2. If symptoms are severe, discuss drug discontinuance with MD

(*continued*)

Chlorambucil (continued)

Nursing Diagnosis	Defining Characteristics	Expected Outcomes	Nursing Interventions

V. Potential for impaired gas exchange related to pulmonary fibrosis	V. A. Alveolar dysplasia and pulmonary fibrosis may occur with long-term use
	B. Infrequent
		V. A. Early dysfunction will be identified	V. A. Assess pts at risk
			  1. Cumulative dose 1 g/m^2
			  2. Preexisting lung disease
			  3. Concurrent cyclophosphamide and thoracic irradiation
			B. Assess breath sounds and assess presence of dyspnea
			C. Monitor pulmonary function studies periodically for evidence of pulmonary dysfunction

VI. Potential for sensory/perceptual alterations (rare)	VI. A. Occular disturbances may occur:
	  1. Diplopia
	  2. Papilledema
	  3. Retinal hemorrhage
		VI. A. Visual disturbances will be identified early	VI. A. Assess vision before giving treatment
			B. Encourage pt to report any visual changes

DRUG

Cisplatin (*Cis*-Platinum, CDDP, Platinum, Platinol)

Class: heavy metal that acts like alkylating agent

MECHANISM OF ACTION

Inhibits DNA synthesis by forming inter- and intrastrand cross-links and by denaturing the double helix, preventing cell replication. Is cell cycle phase nonspecific. Has chemical properties similar to that of bifunctional alkylating agents.

METABOLISM

Rapidly distributed to tissues (predominantly the liver and kidneys) with less than 10% in the plasma 1 hour after infusion. Clearance from plasma proceeds slowly after the first 2 hours due to platinum's covalent bonding with serum proteins. 20%–74% of administered drug is excreted in the urine within 24 hours.

DOSAGE/RANGE

50–120 mg/m^2 every 3–4 weeks
or
15–20 mg/m^2 × 5—repeated every 3–4 weeks

DRUG PREPARATION

10-mg and 50-mg vials. Add sterile water to develop a concentration of 1 mg/ml.

Further dilute solution with 250 ml or more of NS or D$_5$W ½ NS. Never mix with D$_5$W as a precipitate will form.

Refrigerate lyophilized drug, but NOT reconstituted drug, as a precipitate will form.

DRUG ADMINISTRATION

Avoid aluminum needles when administering as precipitate will form.

SPECIAL CONSIDERATIONS

Hydrate vigorously before and after administering drug. Urine output should be at least 100–150 mL/hr. Mannitol or furosemide diuresis may be needed to assure this output.

Hypersensitivity reactions have occurred, manifested by wheezing, flushing, hypotension, tachycardia. Usually occurs within minutes of starting infusion. Treat with epinephrine, corticosteroids, antihistamines.

Decreases the pharmacologic effects of phenytoin.

Drug causes potassium and magnesium wasting. Some ideas to help increase magnesium follow.

To help increase absorption it is recommended that excessive milk, cheese, or other high-calcium products are limited when eating foods high in magnesium. Calcium and magnesium compete to gain entrance to the body in the intestines, so a high-calcium diet increases requirements for dietary magnesium.

Foods high in magnesium: 100 mg or greater per 100 grams.

Nuts:	*Other good sources:*
Almonds	Whole wheat breads and cereals
Cashews	Cornmeal
Peanuts	Shredded wheat
Peanut butter	Oatmeal
Pecans	Wheat germ
Brazil nuts	Brewer's yeast
Walnuts	Cocoa (dry breakfast)
	Chocolate (bitter)
	Instant coffee and tea
	Blackstrap molasses

Peas and Beans:
Split peas
Red beans
White beans

Cisplatin

Nursing Diagnosis	Defining Characteristics	Expected Outcomes	Nursing Interventions
I. *Potential alteration in urinary elimination*	I. A. Drug accumulates in kidney causing necrosis of proximal and distal renal tubules B. Is a dose-limiting toxicity and is cumulative with repeated doses C. Damage to distal renal tubules prevents reabsorption of Mg, Ca, K, with resultant decreased serum levels D. Peak detrimental effect usually occurs 10–20 days after treatment and is reversible E. Hyperuricemia may occur due to impaired tubular transport of uric acid but is reponsive to allopurinol F. Concurrent use of aminoglycosides is not recommended	I. A. Pt will maintain normal renal functions as evidenced by BUN <20, creatinine <1.5 B. Mg, K Ca levels will be normal	I. A. Prevent nephrotoxicity with vigorous hydration and diuresis to produce urinary output of at least 100 cc/hr B. A typical hydration schedule is NS or D$_5$W ½ NS at 250 cc/hr for 3 hrs prior to cisplatin and for 5 hrs after. Outpatient hydration would be over 1–2 hrs. Diuresis is induced by the use of lasix or mannitol given prior to cisplatin administration C. Monitor BUN and creatinine prior to initiating drug dose as drug is excreted by the kidneys D. Check parameters of BUN and creatinine established in protocol E. Dose modifications may be made for renal impairment

II. *Altered nutrition; less than body requirements related to*

A. Nausea and vomiting	II. A. Nausea and vomiting may be severe: begins 1 + hrs after dose, lasting 8–24 hrs and may recur 48–72 hrs after dose	II. A. 1. Pt will be without nausea and vomiting 2. Nausea and vomiting, if they occur, will be minimal	II. A. 1. Premedicate with antiemetics and continue prophylactically × 24 hrs prevent nausea and vomiting, at least for first treatment. Continue antiemetic for 3–5 days 2. Encourage small frequent feedings of cool, bland foods and liquids 3. Infuse cisplatin over at least 1 h to minimize nausea and vomiting 4. Refer to sec. on nausea and vomiting, chap 4
B. Taste alteration	B. Taste alterations can occur with long-term use	B. Pt will eat adequate calories, proteins, minerals	B. 1. Suggest increased use of spices as tolerated 2. Help pt or significant other develop menu based on past favorite foods 3. Dietary consultation as needed
III. *Potential for injury related to anaphylaxis*	III. A. Anaphylactic hypersensitivity reactions have occurred (infrequently) following IV drug administration to previously treated patients B. Tachycardia, wheezing, hypotension, facial edema C. Usually controlled by corticosteroids, epinephrine, antihistamines	III. A. If anaphylaxis occurs, pt will stabilize	III. A. Have anaphylaxis tray with corticosteroids, antihistamines, epinephrine ready in clinic or unit where chemotherapy is administered B. Discuss with physician the development of standing orders in case anaphylaxis occurs C. Monitor and observe patient closely during cisplatin infusions D. Refer to sec. on reactions, chap. 6

(continued)

Cisplatin *(continued)*

Nursing Diagnosis	Defining Characteristics	Expected Outcomes	Nursing Interventions
IV. *Infection and bleeding related to bone marrow depression*	IV. A. Bone marrow suppression mild with low to moderate doses B. High-dose nadir is 2–3 weeks with recovery in 4–5 weeks C. Concurrent low-dose cisplatin radiotherapy may result in bone marrow suppression	IV. A. Patients will be without s/s of infection or bleeding	IV. A. Monitor CBC, platelet count prior to drug administration as well as s/s infection and bleeding B. Refer to sec. on bone marrow depression, chap. 4
V. *Potential for activity intolerance, related to anemia-induced fatigue*	V. A. Cisplatin may interfere with renal erythroprotein causing subsequent late anemia	V. A. Pt will be able to do desired activities B. Early fatigue related to anemia will resolve	V. A. Monitor hemoglobin, hematrocit. Transfuse per MD for Hct <25, s/s of severe anemia. Teach pt diet high in iron
VI. *Potential for sensory/ perceptual alterations related to neurological toxicity*	VI. A. Neurotoxicity and ototoxicity may be severe 1. Neurotoxicity: glove and stocking distribution with numbness, tingling, and sensory loss in arms and legs 2. Ototoxicity: high-frequency hearing loss above frequency of normal speech, affecting >30% of patients	VI. A. Neuropathies and ototoxicities will be identified early	VI. A. Assess motor and sensory function prior to therapy

VII. *Potential for sexual dysfunction*	VI. B. May be preceded by tinnitus C. Appears dose related and can be unilateral or bilateral D. Results from the destruction of hair cells that lining organ of Corti E. Damage is cumulative and may be permanent VII. A. Drug is mutagenic and probably teratogenic	VI. B. If neuropathy occurs, pt will verbalize feelings of discomfort and loss of function, and identify alternate coping strategies VII. A. Pt and significant other will understand needs for contraception B. Pt and significant other will identify strategies to cope with sexual dysfunction	VI. B. Encourage pt to verbalize feelings regarding discomfort and sensory loss C. Help pt discuss alternative coping strategies D. See sec. on neurotoxicity, chap. 4 E. Baseline audiogram if high-dose platinum to be administered F. Repeat audiogram if pt complains of tinnitus, feeling underwater, or auditory discomfort G. If audiogram reveals hearing decline, discuss with pt and MD benefits/risks of further cisplatin therapy VII. A. As appropriate, explore with pt and significant other issues of reproductive and sexuality patterns, and impact chemotherapy may have B. Discuss strategies to preserve sexual and reproductive health (i.e., sperm banking, contraception) C. See sec. on gonadal dysfunction, chap 4

DRUG

Cyclophosphamide (Cytoxan, Endoxan, Endoxana, Neosar)

Class: Alkylating agent

MECHANISM OF ACTION

Causes cross-linkage in DNA strands thus preventing DNA synthesis and cell division. Cell cycle phase nonspecific.

METABOLISM

Inactive until converted by microsomes in liver and serum enzymes (phosphamidases). Both cyclophosphamide and its metabolites are excreted by the kidneys. Plasma half-life: 6–12 hours, with 25% drug excreted by 8 hours. Prolonged plasma half-life in patients with renal failure results in increased myelosuppression.

DOSAGE/RANGE

400 mg/m^2 IV × 5 days

100 mg/m^2 PO × 14 days

500–1500 mg/m^2 IV q 3–4 weeks

DRUG PREPARATION

Dilute vials with sterile water. Shake well. Allow solution to clear if lyophilised preparation is not used. Do not use solution unless crystals are fully dissolved. Available in 25- and 50-mg tablets.

DRUG ADMINISTRATION

PO use—administer in morning or early afternoon to allow adequate excretion time. Should be taken with meals.

IV use—for doses greater than 500 mg pre- and posthydration to total 500–3000 ml is needed to ensure adequate urine output and avoid hemmorhagic cystitis. Administer drug over at least 20 min for doses greater than 500 mg.

Solution is stable for 24 hours at room temperature, 6 days if refrigerated.

Rapid infusion may result in dizziness, nasal stuffiness, rhinorrhea, sinus congestion during or soon after infusion.

SPECIAL CONSIDERATIONS

Metabolic and leukopenic toxicity is increased by simultaneous administration of barbiturates, corticosteroids, phenytoin, and sulfonamides.

Activity and toxicity of both cyclophosphamide and the specific drug may be altered by allopurinol, chloroquine, phenothiazides, potassium iodide, chloramphenicol, imipramine, vitamin A, warfarin, succinylcholine, digoxin, thiazide diuretics.

Test urine for occult blood.

High-dose cyclophosphamide therapy may require catheterization and constant bladder irrigation.

Cyclophosphamide

Nursing Diagnosis	Defining Characteristics	Expected Outcomes	Nursing Interventions
I. *Alterated nutrition; less than body requirements related to*			
A. Nausea and vomiting	I. A. Nausea and vomiting begins 2–4 hrs after dose, peaks in 12 hrs, and may last 24 hrs	I. A. 1. Pt will be without nausea and vomiting 2. Nausea and vomiting, if they occur, will be minimal	I. A. 1. Premedicate with antiemetics and continue prophylactically × 24 hrs to prevent nausea and vomiting, at least for first treatment 2. Encourage small frequent feedings of cool, bland foods and liquids
B. Anorexia	B. Commonly occurs	B. Pt will maintain baseline weight ± 5%	B. 1. Encourage small, frequent feedings of favorite foods, especially high-calorie, high-protein foods 2. Encourage use of spices 3. Weekly weights 4. Nutritional consultation as needed
C. Stomatitis	C. Mild	C. Oral mucous membranes will remain intact without infection	C. 1. Teach pt oral assessment 2. Encourage pt to report early stomatitis 3. Teach pt oral hygiene regimen 4. See sec. on stomatitis, chap. 4
D. Diarrhea	D. Infrequent and mild	D. Pt will have minimal diarrhea	D. 1. Encourage pt to report onset of diarrhea 2. Administer, or teach pt to self administer, antidiarrheal medications 3. See sec. on diarrhea, chap. 4
E. Hepatotoxicity	E. Rare	E. Early hepatotoxicity will be identified	E. 1. Monitor LFTs, i.e., alkaline phosphatase and bilirubin, periodically during treatment 2. Monitor pt for any elevations 3. Dose modifications may be necessary if elevation occurs

(continued)

Cyclophosphamide (continued)

Nursing Diagnosis	Defining Characteristics	Expected Outcomes	Nursing Interventions
II. Infection and bleeding related to bone marrow depression	II. A. Leukopenia nadir 7–14 days with recovery in 1–2 weeks B. Less frequent thrombocytopenia C. Mild anemia D. Potent immunosuppressant	II. A. Pts will be without s/s of infection or bleeding B. Early s/s of infection or bleeding will be identified	II. A. Monitor CBC, platelet count prior to drug administration and monitor for s/s of infection and bleeding B. Instruct pt in self-assessment of s/s of infection and bleeding C. Dose reduction often necessary (35%–50%) if compromised bone marrow function D. See sec. on bone marrow depression, chap. 4
III. Potential for injury related to A. Acute water intoxication (SIADH) B. Second malignancy (bladder CA, acute leukemia)	III. A. May occur with high-dose administration (> 50 mg/kg) B. Prolonged therapy may cause bladder cancer (related to local toxicity of drug metabolites) and acute leukemia (related to prolonged bone marrow toxicity)	III. A. SIADH will be identified early B. Malignancy, if it occurs, will be identified early	III. A. 1. If high-dose cytoxan administered, monitor serum sodium, osmolality, and urine electrolytes and osmolality 2. Strictly monitor I/O and total body balance 3. Qd weights 4. Water restrictions as ordered B. Pts receiving prolonged therapy should be screened

Nursing Diagnosis	Analysis	Desired Outcome	Interventions
IV. *Altered urinary elimination, related to hemorrhagic cystitis*	IV. A. Metabolites of cyclophosphamide, if allowed to accumulate in bladder, irritate bladder wall capillaries causing hemorrhagic cystitis B. Sterile chemical cystitis occurs 5%–10% C. Evidenced by hematuria, gross or microscopic (>20 rbc) D. Is preventable E. Another potential side effect is bladder fibrosis	IV. A. Pt will be without hemorrhagic cystitis	IV. A. Monitor BUN and creatinine prior to drug dose as drug is excreted by kidneys B. Provide or instruct pt in hydration of at least 3 L of fluid/day C. Encourage voiding to empty bladder at least q 2–3 hours, and at bedtime D. Assess pt for signs and instruct pt to report signs of hematuria, urinary frequency, dysuria E. Instruct pt that oral cyclophosphamide should be taken early in day to prevent accumulation of drug in the bladder
V. *Alteration in cardiac output, related to high-dose cyclophosphamide*	V. A. Cardiomyopathy may occur with high doses; also, potentiates cardiotoxicity of doxorubicin (Adriamycin)	V. A. Early s/s of cardiomyopathy will be identified	V. A. If pt is receiving high-dose cyclophosphamide, assess for s/s of cardiomyopathy B. Discuss GBPS with MD C. Assess quality and regularity of heartbeat D. Instruct pt to report dyspnea, shortness of breath
VI. *Potential for impaired gas exchange, related to pulmonary toxicity*	VI. A. Rare, but may occur with prolonged, high-dose therapy or continuous low-dose Rx B. Appears as interstitial pneumonitis and onset insidious C. May respond to steroids	VI. A. Early s/s of pulmonary toxicity will be identified	VI. A. If pt is receiving high-dose or continuous low-dose cyclophosphamide, assess for s/s of pulmonary dysfunction B. Discuss pulmonary function studies to be performed periodically with MD C. Assess lung sounds prior to drug administration D. Instruct pt to report cough or dyspnea

(continued)

Cyclophosphamide *(continued)*

Nursing Diagnosis	Defining Characteristics	Expected Outcomes	Nursing Interventions
VII. *Altered body image related to*			
A. Alopecia	VII. A. 1. Occurs in 30%–50% of pts, especially with IV dosing 2. Some degree of hair loss expected in all pts 3. Begins after 3+ weeks and may grow back while on therapy 4. May be slight to diffuse thinning	VII. A. Pt will verbalize feelings re hair loss, and identify strategies to cope with change in body image	VII. A. 1. Assess pt for s/s of hair loss 2. Discuss with pt impact of hair loss, and strategies to minimize distress: i.e., wig, scarf, cap 3. Begin discussion before therapy has been initiated 4. See sec. on alopecia, chap. 4
B. Changes in nails, skin	B. Hyperpigmentation of nails and skin, transverse ridging of nails ("banding") may occur	B. Pt will verbalize feelings re changes in nail or skin color or texture, and identify strategies to cope with change in body image	B. 1. Assess pt for changes in skin, nails 2. Discuss with pt impact of changes, and strategies to minimize distress; i.e., wearing nail polish (women), long sleeved tops
VIII. *Sexual dysfunction*	VIII. A. Drug is mutagenic and teratoginic B. Testicular atrophy sometimes with reversible oligo- and azoospermia C. Amenorrhea often occurs in females D. Drug is excreted in breast milk	VIII. A. Pt and significant other will understand need for contraception B. Pt and significant other will identify strategies to cope with sexual dysfunction	VIII. A. As appropriate, explore with pt and significant other issues of reproductive and sexuality patterns, and the impact chemotherapy will have on these activities B. Discuss strategies to preserve sexual and reproductive health (i.e., sperm banking, contraception) C. See sec. on gonadal dysfunction, chap. 4

DRUG

Cytarabine, Cytosine arabinoside (Ara-C, Cytosar-U, Arabinosyl Cytosine)

Class: Antimetabolite

MECHANISM OF ACTION

Antimetabolite (pyrimidine analogue) that is incorporated into DNA, slowing its synthesis and causing defects in the linkages in new DNA fragments. Also, cells exposed to cytarabine in the S phase reinitiate DNA synthesis when the drug is removed, resulting in erroneous duplication of the early portions of the DNA strands. Most effective when cells are undergoing rapid DNA synthesis.

METABOLISM

Inactivated by liver enzymes in biphasic manner: half-lives 10–15 minutes and 2–3 hours. Crosses the blood-brain barrier with CSF concentration of 50% that of plasma. 70% of dose excreted in urine as Ara-U. 4%–10% excreted 12–24 hours after administration.

DOSAGE/RANGE

(varies depending upon disease)

Leukemia: 100 mg/m^2 day IV continuous infusion × 5–10 days
100 mg/m^2 every 12 hours × 1–3 weeks IV or SQ
Head and Neck: 1 mg/kg every 12 hours × 5–7 days IV or SQ
High Dose: 2–3 g/m^2 IV
Differentiation: 10 mg/m^2 SQ every 12 hours × 15–21 days
Intrathecal: 20–30 mg/m^2

DRUG PREPARATION

100-mg vials: Add water with benzyl alcohol then dilute with NS or D$_5$W.

500-mg vials: Add water with benzyl alcohol then dilute with NS or D$_5$W.

For intrathecal use and high dose: Use preservative-free diluent.

Reconstituted drug is stable 48 hours at room temperature and 7 days refrigerated.

DRUG ADMINISTRATION

Doses of 100–200 mg can be given SQ.

Doses less than 1 gm: Administer via volutrol over 10–20 minutes.

Doses over 1 gm: Administer over 2 hours.

SPECIAL CONSIDERATIONS

Thrombophlebitis, pain at the injection site, should be treated with warm compresses.

Dizziness has occurred with too rapid IV infusions.

Use with caution if hepatic dysfunction exists.

May be decreased bioavailability of digoxin when given in combination.

Cytarabine, Cytosine Arabinoside

Nursing Diagnosis	Defining Characteristics	Expected Outcomes	Nursing Interventions
I. *Altered nutrition: less than body requirements related to*			
A. Nausea and vomiting	I. A. 1. Occurs in 50% of patients 2. Dose related 3. Lasts for several hours	I. A. 1. Pt will be without nausea or vomiting 2. Nausea and vomiting, if they occur, will be minimal	I. A. 1. Premedicate with antiemetics and continue prophylactically × 24 hrs to prevent nausea and vomiting, at least for first teatment 2. Encourage small, frequent feedings of cool, bland foods and liquids 3. I/O, daily wts if administered inpatient (assess for s/s of fluid and electrolyte imbalance) 4. Refer to sec. on nausea and vomiting, chap. 4
B. Anorexia	B. Commonly occurs	B. Pt will maintain baseline wt ±5%	B. 1. Encourage small, frequent feedings of favorite foods, especially high-calorie, high-protein foods 2. Encourage use of spices 3. Weekly weights, daily if inpatient
C. Stomatitis	C. Occurs 7–10 days after therapy is initiated in about 15% of pts	C. Oral mucous membranes will remain intact and without signs of infection	C. 1. Assess oral cavity every day: teach pt to do own oral assessment and oral hygiene regimen 2. Encourage pt to report early stomatitis 3. Pain relief measures, if indicated 4. See sec. on stomatitis/mucositis, chap. 4
D. Diarrhea	D. Infrequent and mild	D. Pt will have minimal diarrhea	D. 1. Encourage pt to report onset of diarrhea 2. Administer or teach pt to administer antidiarrheal medication 3. See sec. on diarrhea, chap. 4

I. E. Hepatoxicity	I. E. Usually mild and reversible, but drug should be used cautiously in patients with hepatic dysfunction	I. E. Early hepatotoxicity will be identified	I. E. 1. Monitor LFTs prior to drug dose, especially with high drug doses 2. Assess pt prior to, and during, treatment, for s/s hepatotoxicity
II. *Infection and bleeding related to bone marrow depression*	II. A. Related to dose and duration of therapy B. Leukopenic nadir 7–14 days after drug administration; recovery in 3 weeks C. Thrombocytopenia common D. Megaloblastic changes in the marrow are common E. Anemia seen frequently F. Potent but transient suppression of primary and secondary antibody responses	II. A. Pt will be without s/s of infection or bleeding B. Early s/s of bleeding and infection will be identified	II. A. Monitor CBC, platelet count prior to drug administration as well as s/s of infection and bleeding B. Assess pt q day for s/s of infection and bleeding. Instruct pt in self-assessment C. Refer to sec. on bone marrow depression, chap. 4
III. *Impaired skin integrity, related to alopecia*	III. A. Occurs infrequently	III. A. Pt will verbalize feelings re: hair loss, and identify strategies to cope with change in body image	III. A. 1. Assess pt for s/s of hair loss 2. Discuss with pt impact of hair loss, and strategies to minimize distress; i.e., wig, scarf, cap (begin before therapy is initiated) 3. See sec. on alopecia, chap. 4

(continued)

Cytarabine, Cytosine Arabinoside *(continued)*

Nursing Diagnosis	Defining Characteristics	Expected Outcomes	Nursing Interventions
IV. *Potential for injury related to*			
A. Neurotoxicity	IV. A. 1. Can occur with high doses 2. Cerebellar toxicity is indication for immediate cessation of therapy 3. Lethargy, somnolence have resulted from too-rapid infusions of drug	IV. A. 1. Early cerebellar toxicity will be recognized and reported 2. Neurotoxicity will be minimized	IV. A. 1. Assess pt q shift and before administering drug for cerebellar toxicity 2. Instruct pt in self-assessment of cerebellar function: Encourage pt to report changes 3. Report changes in cerebellar function 4. Administer drug according to established guidelines. Monitor pt during infusion for lethargy, somnolence 5. See sec. on neurotoxicity, chap. 4
B. Tumor lysis syndrome (TLS) hyperuricemia	B. 1. TLS may develop secondary to rapid lysis of tumor cells 2. Usually begins 1–5 days after initiation of chemotherapy	B. Serum uric acid, potassium, and phosphorus will remain within normal limits	B. 1. Monitor BUN, creatinine, potassium, phosphorous, uric acid, and calcium 2. Monitor I/O 3. Monitor for renal, cardiac, neuromuscular s/s of TLS 4. Administer allopurinol, fluids as ordered 5. See sec. on nephrotoxicity, chap. 4

DRUG

Dacarbazine (DTIC-Dome, Imidazole carboximide)

Class: Alkylating agent

MECHANISM OF ACTION

Unclear, but appears to be an agent that methylates nucleic acids (particularly DNA) causing cross-linkage and breaks in DNA strands. This inhibits RNA and DNA synthesis. Also interacts with sulfhydryl groups in proteins. Generally, cell cycle phase nonspecific.

METABOLISM

Thought to be activated by liver microsomes. Excreted renally, with a plasma half-life of 0.65 hour, and terminal half-life of 5 hours.

DOSAGE/RANGE

375 mg/m^2 every 3–4 weeks
or 150–250 mg/m^2 day $\times$ 5 days repeat every 3–4 weeks
or 800–900 mg/m^2 as a single dose every 3–4 weeks

DRUG PREPARATION

Add sterile water or NS to vial.

DRUG ADMINISTRATION

Administer via volutrol over 20 minutes or can give via IV push over 2–3 minutes.

Stable for 8 hours at room temperature: 72 hours if refrigerated. Store lyophilized drug in refrigerator and protected from light. Drug decomposition is denoted by a change in color from yellow to pink.

SPECIAL CONSIDERATIONS

Irritant—avoid extravasation.

Pain may occur above site: usually unrelieved by slowing IV, but may be relieved by applying ice to painful area. May cause venospasm; slow rate if this occurs.

Anaphylaxis has occurred with infusion of dacarbazine.

Drug interactions: increased drug metabolism with concurrent administration of dilantin, phenobarbital; potential increased toxicity with Imuran and 6-MP.

Dacarbazine

Nursing Diagnosis	Defining Characteristics	Expected Outcomes	Nursing Interventions
I. *Altered nutrition, less than body requirements related to*			
A. Nausea and vomiting	I. A. 90% incidence of nausea and vomiting, moderate to severe, beginning 1–3 hrs after dose. Tolerance develops when given over several days, so that nausea and vomiting are less severe	I. A. 1. Pt will be without nausea and vomiting 2. Nausea and vomiting, if they occur, will be minimal	I. A. 1. Premedicate with antiemetic (Ativan/metoclopramide/ Decadron has been successful in preventing nausea and vomiting caused by DTIC) 2. Help pt relax using distraction, progressive muscle relaxation, imagery, and teach pt how to induce relaxation 3. *Infuse drug slowly over 1 hr to decrease nausea and vomiting* 4. Refer to sec. on nausea and vomiting, chap. 4
B. Diarrhea	B. Uncommon	B. Diarrhea, if it occurs, will abate	B. 1. Assess pt for evidence of diarrhea 2. Administer antidiarrheal medication or teach pt to self administer
C. Anorexia	C. Commonly occurs; may also cause metallic taste sensation	C. Pt will maintain baseline weight ± 5%	C. 1. Encourage small, frequent feedings of favorite foods, especially high-calorie, high-protein foods 2. Encourage use of spices 3. Weekly weights
D. Hepatotoxicity	D. Rare; however, hepatic veno-occlusive disease has been described (hepatic vein thrombosis and hepatocellular necrosis)	D. Hepatocellular dysfunction, if it occurs, will be identified early	D. 1. Monitor LFTs prior to treatment 2. If LFTs are elevated discuss holding medication with MD

II. *Infection and bleeding, related to bone marrow depression*	II. A. Nadir 14–28 days following treatment B. Anemia may occur with long-term treatment	II. A. Pt will be without s/s of infection or bleeding B. Early s/s of infection or bleeding will be identified	II. A. Monitor CBC, platelet count prior to drug administration, as well as s/s of infection and bleeding B. Instruct pt in self-assessment of s/s of infection and bleeding C. Transfuse with red cells, platelets per MD order D. Refer to sec. on bone marrow depression, chap. 4
III. *Potential for injury related to anaphylaxis*	III. A. Anaphylaxis may occur rarely, with fever, confusion, urticaria, wheezing, or hypotension	III. A. Allergic reaction or anaphylaxis, if it occurs, will be detected early B. Airway will remain patent C. BP will remain within 20 mm Hg of baseline D. Future allergic responses will be prevented	III. A. Review standing orders for management of pt in anaphylaxis or identify location of anaphylaxis kit containing epinephrine 1:1000, hydrocortisone sodium succinate (SoluCortef), diphenhydramine HCl (Benadryl), Aminophylline, and others B. Prior to drug administration, obtain baseline vital signs and record mental status C. Observe for following s/s during infusion, usually occurring within first 15 mins of start of infusion *Subjective* generalized itching chest tightness difficulty speaking agitation uneasiness dizziness nausea crampy abdominal pain anxiety sense of impending doom desire to urinate/defecate chills

(*continued*)

Dacarbazine *(continued)*

Nursing Diagnosis	Defining Characteristics	Expected Outcomes	Nursing Interventions
			III. C. *Objective* flushed appearance (angioedema of face, neck, eyelids, hands, feet) localized or generalized urticaria respiratory distress ± wheezing hypotension cyanosis
			D. If reaction occurs, stop infusion and notify MD
			E. Place pt in supine position to promote perfusion of visceral organs
			F. Monitor vital signs until stable
			G. Provide emotional reassurance to pt and family
			H. Maintain patent airway, and have ready equipment for CPR if needed
			I. Document incident
			J. Discuss with MD desensitization, versus drug discontinuance for further dosing
			K. See sec. on reactions, chap. 6
IV. *Alteration in comfort related to* A. "Flu-like syndrome"	IV. A. 1. Influenza-like syndrome characterized by malaise, headache, myalgia, chills, and hypotension 2. May occur up to 7 days after first dose, last 7–21 days and recur with subsequent doses	IV. A. Pt will verbalize increased comfort	IV. A. 1. Discuss possibility of flulike syndrome occurring 2. Suggest symptom management of acetaminophen as needed 3. Encouraging fluids orally ≥ 3 L/day, rest 4. Encourage pt to verbalize feelings, and give other emotional support

Nursing Diagnosis	Defining Characteristics	Expected Outcomes	Nursing Interventions

IV. B. Pain at injection site	IV. B. Drug is an *irritant* and may cause phlebitis of vein	IV. B. Pain will be minimized	IV. B. 1. Assess pt for appropriateness of central venous access device, especially if pt will receive successive treatments
			2. Administer DTIC in 100–250 cc IV fluid and infuse slowly over 1 hr
			3. Consider premedication, and discuss with MD:
			  a. Apply ice or heat above injection site to reduce venous burning
			  b. Premedicate with hydrocortisone IVP, lidocaine 1%–2% IVP, or heparin IVP to minimize trauma to vein prior to DTIC infusion (DTIC forms precipitate with hydrocortisone sodium succinate (solucortef) but not with hydrocortisone)

V. *Impaired skin integrity related to*

Nursing Diagnosis	Defining Characteristics	Expected Outcomes	Nursing Interventions
A. Alopecia	V. Causes alopecia in 90% of pts, with obvious impact on body image	V. A. Pt will verbalize expected side effects relating to hair loss, and strategies to minimize distress related to these side effects	V. A. 1. Encourage pt to obtain wig prior to hair loss 2. Encourage pt to verbalize feelings re: anticipated, actual hair loss, and discuss strategies to minimize impact of alopecia 3. Provide emotional support 4. Refer to sec. on alopecia, chap. 4
B. Facial flushing, erythema, and urticaria	B. Facial flushing occurs rarely, and is self-limiting. Erythema and urticaria are rare, and if occur, occur around injection site	B. Pt will verbalize feelings re: skin changes in skin and identify strategies to cope with these changes	B. 1. Assess pt for changes in skin 2. Discuss with pt impact of changes and strategies to minimize distress

(continued)

Dacarbazine *(continued)*

Nursing Diagnosis	Defining Characteristics	Expected Outcomes	Nursing Interventions
VI. *Potential for sensory/perceptual alterations*	VI. A. Facial paresthesia, photosensitivity	VI. A. Pt will verbalize expected side effects and self-care measures	VI. A. Instruct pt in self-care measures if sensory changes occur: 1. Report facial paresthesias to nurse 2. Avoid strong sunlight, wear sunscreens on skin, and protective clothing and hat
VII. *Potential for sexual dysfunction*	VII. A. Drug is teratoginic	VII. A. Pt and significant other will verbalize importance and need for contraception	VII. A. As appropriate, discuss birth control measures: 1. Discuss reproductive goals, hopes, and impact contraception will have 2. Provide teaching booklets 3. See sec. on gonadal dysfunction, chap. 4

DRUG

Dactinomycin (Actinomycin D, Cosmegan)

Class: antitumor antibiotic isolated from *streptomyces* fungus

MECHANISM OF ACTION

Binds to guanine portion of DNA and blocks the ability of DNA to act as a template for both DNA and RNA. At lower drug doses, the predominate action inhibits RNA whereas at higher doses both RNA and DNA are inhibited. Cell cycle specific for G_1 and S phases.

METABOLISM

Most of drug is excreted unchanged in bile and urine. There is a rapid clearance of drug from plasma (approximately 36 hrs). Dose reduction in the presence of liver or renal failure may be needed.

DOSAGE/RANGE

10–15 mcg/kg/day × 5 days every 3–4 weeks
15–30 mcg/kg/week 400–600 mcg/m^2/day for 5 days IV

Frequency and schedule may vary according to protocol and age.

DRUG PREPARATION

Add Sterile water for a concentration of 500 mcg/mL. Use preservative-free water as precipitate may develop otherwise.

DRUG ADMINISTRATION

IV. This is a vesicant and should be given through a running IV so as to avoid extravasation which can lead to ulceration, pain, and necrosis. Be sure to check the nursing policy and procedure for administration of vesicants.

SPECIAL CONSIDERATIONS

Drug is a vesicant. Give through a running IV to avoid an extravasation which may develop into ulceration, necrosis and pain.

Nausea and vomiting are moderate to severe. Usually occurring 2–5 hours after administration; may persist up to 24 hours.

Potent myelosuppressive agent—severity of nadir is dose-limiting toxicity.

Gastrointestinal toxicity—mucositis, diarrhea, and abdominal pain.

Skin changes—radiation recall phenomenon. Skin discoloration along vein used for injection.

Alopecia.

Malaise, fatigue, fever, mental depression.

Hypocalcemia has been noted as a side effect.

Dactinomycin

Nursing Diagnosis	Defining Characteristics	Expected Outcomes	Nursing Interventions
I. *Potential for infection and bleeding related to bone marrow depression*	I. A. Onset 7–10 days, nadir 14–21 days with recovery 21–28 days B. Anemia is delayed C. Myelosuppression may be dose limiting and severe	I. A. Pt will be without infection or bleeding B. Early s/s of infection and bleeding will be identified	I. A. Monitor CBC, platelet count prior to drug administration B. Assess pt and teach pt self-assessment for s/s of infection and bleeding C. Transfuse red cells, platelets per MD order D. Drug dosage should be reduced for lower than normal blood values E. See sec. on bone marrow depression, chap. 4
II. *Alteration in nutrition* A. Nausea and vomiting	II. A. Beginning 2–5 hrs after dose, may last 24 hrs	II. A. 1. Pt will be without nausea and vomiting 2. Nausea and vomiting, if they occur, will be minimal	II. A. 1. Premedicate with antiemetics and continue prophylactically × 24 hrs to prevent nausea and vomiting, at least first treatment 2. Encourage small, frequent feedings of cool, bland foods and liquids 3. Administer oral dose on an empty stomach 4. Refer to sec. on nausea and vomiting, chap. 4
B. Diarrhea, cramps	B. 30% incidence	B. Pt will have minimal diarrhea	B. 1. Encourage pt to report onset of diarrhea 2. Administer or teach pt to self-administer antidiarrheal medication 3. See sec. on diarrhea, chap. 4
C. Anorexia	C. Occurs frequently	C. Pt will maintain baseline weight ± 5%	C. 1. Encourage small, frequent feedings of favorite foods, especially high-calorie, high-protein foods 2. Encourage use of spices 3. Weekly weights

| III. Alteration in mucous membranes, including stomatitis, esophagitis, proctitis | III. A. There is an incidence of irritation of mucous membranes lining the entire gastrointestinal tract | III. A. 1. Oral mucous membranes will remain intact without infection
2. The gastrointestinal toxicity will be minimal | III. A. Teach pt oral assessment and oral hygiene regimen
B. Encourage pt to report early stomatitis
C. Teach pt importance of stomatitis and the entire gastrointestinal system
D. Refer to sec. on stomatitis, mucositis, chap. 4 |
| IV. Impaired skin integrity | IV. A. Radiation recall at previously irradiated skin site
B. Acne-like rash and alopecia can occur in 47% of pts
C. Drug is a vesicant | IV. A. Pt will verbalize feelings re changes in nail or skin color, texture
B. Identify strategies to cope with change in body image
C. Extravasation, if it occurs, is detected early with early intervention
D. Skin and underlying tissue damage is minimized | IV. A. 1. Assess pt for changes in skin, nails, and hair loss
2. Discuss with pt impact of changes and strategies to minimize distress
3. See sec. on reactions, chap. 6
B. 1. Discuss skin changes as they relate to changes in body image
2. See sec. on alopecia, chap. 4
C. 1. Careful technique is used during venipuncture. See sec. on intravenous administration, chap. 7
2. Administer vesicant through freely flowing IV, constantly monitoring IV site and pt response
3. Nurse should be THOROUGHLY familiar with institutional policy and procedure for administration of a vesicant agent
4. If vesicant drug is administered as a continuous infusion, drug must be given through a patent central line |

(continued)

Dactinomycin (continued)

Nursing Diagnosis	Defining Characteristics	Expected Outcomes	Nursing Interventions
			IV. C. 5. If extravasation is suspected: a. Stop drug administered b. Aspirate any residual drug and blood from IV tubing, IV catheter/needle, and IV site if possible c. Instill antidote into area of apparent infiltration, IF ANTIDOTE EXISTS, as per MD orders and institutional policy and procedure d. Apply cold or topical medication as per MD order and institutional policy and procedure
			6. Assess site regularly for pain, progression of erythema, induration, and for evidence of necrosis
			7. When in doubt about whether drug is infiltrating, TREAT AS AN INFILTRATION
			8. Teach pt to assess site and notify MD if condition worsens
			9. Arrange next clinic visit for assessment of site depending on drug, amount infiltrated, extent of potential injury, and pt variables
			10. Document in pt's record as per institutional policy and procedure. See sec. on reactions, ch. 6
V. Alteration in comfort	V. A. Flu-like symptoms can occur including symptoms of malaise, myalgia, fever, depression	V. A. Pt will remain comfortable during therapy	V. A. Assess pt for symptoms during and after treatment B. Premedicate with acetaminophen, antihistamine, or steroids as per MD order C. Evaluate the effectiveness of the symptomatic relief that is prescribed and administered

VI. Alteration in metabolism			
A. Hepatotoxicity	VI. A. Drug is metabolized rapidly by the liver	VI. A. Hepatic dysfunction will be identified early	VI. A. 1. Establish a baseline for liver function tests 2. Monitor SGOT, SGPT, LDH, alkaline phosphatase, and bilirubin on a regular basis 3. Notify MD of any elevations 4. Refer to sec. on hepatotoxicity, chap. 4
B. Renal toxicity	B. Drug is metabolized rapidly by the kidneys	B. Renal toxicity will be minimal	B. 1. Monitor BUN and creatinine prior to drug dose 2. Provide fluid and teach pt the importance of hydration 3. See sec. on nephrotoxicity, chap. 4
VII. Alteration in sexual dysfunction	VII. A. Drug is mutagenic and teratogenic	VII. A. Pt and significant other will understand need for contraception B. Pt and significant other will identify strategies to cope with sexual dysfunction	VII. A. As appropriate, explore with pt and significant other reproductive patterns and impact chemotherapy will have B. Discuss strategies to preserve sexuality and reproductive health (sperm banking, contraception) C. See sec. on gonadal dysfunction, chap. 4

DRUG

Daunorubicin hydrochloride (Cerubidine, Daunomycin)

Class: Anthracycline antibiotic isolated from streptomycin products, in particular the rhodomycin products.

MECHANISM OF ACTION

No clearly defined mechanism. Intercalates DNA, therefore blocking DNA, RNA, and protein synthesis. Binds to DNA and inhibits DNA replication and DNA-dependent RNA synthesis.

METABOLISM

Site of significant metabolism is in the liver. Doses need to be modified in presence of abnormal liver function. Excreted in urine and bile.

DOSAGE/RANGE

30–60 mg/m^2/day IV for 3 consecutive days.

DRUG PREPARATION

Add sterile water to produce liquid. Drug will form a precipitate when mixed with heparin and is incompatible with dexamethasone.

DRUG ADMINISTRATION

IV. This drug is a potent vesicant. Give through a running IV so as to avoid extravasation which can lead to ulceration, pain, and necrosis. Check individual hospital policy and procedure on administration of a vesicant.

SPECIAL CONSIDERATIONS

Drug is a potent vesicant. Give through running IV to avoid extravasation.

Moderate to severe nausea and vomiting occur in 50% of patients within first 24 hours.

Causes discoloration of urine (pink to red for up to 48 hours after administration).

Potent myelosuppressive agent. Nadir occurs within 10–14 days.

Alopecia.

Cardiac Toxicity—dose limit at 550 mg/m^2. Patients may exhibit irreversible congestive heart failure. Acute toxicity may be seen within hours after administration. This is unrelated to cumulative dose and may manifest symptoms of pump or conduction function. Rarely, transient EKG abnormalities, CHF, pericardial effusion (whole syndrome referred to as myocarditis-pericarditis syndrome) may occur, which may lead to demise of patient.

Daunorubicin hydrochloride

Nursing Diagnosis	Defining Characteristics	Expected Outcomes	Nursing Interventions
I. Potential for infection and bleeding related to bone marrow depression	I. A. Leukopenia onset in 7 days; nadir 10–14 days; recovery 21–28 days B. Thrombocytopenia occurs with BMD	I. A. 1. Pt will be without s/s of infection or bleeding 2. Early s/s of infection and bleeding will be identified	I. A. 1. Monitor CBC, platelet count prior to drug administration 2. Monitor s/s of infection and bleeding 3. Instruct pt in self-assessment of s/s of infection and bleeding 4. Dose reduction may be necessary 5. Transfuse with red cells, platelets per MD order 6. Refer to sec. on bone marrow depression, chap. 4
II. Potential for altered cardiac output	II. A. Acute: 6%–30% of pts develop transient EKG changes 1–3 days after dose B. Chronic: Cumulative, dose-related cardiomyopathy C. CHF may develop 1–16 mos after therapy ceases	II. A. Early s/s of cardiomyopathy will be identified	II. A. Assess for s/s of cardiomyopathy B. Assess quality and regularity of heartbeat C. Baseline EKG D. Instruct pt to report dyspnea, shortness of breath, swelling of extremities, orthopnea E. Chronic cardiomyopathy: Monitor GBPS, and ejection fraction, baseline and periodically through treatment as cumulative dosages approach maximum F. See sec. on cardiotoxicity, chap. 4

(continued)

Daunorubicin hydrochloride (continued)

Nursing Diagnosis	Defining Characteristics	Expected Outcomes	Nursing Interventions
III. Alteration in nutrition, less than body requirements	III. A. Mild nausea, vomiting day of therapy (50% incidence)	III. A. Pt will be without nausea and vomiting, or, if they occur, they will be minimal	III. A. 1. Premedicate with antiemetic, as ordered, and continue prophylactically to prevent nausea and vomiting 2. Encourage small, frequent feedings of cool, bland foods and liquids 3. Refer to sec. on nausea and vomiting, chap. 4
	B. Stomatitis infrequent, 3–7 days after dose	B. Oral mucous membranes will remain intact	B. 1. Encourage small, frequent feedings of favorite foods, especially high-calorie, high-protein foods 2. Encourage use of spices 3. Weekly weights 4. Assess oral mucous membranes 5. Instruct pt in oral assessment and mouth care 6. See sec. on stomatitis, chap. 4
IV. Potential for impaired skin integrity	IV. A. Extravasation of drug can cause tissue necrosis	IV. A. Extravasation, if it occurs, is detected early with early intervention. Skin and underlying tissue damage is minimized	IV. A. 1. Careful technique is used during venipuncture. See sec. on intravenous administration, chap. 7 2. Administer vesicant through freely flowing IV, constantly monitoring IV site and pt response 3. Nurse should be THOROUGHLY familiar with institutional policy and procedure for administration of a vesicant agent 4. If vesicant drug is administered as a continuous infusion, drug must be given through a patent central line

IV. A.

5. If extravasation is suspected:

   a. Stop drug administered

   b. Aspirate any residual drug and blood from IV tubing, IV catheter/needle, and IV site if possible

   c. Instill antidote into area of apparent infiltration, IF ANTIDOTE EXISTS, as per MD orders and institutional policy and procedure

   d. Apply cold or topical medication as per MD order and institutional policy and procedure

6. Assess site regularly for pain, progression of erythema, induration, and for evidence of necrosis

7. When in doubt about whether drug is infiltrating, TREAT AS AN INFILTRATION

8. Teach pt to assess site and notify MD if condition worsens

9. Arrange next clinic visit for assessment of site depending on drug, amount infiltrated, extent of potential injury, and pt variables

10. Document in pt's record as per institutional policy and procedure. See sec. on reactions, ch. 6

(continued)

Daunorubicin hydrochloride (continued)

Nursing Diagnosis	Defining Characteristics	Expected Outcomes	Nursing Interventions
	IV. B. Alopecia (complete) in 3–4 weeks after treatment begins	IV. B. Pt will verbalize feelings re hair loss and identify strategies to cope with changes in body image	IV. B. 1. Discuss with pt impact of hair loss 2. Suggest wig as appropriate prior to actual hair loss 3. Explore with pt response to actual hair loss and plan strategies to minimize distress; i.e., wig, scarf, cap 4. Refer to sec. on alopecia, chap. 4
	C. Reactivation of radiation-induced lesions (radiation recall); hyperpigmentation, rash; Onycholysis (nail loosening from nail bed)	C. Skin discomfort will be minimized and skin will remain intact. Pt will verbalize feelings re skin changes	C. 1. This is not an indication to stop drug 2. Discuss with MD symptomatic management 3. Reinforce pt teaching on the action and side effects of daunorubicin 4. Offer emotional support
V. Potential for alteration in sexual dysfunction	V. A. Drug is mutagenic and teratogenic	V. A. Pt and significant other will understand the need for contraception B. Pt and significant other will identify strategies to cope with sexual dysfunction	V. A. As appropriate, explore with pt and significant other reproductive and sexuality patterns and impact chemotherapy will have B. Discuss strategies to preserve sexuality and reproductive health (i.e., sperm banking, contraception) C. See sec. on gonadal dysfunction, chap. 4
VI. Potential for alteration in comfort, i.e., pain	VI. A. Abdominal pain may occur	VI. A. Pt will be supported during therapy	VI. A. Offer emotional support to pt B. Reinforce information on the action and side effects of daunorubicin hydrochloride C. Discuss with MD medicating for the pain

DRUG

Doxorubicin hydrochloride (Adriamycin, Rubex)

Class: Anthracycline antibiotic isolated from streptomycin products, in particular from the rhodomycin products.

MECHANISM OF ACTION

Antitumor antibiotic—no clearly defined mechanism. Binds directly to DNA base pairs (intercalates) and inhibits DNA and DNA-dependent RNA synthesis, as well as protein synthesis. Cell cycle specific for S-phase.

METABOLISM

Excretion of drug predominates in the liver; renal clearance is minor. Alteration in liver function refuses modification of doses, whereas with renal failure no need to alter doses. Drug excreted through urine and may discolor urine from 1–48 hours after administration.

DOSAGE/RANGE

30–75 mg/m^2 IV every 3–4 weeks

20–45 mg/m^2 IV for 3 consecutive days

For bladder instillation: 3–60 mg/m^2

For interperitoneal instillation: 40 mg in 2 L dialysate (no heparin)

Continuous infusion: varies with individual protocol

DRUG PREPARATION

Drug will form a precipitate if mixed with heparin or 5-fluorouracil. Dilute with Sodium Chloride (preservative free) to produce 2 mg/mL concentration.

DRUG ADMINISTRATION

IV. This drug is a potent vesicant. Give through a running IV so as to avoid extravasation which can lead to ulceration, pain, and necrosis. Be sure to check nursing procedure for administration of a vesicant.

SPECIAL CONSIDERATIONS

Drug is a potent vesicant. Give through running IV to avoid extravasation and tissue necrosis.

Give through central line if drug is to be given by continuous infusion.

Nausea and vomiting is dose related. Occurs in 50% of patients. Begins 1–3 hours after administration.

Causes discoloration of urine (from pink to red for up to 48 hours).

Skin changes: may cause "recall phenomenon"—recalls reaction to previously irradiated tissue.

Potent myelosuppressive agent causes gastrointestinal toxicities: mucositis, esophagitis, and diarrhea.

Cardiac Toxicity—dose limit at 550 mg/m^2. Patients may exhibit irreversible congestive heart failure. May see acute toxicity in hours or days after administration. This is unrelated to cumulative dose and may manifest symptoms of pump or conduction function. Rarely, transient EKG abnormalities, CHF, pericardial effusions (whole syndrome referred to as myocarditis-pericarditis syndrome) may occur, which may lead to demise of patient.

Vein discoloration.

Increased pigmentation in black patients.

When given with barbiturates there is increased plasma clearance of doxorubicin.

When given with cyclophosphamide there is risk of hemorrhage and cardiotoxicity.

When given with mitomycin there is increased risk of cardiotoxicity.

There is decreased oral bioavailability of digoxin when given together.

When given with mercaptopurine there is increased risk of hepatotoxicity.

Doxorubicin hydrochloride

Nursing Diagnosis	Defining Characteristics	Expected Outcomes	Nursing Interventions
I. Potential for infection and bleeding related to bone marrow depression	I. A. Nadir 10–14 days with recovery 15–21 days B. Myelosuppression may be severe; overall incidence of occurrence 60%–80%, less common with weekly dosing	I. A. Pt will be without s/s of infection or bleeding B. Early s/s of infection or bleeding will be identified	I. A. 1. Monitor CBC, platelet count prior to drug administration, as well as s/s of infection and bleeding 2. Instruct pt in self-assessment of s/s of infection and bleeding 3. Dose reduction may be necessary; discuss with MD 4. Transfuse with red cells and platelets per MD order 5. Refer to sec. on bone marrow depression, chap. 4
II. Potential for alteration in nutrition, less than body requirements			
A. Nausea and vomiting	II. A. 1. Moderate to severe; 50% incidence as single agent with increased incidence in combination with Cytoxan 2. Onset 1–3 hours after drug administration lasting up to 24 hours	II. A. 1. Pt will be without nausea and vomiting 2. Nausea and vomiting, if they occur, will be minimal	II. A. 1. Premedicate with antiemetics and continue prophylactically × 24 hrs to prevent nausea and vomiting, at least first treatment 2. Encourage small, frequent feedings of cool, bland food and liquids 3. Refer to sec. on nausea and vomiting, chap. 4
B. Anorexia	B. Occurs frequently	B. Pt will maintain baseline weight ± 5%	B. 1. Encourage small, frequent feedings of favorite foods, especially high-calorie, high-protein foods 2. Encourage use of spices 3. Weekly weights
C. Stomatitis	C. 10% incidence esophagitis	C. Oral mucous membrane will remain intact without infection	C. 1. Teach pt oral assessment 2. Encourage pt to report early signs of stomatitis 3. See sec. on stomatitis/ mucositis, chap. 4

III. *Potential for alteration in cardiac output*	III. A. Early s/s of cardiomyopathy will be identified	III. A. If pt is receiving cyclophosphamide in addition to doxorubicin assess for s/s of cardiomyopathy
	A. Acute: Pericarditis-myocarditis syndrome with nonspecific EKG changes (flat Twaves, ST, PVCs) during infusion or immediately after (nonlife threatening)	B. Cardiac evaluation on a regular basis
		C. Discuss gated blood pools scans with MD baseline and periodically
		D. Assess pt's baseline prior to beginning chemotherapy
	B. Cumulative dose cardiomyopathy; risk if dose > 550 mg/m² or >450 mg/m² receiving chest XRT or Cytoxan	E. Assess quality and regularity of heartbeat
		F. Instruct pt to report dyspnea, shortness of breath
		G. See sec. on cardiotoxicity, chap. 4
IV. *Potential for alteration in sexual dysfunction*	IV. A. Pt and significant other will understand need for contraception	IV. A. As appropriate, explore with pt and significant other reproductive and sexuality patterns and impact chemotherapy will have
	IV. Drug is teratogenic and mutagenic	
	B. Pt and significant other will identify strategies to cope with sexual dysfunction	B. Discuss strategies to preserve sexuality and reproductive health
		C. See sec. on gonadal dysfunction, chap. 4
V. *Alteration in skin integrity* A. Alopecia	V. A. Pt will verbalize feelings re hair loss and identify strategies to cope with change in body image	V. A. 1. Assess pt for s/s of hair loss
	V. A. Complete hair loss with 60–75 mg/m² dosing	2. Discuss with pt impact of hair loss and strategies to minimize distress; i.e., wig, scarf, cap
	1. Occurs 2–5 weeks after therapy begins	3. See sec. on alopecia, chap. 4
	2. Regrowth usually begins a few months after drug is stopped	

(continued)

Doxorubicin hydrochloride (continued)

Nursing Diagnosis	Defining Characteristics	Expected Outcomes	Nursing Interventions
V. B. Changes in nails and skin, radiation recall reaction, flare reaction	V. B. 1. Nail beds and dermal creases (especially in black pts) become hyperpigmented 2. Reactivation of the erythema and skin damage of prior sites of skin irradiation 3. Erythematous streaking along vein during drug administration, often with urticaria and pruritis. This condition is self-limiting, usually within 30 mins with or without use of antihistamines	V. B. Pt will verbalize feelings re changes in nail or skin color, texture and identify strategies to cope with change in body image	V. B. 1. Assess pt for changes in skin and nails 2. Discuss with pt impact of changes and strategies to minimize distress; i.e., wearing nail polish (women) or long sleeve tops
C. Extravasation	C. Avoid extravasation as tissue necrosis may occur	C. 1. Extravasation, if it occurs, is detected early with early intervention 2. Skin and underlying tissue damage is minimized	C. 1. Careful technique is used during venipuncture. See sec. on intravenous administration, chap. 7 2. Administer vesicant through freely flowing IV, constantly monitoring IV site and pt response 3. Nurse should be THOROUGHLY familiar with institutional policy and procedure for administration of a vesicant agent 4. If vesicant drug is administered as a continuous infusion, drug must be given through a patent central line

V. C. 5. If extravasation is suspected:

    a. Stop drug administered

    b. Aspirate any residual drug and blood from IV tubing, IV catheter/needle, and IV site if possible

    c. Instill antidote into area of apparent infiltration, IF ANTIDOTE EXISTS, as per MD orders and institutional policy and procedure

    d. Apply cold or topical medication as per MD order and institutional policy and procedure

    6. Assess site regularly for pain, progression of erythema, induration, and for evidence of necrosis

    7. When in doubt about whether drug is infiltrating, TREAT AS AN INFILTRATION

    8. Teach pt to assess site and notify MD if condition worsens

    9. Arrange next clinic visit for assessment of site depending on drug, amount infiltrated, extent of potential injury, and pt variables

    10. Document in pt's record as per institutional policy and procedure. See sec. on reactions, chap. 6

DRUG

Estramustine phosphate (Estracyte, Emcyt)

Class: Alkylating agent

MECHANISM OF ACTION

At usual therapeutic concentrations, act as a weak alkylator. A chemical combination of mechlorethamine and estradiol phosphate, estramustine is believed to selectively enter cells with estrogen receptors where the drug acts as an alkylating agent due to bischlorethyl sidechain and liberated estrogens.

METABOLISM

Well absorbed orally, metabolized in liver, partly excreted in urine. Induces a marked decline in serum calcium and phosphate levels.

DOSAGE/RANGE

600 mg/m^2 (15 mkg/kg) orally daily in 3 divided doses (range 10–16 mg/kg/day in most studies with evaluation after 30–90 days).

DRUG PREPARATION

Available in 140-mg capsules

DRUG ADMINISTRATION

Oral

SPECIAL CONSIDERATIONS

Administer with food or antacids to decrease gastrointestinal side effects.

IV preparation is a *vesicant*: avoid extravasation.

Transient perineal itching and pain after IV administration.

Estramustine phosphate

I. *Potential for alteration in nutrition, less than body requirements related to*

Nursing Diagnosis	Defining Characteristics	Expected Outcomes	Nursing Interventions
A. Nausea and vomiting	I. A. Occurs at higher dosing 1. Pt may develop tolerance 2. Dose may need to be reduced or temporarily stopped for moderate to severe nausea and vomiting 3. Delayed (6–8 weeks) and intractable nausea and vomiting may occur requiring discontinuance of therapy	I. A. 1. Nausea and vomiting will be prevented 2. Nausea and vomiting, if they occur, will be minimal	I. A. 1. Premedicate with antiemetic (e.g., phenothiazine) and instruct pt in self-administration of antiemetic, especially for high doses 2. Refer to sec. on nausea and vomiting, chap. 4
B. Diarrhea	B. Occurs occasionally	B. Pt will have minimal diarrhea	B. 1. Encourage pt to report onset of diarrhea 2. Administer or teach pt to self-administer antidiarrheal medications 3. Teach pt diet modifications 4. Refer to sec. on diarrhea, chap. 4
C. Hepatic dysfunction	C. Mild elevations in liver function studies may occur 1. LDH, SGOT especially 2. Usually are transient and self-limiting 3. Jaundice	C. Hepatic dysfunction will be identified early	C. 1. Monitor SGOT, LDH as well as SGPT, alkaline phosphatase, bilirubin periodically during treatment 2. Notify MD of any elevations
D. ↓ Ca^{++} and P levels	D. Serum Ca^{++} and phosphorus may occur related to changes in metabolism of bone	D. Abnormalities in Ca^{++}, P levels will be identified and corrected	D. Monitor Ca^{++}, P levels

(continued)

Estramustine phosphate *(continued)*

Nursing Diagnosis	Defining Characteristics	Expected Outcomes	Nursing Interventions
II. *Body image disturbance, related to gynecomastia*	II. A. Occurs less frequently than with DES B. Nipple tenderness may occur initially	II. A. Pt will verbalize feelings re changes in body image B. Pt will identify strategies to cope with changes in body image	II. A. Instruct pt in potential drug side effect of gynecomastia and breast tenderness B. Encourage pt to verbalize feelings re breast enlargement C. Discuss with pt potential coping strategies to deal with these changes
III. *Alteration in cardiac output*	III. A. CHF may occur rarely, possibly related to estrogen property of salt retention	III. A. Early CHF or worsening CHF will be detected	III. A. Drug should be used cautiously in pts with history of congestive heart failure or myocardial infarction B. Assess cardiac function (i.e., heartrate and heart sounds—S3, BP, RR, breath sounds) and symptoms of edema, dyspnea, SOB at each visit C. Instruct pt to report any changes in health; i.e., symptoms of dyspnea, SOB, edema
IV. *Altered tissue perfusion*	IV. Circulatory changes may occur —Thrombophlebitis, thrombosis	IV. Early changes in circulation will be detected	IV. A. Drug should be used cautiously in pts with a history of thrombophlebitis, thrombosis, cerebrovascular or coronary artery disease, other thromboembolic states B. Assess circulatory function (pulses, temperature of extremities, etc.) and for s/s of thrombophlebitis, thrombosis C. Instruct pt to report any changes in health (e.g., coolness of extremities, redness/warmth of extremities, leg cramps) D. Instruct pt to avoid crossing legs

V. *Potential for alteration in comfort*	V. A. Perineal symptoms, headache, rash, urticaria may occur B. Transient paresthesias of mouth with IV administration	V. A. Pt will be comfortable	V. A. Assess for occurrence of perineal itching and pain after IV administration, and headaches, rash, urticaria, and discuss with MD symptomatic treatment B. Use careful IV administration technique as drug may cause severe thrombophlebitis
VI. *Potential for infection and bleeding related to bone marrow depression*	VI. A. Approximately 5% of pts experience	VI. A. Pt will be without infection and bleeding B. Early s/s of infection or bleeding will be identified	VI. A. Monitor CBC and platelet count prior to drug administration B. Assess pt for and teach pt self-assessment for s/s of infection and bleeding C. Transfuse with red cells, platelets per MD order D. Drug dosage should be reduced for lower than normal blood values E. See sec. on bone marrow depression, chap. 4
VII. *Alteration in skin integrity related to extravasation potential*	VII. A. Estramustine is a potent vesicant B. Vesicant drugs cause erythema, burning, tissue necrosis, and tissue sloughing, if extravasated	VII. A. Extravasation, if it occurs, is detected early with early intervention B. Skin and underlying tissue damage is minimized	VII. A. Careful technique is used during venipuncture. See sec. on intravenous administration, chap. 7 B. Administer vesicant through freely flowing IV, constantly monitoring IV site and pt response C. Nurse should be THOROUGHLY familiar with institutional policy and procedure for administration of a vesicant agent D. If vesicant drug is administered as a continuous infusion, drug must be given through a patent central line

(continued)

Estramustine phosphate *(continued)*

Nursing Diagnosis	Defining Characteristics	Expected Outcomes	Nursing Interventions
			VII. E. If extravasation is suspected: 1. Stop drug administered 2. Aspirate any residual drug and blood from IV tubing, IV catheter/needle, and IV site if possible 3. Instill antidote into area of apparent infiltration, IF ANTIDOTE EXISTS, as per MD orders and institutional policy and procedure 4. Apply cold or topical medication as per MD order and institutional policy and procedure F. Assess site regularly for pain, progression of erythema, induration, and for evidence of necrosis G. When in doubt about whether drug is infiltrating, TREAT AS AN INFILTRATION H. Teach pt to assess site and notify MD if condition worsens I. Arrange next clinic visit for assessment of site depending on drug, amount infiltrated, extent of potential injury, and pt variables J. Document in pt's record as per institutional policy and procedure. See sec. on reactions, chap. 6

DRUG

Estrogens: Diethylstilbestrol (DES), Diethystilbestrol diphosphate (Stilphostrol, Stilbestrol diphosphate), Ethinyl estradiol (Estinyl), Conjugated equine estrogen (Premarin), Chlorotriarisene (Tace)

Class: Hormones

MECHANISM OF ACTION

Unknown
 Estrogens change the hormonal milieu of the body

METABOLISM

Metabolized mainly in the liver. Undergoes enterohepatic recirculation. DES is metabolized more slowly than natural estrogens.

DOSAGE/RANGE

DES—prostate cancer: 1–3 mg orally daily; breast cancer: 5 mg orally TID

Diethylstilbestrol diphosphate—prostate cancer: 50–200 orally TID, 0.5–1.0 gm IV daily × 5 days then 250–1000 mg each week

Chlorotrianisene—1–10 orally TID

Ethinyl estradiol—0.5–1.0 mg orally TID

DRUG PREPARATION

None

DRUG ADMINISTRATION

Oral

SPECIAL CONSIDERATIONS

Long-term dosage of DES in males has been associated with cardiovascular deaths. Maximum dose should be 1 mg TID for prostate cancer.

Can cause inaccurate laboratory results (liver, adrenal, thyroid).

Causes rapid rise in serum calcium in patients with bony metastases—watch for symptoms of hypercalcemia.

Estrogens

Nursing Diagnosis	Defining Characteristics	Expected Outcomes	Nursing Interventions
I. *Altered nutrition: less than body requirements related to nausea and vomiting*	I. A. 1. Occurs in 25% of pts on estrogens B. Degree of nausea varies depending on the specific drug, and is usually dose-dependent C. Nausea tends to decrease after a few weeks of therapy	I. A. 1. Pt will be without nausea or vomiting B. Nausea and vomiting, should they occur, will be minimal	I. A. Inform pt that nausea and vomiting can occur; encourage pt to report nausea or vomiting B. Instruct pt to take estrogens at bedtime to decrease nausea C. Consider starting pt at a low dose and increase dose as tolerated D. Refer to sec. on nausea and vomiting, chap. 4
II. *Potential for injury, related to*			
A. Sodium and water retention	II. A. 1. May occur 2. Estrogens should be used with great caution in pts with underlying cardiac, renal, hepatic disease	II. A. 1. Fluid and electrolyte balance will be maintained	II. A. 1. Identify pt with underlying cardiac, hepatic, and renal disease 2. Inform pts of potential for sodium and water retention, of s/s to watch for and report to MD 3. Assess pts for s/s of fluid overload
B. Hypercalcemia	B. 1. Occurs in 5%–10% of women with breast cancer metastatic to bone 2. Particular risk of hypercalcemia in first 2 weeks of therapy 3. Renal disease can aggravate hypercalcemia	B. 1. Serum calcium will remain within normal limits 2. Hypercalcemia will be identified and treated early	B. 1. Identify pts at risk and monitor serum calcium closely during the first few weeks of treatment 2. Teach pts s/s of hypercalcemia (drowsiness, increased thirst, constipation, increased urine output). Instruct pt to notify MD if s/s occur

C. Cardiotoxicity	C. 1. Increased incidence of cardiovascular-associated death, especially in men on high-dose estrogens for prostate cancer 2. Effects of digitalis are potentiated by estrogens	C. Cardiotoxicity will be avoided	C. 1. Identify pts at risk for cardiotoxicity 2. Inform pts of risk, s/s to report 3. Monitor cardiac drug levels; alert cardiologist that pt is on estrogen
D. Thromboembolic complications	D. Occurrence infrequent, but more common with long-term use and high doses	D. Pt will avoid injury related to abnormal blood clotting	D. 1. Teach pt s/s of thromboemboli: i.e., Positive Homan's sign, localized swelling, pain, tenderness, erythema, sudden CNS changes, shortness of breath 2. Instruct pt to notify MD if any of above occur

III. *Potential for sexual dysfunction, related to*

A. Gynecomastia, loss of libido, impotence, and voice changes	III. A. 1. May occur in men 2. Gynecomastia may be prevented by pretreating each breast with radiation therapy 3. Feminine characteristics disappear when therapy is stopped	III. A. 1. Pt and significant other will verbalize understanding of changes in sexuality that may occur 2. Pt and significant other will identify strategies to cope with sexual dysfunction	III. A. 1. As appropriate, explore with pt and significant other reproductive and sexuality patterns, and impact that therapy may have on them 2. Discuss strategies to preserve sexuality and reproductive health 3. See sec. on gonadal dysfunction, chap. 4

(continued)

Estrogens (*continued*)

Nursing Diagnosis	Defining Characteristics	Expected Outcomes	Nursing Interventions
III. B. Breast tenderness, engorgement in women	III. B. Engorgement may occur in postmenopausal women	III. B. Pt will be supported throughout treatment	III. B. 1. As appropriate, explore with pt and significant other reproductive and sexuality patterns, and impact that therapy may have on them 2. Application of heat for local decrease of breast tenderness
C. Uterine prolapse, exacerbation of preexisting uterine fibroids with possible uterine bleeding	C. May occur	C. Pt will identify the side effects of treatment	C. 1. Discuss with MD symptomatic management 2. Reinforce pt teaching on the action and side effects of estrogen therapy 3. Offer emotional support
D. Urinary incontinence	D. May occur in women	D. Pt will be made comfortable	D. 1. Reinforce information on the action and side effects of estrogen therapy 2. Offer emotional support 3. Offer specific suggestions (pads, Attends)

DRUG

Etoposide (VP-16, Vepesid)

Class: Plant alkaloid, a derivative of the mandrake plant (may apple plant)

MECHANISM OF ACTION

Inhibits DNA synthesis in S and G_2 so that cells do not enter mitosis. Causes single-strand breaks in DNA. Cell cycle specific for S and G_2 phases.

METABOLISM

VP-16 is rapidly excreted in the urine, and to a lesser extent, the bile. About 30% of drug is excreted unchanged. Binds to serum albumin (94%), then becomes extensively tissue bound.

DOSAGE/RANGE

50–100 mg/m^2 IV qd $\times$ 5 (testicular cancer) q 3–4 weeks

75–200 mg/m^2 IV qd $\times$ 3 (small cell lung cancer) q 3–4 weeks

Oral dose is twice the intravenous dose.

DRUG PREPARATION

Available in 5 cc (100-mg) vials

Oral capsules available in 50-mg and 100-mg capsules

DRUG ADMINISTRATION

Intravenous infusion: over 30–60 minutes to minimize risk of hypotension and bronchospasm (wheezing). In some instances, a test dose may be infused slowly (0.5 ml in 50 NS) and the remaining drug infused if no untoward reaction after 5 minutes.

Stability: Drug must be diluted with either 5% Dextrose Injection USP or 0.9% Sodium Chloride solution and is stable 96 hours in glass and 48 hours in plastic containers at room temperature (25°C) under normal fluorescent light at a concentration of 0.2 mg/ml.

Inspect for clarity of solution prior to administration.

Oral Administration: may give as a single dose if ≤ 400 mg; otherwise divide dose.

SPECIAL CONSIDERATIONS

Nadir 7 to 14 days after treatment.

Reduce drug dose by 50% if bilirubin > 1.5 mg/dl, by 75% if bilirubin > 3.0 mg/dl.

Synergistic drug effect in combination with cisplatin.

Radiation recall may occur when combined therapies are used.

Etoposide

Nursing Diagnosis	Defining Characteristics	Expected Outcomes	Nursing Interventions
I. *Potential for injury during drug administration related to*			
A. Allergic reaction	I. A. Bronchospasm as evidenced by wheezing may occur; may experience fever, chills	I. A. 1. Bronchospasm will be prevented 2. Bronchospasm will be identified early and terminated, if it occurs	I. A. 1. Test dose of 0.5 mL/50 NS IV, may be given, then waiting 5 mins before slowly administering remainder of drug 2. Infuse drug slowly over *at least* 30–60 mins 3. Discontinue drug and notify MD if bronchospasm occurs; have antihistamines ready (e.g., diphenhydramine)
B. Hypotension	B. Hypotension may occur during rapid infusion	B. Hypotension will be prevented	B. 1. Monitor BP prior to drug administration and periodically during infusion, at least during first drug administration 2. Infuse drug over *at least* 30–60 mins
C. Anaphylaxis	C. Anaphylaxis may occur but is rare	C. Anaphylaxis, if it occurs, will be managed successfully	C. 1. Monitor pt closely during infusion 2. Review standing orders for management of pt in anaphylaxis and identify location of anaphylaxis kit containing epinephrine 1:1000, hydrocortisone sodium succinate (Solucortef), diphenhydramine HCL (Benadryl), Aminophylline, and others 3. Prior to drug administration, obtain baseline vital signs and record mental status

I. C. 4. Observe for following s/s during infusion usually occuring within first 15 mins of start of infusion:

Subjective

generalized itching

nausea

chest tightness

crampy abdominal pain

difficulty speaking

anxiety

agitation

sense of impending doom

uneasiness

desire to urinate or defecate

dizziness

chills

Objective

flushed appearance (angioedema of face, neck, eyelids, hands, feet)

localized or generalized urticaria

respiratory distress ± wheezing

hypotension

cyanosis

5. Stop infusion if reaction occurs and notify MD

6. Place pt in supine position to promote perfusion of visceral organs

7. Monitor vital signs until stable

8. Provide emotional reassurance to pt and family

9. Maintain patent airway, and have CPR equipment ready if needed

10. Document incident

11. Discuss with MD desensitation versus drug discontinuance for further dosing

12. See sec. on reactions, chap. 6

(continued)

Etoposide *(continued)*

Nursing Diagnosis	Defining Characteristics	Expected Outcomes	Nursing Interventions
II. *Potential for infection and bleeding related to bone marrow depression*	II. A. Nadir 7–14 days B. Dose-limiting toxicity C. Granulocytopenia can be severe D. Neutropenia, thrombocytopenia, anemia can all occur E. Recovery 20–22 days	II. A. Pt will be without s/s of infection or bleeding B. Early s/s of infection or bleeding will be identified	II. A. Monitor CBC, platelet count prior to drug administration, and at time of expected nadir B. Assess for s/s of infection and bleeding C. Instruct pt in self-assessment of s/s of infection and bleeding D. Dose reduction may be necessary if compromised bone marrow function, low nadir counts, or hepatic dysfunction E. Refer to sec. on bone marrow depression, chap. 4
III. *Altered nutrition: less than body requirements related to*			
A. Nausea and vomiting	III. A. 1. Usually mild, occurring soon after infusion 2. Intensity and frequency increases with oral dosing and may be severe	III. A. 1. Pt will be without nausea and vomiting 2. If nausea and vomiting occur, they will be minimal	III. A. 1. Premedicate with antiemetics and continue prophylactically for at least 4–6 hrs after drug administration, at least first treatment 2. Encourage small, frequent feedings of cool, bland food and liquids 3. Refer to sec. on nausea and vomiting, chap. 4
B. Anorexia	B. Usually mild but may be severe with oral dosing	B. Pt will maintain baseline weight within ± 5% baseline	B. 1. Encourage small, frequent feedings of favorite foods, especially high-calorie, high-protein foods 2. Encourage use of spices 3. Weekly weights in ambulatory setting
IV. *Body image disturbance related to alopecia*	IV. Incidence 20%–90% depending on dose; regrowth may occur between drug cycles	IV. Pt will verbalize feelings re hair loss, and identify strategies to cope with change in body image	IV. A. Discuss with pt anticipated impact of hair loss—suggest wig as appropriate prior to actual hair loss B. Explore with pt response to hair loss, and whether strategies used to minimize distress (wig, scarf, cap) are effective C. Refer to sec. on alopecia, chap. 4

Nursing Diagnosis	Defining Characteristics	Expected Outcomes	Nursing Interventions
V. Potential for sexual dysfunction	V. A. Drug is teratogenic and embryocidal in rats B. Drug is mutagenic	V. A. Pt and significant other will understand need for contraception B. Pt and significant other will identify strategies to cope with sexual dysfunction	V. A. As appropriate, explore with pt and significant other issues of reproductive and sexual patterns, and expected impact chemotherapy will have B. Discuss strategies to preserve sexuality and reproductive health (i.e., sperm banking, contraception) C. See sec. on gonadal dysfunction, chap. 4
VI. Altered skin integrity related to			
A. Radiation recall	VI. A. Radiation sensitizer: may reactivate skin reactions from prior radiation therapy	VI. A. Skin surface will remain intact or heal following injury	VI. A. 1. Assess skin in area of prior XRT when combined therapies are given 2. Drug may need to be withheld until skin healing occurs if radiation recall results in skin breakdown 3. Wound management based on type of skin reaction
B. Irritation	B. Perivascular irritation may occur if drug extravasates	B. Skin irritation will be minimal	B. 1. Use careful venipuncture techniques, and administer drug over 30–60 mins, diluted as directed by manufacturer 2. Refer to sec. on reactions, chap. 6
VII. Alteration in cardiac output	VII. A. Rare B. Myocardial infarction has been reported after prior mediastinal XRT, and in pts receiving VP-16–containing combination chemotherapy C. Arrhythmias have been reported but are rare	VII. A. Early cardiac dysfunction will be identified	VII. A. Monitor pt closely during treatment, especially if coexisting cardiac dysfunction B. Notify MD of any abnormalities C. Document any irregular cardiac rhythm on EKG D. Refer to sec. on cardiotoxicity, chap. 4

(continued)

Etoposide *(continued)*

Nursing Diagnosis	Defining Characteristics	Expected Outcomes	Nursing Interventions
VIII. *Sensory/perceptual alterations related to neurological toxicities*	VIII. A. Peripheral neuropathies may occur, but are rare and mild	VIII. A. Peripheral neuropathies will be identified early B. Pt will verbalize feelings re discomfort and dysfunction related to neuropathies, and will identify alternate coping strategies	VIII. A. Assess motor and sensory function prior to therapy B. Encourage pt to verbalize feelings re discomfort and sensory loss if these occur C. Assist pt to discuss alternate coping strategies D. Refer to sec. on neurotoxicity, chap. 4

DRUG

Floxuridine (FUDR, 5-FUDR, 5-fluoro-2'-deoxyuridine)

Class: Antimetabolite

MECHANISM OF ACTION

Antimetabolite (fluorinated pyrimidine) which is metabolized to 5-fluorouracil when given by IV bolus, or metabolized to 5-FUDR-MP when smaller doses are given, by continuous infusion intra-arterially. FUDR-MP is four times more effective in inhibiting the enzyme thymidine synthetase than 5-FU, and this prevents the synthesis of thymidine, an essential component of DNA, resulting in interruption of DNA synthesis and cell death. Other FUDR metabolites inhibit RNA synthesis. Drug is cell cycle specific, with activity during the S phase.

METABOLISM

When given IV, drug is transformed to 5-FU. 70%–90% of drug is extracted by liver on first pass. Metabolites are excreted by kidneys and lungs. Continuous infusion decreases metabolisms of drug with more of the drug being converted to the active metabolite FUDR-MP.

DOSAGE/RANGE

Intra-arterially by slow infusion pump: 0.3 mg/kg/day (range 0.1–0.6 mg/kg/day)
or
5–20 mg/m^2/day every day $\times$ 14–21 days

DRUG PREPARATION

Reconstitute 500-mg vial of lyophilized powder with sterile water, then dilute with NS.

DRUG ADMINISTRATION

Usually administered by slow intra-arterial infusion using a surgically placed catheter or percutaneous catheter in a major artery.

SPECIAL CONSIDERATIONS

Drug usually given for 14 days then heparinized saline for 14 days to maintain line patency.

Dose reductions or infusion breaks may be necessary depending on toxicity.

FDA approved for intrahepatic arterial infusion only.

Floxuridine

I. *Altered nutrition: less than body requirements related to*

Nursing Diagnosis	Defining Characteristics	Expected Outcomes	Nursing Interventions
A. Nausea and vomiting	I. A. Occurs infrequently and is mild	I. A. 1. Pt will be without nausea and vomiting 2. Nausea and vomiting, if they occur, will be mild	I. A. 1. Premedicate with antiemetics, and continue prophylactically as needed 2. Instruct pt in self-assessment and self-administration of antiemetics at home 3. Encourage small, frequent feedings of cool, bland foods and liquids 4. If intractable nausea and vomiting occur, stop drug and infuse heparinized saline—*Notify MD* 5. Refer to sec. on nausea and vomiting, chap. 4
B. Anorexia	B. Occurs commonly	B. Pt will maintain baseline weight ±5%	B. 1. Encourage small, frequent feedings of favorite foods, especially high-calorie, high-protein foods 2. Encourage use of spices 3. Weekly weights
C. Stomatitis/esophopharyngitis	C. 1. Milder than 5-FU induced stomatitis when drug is given as hepatic artery infusion 2. More severe when administered intracarotid (external) arterial infusion	C. Oral mucous membranes will remain intact without infection	C. 1. Teach pt oral assessment and mouth care 2. Assess oral mucosa prior to and during therapy 3. Encourage pt to report early stomatitis 4. If stomatitis occurs in pt receiving hepatic artery infusion, stop drug, infuse with heparinized saline, and notify MD 5. Refer to sec. on stomatitis, mucositis, chap. 4

I. D. Diarrhea	I. D. Occurs occasionally and is mild to moderately severe	I. D. Pt will have minimal diarrhea	I. D. 1. Encourage pt to report onset of diarrhea 2. Administer or teach pt to administer antidiarrheal medication 3. Teach pt diet modifications 4. Stop drug and infuse heparinized saline if moderate to severe diarrhea occurs; notify MD 5. Refer to sec. on diarrhea, chap. 4
E. Gastritis	E. 1. Epigastric distress (mild to moderately severe) with abdominal pain and cramping may occur 2. Moderately severe gastritis may occur 3. Incidence greater in pts receiving hepatic artery infusions 4. Duodenal ulcer occurs in 10% of pts, may be painless, and may lead to gastric outlet obstruction and vomiting 5. Biliary sclerosis may occur	E. 1. Gastric distress and injury will be detected early and minimized 2. Gastric complications will be prevented	E. 1. Assess for s/s of abdominal distress, cramping prior to and during infusion 2. Discuss with MD use of antacids and antisecretory agents 3. Stop drug for moderate to severe symptoms, infuse heparinized saline, and notify MD 4. Catheter placement should be verified prior to each infusion cycle, and inadvertent drug infusion into gastric/duodenal-supplying arteries should be investigated

(continued)

Floxuridine *(continued)*

Nursing Diagnosis	Defining Characteristics	Expected Outcomes	Nursing Interventions

I. F. Hepatic dysfunction	I. F. 1. Chemical hepatitis may be severe, with ↑ alkaline phosphatase, liver enzymes, and finally bilirubin
	2. Incidence greater in pts receiving hepatic artery infusions
	3. Drug interruption allows healing of injured hepatocytes
		I. F. 1. Early hepatic dysfunction will be identified
		2. Injury to liver will be temporary
			I. F. 1. Monitor LFTs prior to drug initiation, during therapy, and at end of 14-day cycle
			2. Discuss dose modifications if LFTs are elevated and if symptoms occur:
			  a. If SGOT/SGPT ↑ by 100% at end of 2-week treatment cycle, dose reduced 25% of original dose at next cycle
			  b. If AST increases by 3 ×, hold cycle until AST normal
			3. Assess for s/s of liver dysfunction: lethargy, weakness, malaise, ↓ appetite, fever, presence of jaundice, icterus
			4. Discuss with MD ultrasound study if pt becomes jaundiced to evaluate obstruction versus parenchymal liver injury

II. Infection and bleeding, related to bone marrow depression	II. A. Occurs rarely when FUDR given as single agent by continuous intra-arterial infusion	II. A. Pt will be without s/s of infection or bleeding B. Early s/s of infection or bleeding will be detected	II. A. Monitor CBC, platelet count prior to drug administration, assess for s/s of infection or bleeding B. Instruct pt in self-assessment of s/s of infection or bleeding C. Stop drug if WBC <3500, platelet count <100,000, infuse heparinized saline, and notify MD D. Refer to sec. on bone marrow depression, chap. 4

Nursing Diagnosis		Expected Outcomes	Interventions
III. *Potential for injury, related to intraarterial catheter*	III. A. Catheter-related problems that can occur include 1. Leakage 2. Arterial ischemia or aneurysm 3. Catheter occlusion 4. Bleeding at catheter site 5. Thrombosis or embolism of artery 6. Vessel perforation or dislodgement of catheter 7. Infection 8. Biliary sclerosis	III. A. Catheter-related problems will be identified early B. Further injury will be prevented	III. A. Carefully assess catheter prior to each cycle of therapy: patency, access site of implanted port or pump for s/s of infection or bleeding, and pt comfort during palpation of device and abdomen B. Catheter position and patency should be determined prior to each cycle of chemotherapy (radionucleotide scan) as catheter may migrate and develop clot—flow study will evaluate this C. Do not force flush into catheter if unable to infuse drug or flush solution—reaccess and if still unsuccessful notify MD and arrange for flow study
IV. *Sensory perceptual alterations*	IV. A. Hand and foot syndrome occurs in 30%–40% of pts, characterized by numbness, sensory changes in hands and feet	IV. A. Syndrome will be prevented B. If syndrome occurs, pt will identify strategies to minimize distress	IV. A. Discuss with MD use of pyridoxine 50 mg TID to prevent occurrence of this syndrome B. Assess for occurrence of syndrome, and impact on pt in performing ADLs and level of comfort
V. *Alteration in skin integrity*	V. A. May be manifested as localized erythema, dermatitis, nonspecific skin toxicity, or rash	V. A. Skin will remain intact	V. A. Assess for skin changes B. Assess impact of skin changes on patient: self-image, comfort, ability to perform ADLs C. Treat symptomatically

DRUG

5-Fluorouracil (Fluorouracil, Adrucil, 5-FU, Efudex (topical))

Class: Pyrimidine Antimetabolite

MECHANISM OF ACTION

Acts as a "false" pyrimidine, inhibiting the formation of an enzyme (thymidine synthetase) necessary for the synthesis of DNA. Also incorporates into RNA, causing abnormal synthesis. Methotrexate given prior to 5-Fluorouracil results in synergism and enhanced efficacy.

METABOLISM

Metabolized by the liver, most is excreted as respiratory CO_2; remainder is excreted by the kidneys. Plasma half-life is 20 minutes.

DOSAGE/RANGE

12–15 mg/kg IV once per week
or
12 mg/kg IV every day × 5 days every 4 weeks
or
500 mg/m^2 every week or every week × 5

Hepatic infusion: 22 mg/kg in 100 mL. D_5W infused into hepatic artery over 8 hours for 5–21 consecutive days

Head and neck: 1000 mg/m^2 day × 4–5 days as continuous infusion

DRUG PREPARATION

No dilution required. Can be added to NS or D_5W.

Store at room temperature; protect from light. Solution should be clear: if crystals do not disappear after holding vial under hot water, discard vial.

DRUG ADMINISTRATION

Given IV push or bolus (slow drip), or as continuous infusion.

Topical: as cream.

SPECIAL CONSIDERATIONS

Cutaneous side effects occur, e.g., skin sensitivity to sun, splitting of fingernails, dry flaky skin, and hyperpigmentation on face, palms of hands

Patients who have had adrenalectomy may need higher doses of prednisone while receiving 5-FU or dose of 5-FU may be reduced in postadrenalectomy patients.

Reduce dose in patients with compromised hepatic, renal, or bone marrow function and malnutrition.

Inspect solution for precipitate prior to continuous infusion.

When given with cimetidine there are increased pharmacologic effects of fluorouracil.

When given with thiazide diuretics there is increased risk of myelosuppression.

5-Fluorouracil

I. Altered nutrition: less than body requirements related to

Nursing Diagnosis	Defining Characteristics	Expected Outcomes	Nursing Interventions
A. Nausea and vomiting	I. A. 1. Occur occasionally, may last 2–3 days, usually preventable with antiemetics	I. A. 1. Pt will be without nausea or vomiting 2. Nausea and vomiting, if they occur, will be minimal	I. A. 1. Premedicate with antiemetics and continue prophylactically × 24 hrs to prevent nausea and vomiting, at least with the first treatment 2. Encourage small, frequent feedings of cool, bland foods and liquids 3. Assess for s/s of fluid and electrolyte imbalance: monitor I/O and daily weights if administered in patient 4. Refer to sec. on nausea and vomiting, chap. 4
B. Stomatitis	B. 1. Onset 5–8 days 2. May herald severe bone marrow depression 3. Is an indication to interrupt therapy	B. Oral mucous membranes will remain intact and free of infection	B. 1. Assess mouth prior to each dose: stomatitis is sometimes preceded by a beefy, painful tongue or small, shallow ulcers on the inner lip 2. Report stomatitis to MD; may need to interrupt therapy 3. Teach pt oral assessment and mouth care 4. Use pain relief measures 5. Refer to sec. on stomatitis/mucositis, chap. 4
C. Diarrhea	C. 1. Indication to interrupt treatment 2. May occur with esophagopharyngitis—sore throat with dysphagia	C. 1. Pt will have minimal diarrhea 2. Early s/s of esophagophgaryngitis will be identified and treated	C. 1. Encourage pt to report onset of diarrhea 2. Administer or teach pt to self-administer antidiarrheal medication 3. Guaiac all stools 4. Encourage adequate hydration 5. Refer to sec. on diarrhea, chap. 4 6. Assess pt for sore throat, dysphagia 7. Treat with topical anesthetics

(continued)

5-Fluorouracil (continued)

Nursing Diagnosis	Defining Characteristics	Expected Outcomes	Nursing Interventions
II. *Infection and bleeding, related to bone marrow depression*	II. A. Common B. Neutropenia, thrombocytopenia are most significant C. Nadir 7–14 days after first dose	II. A. Pt will be without s/s of infection or bleeding B. Early s/s of infection or bleeding will be identified	II. A. Monitor CBC, platelet count prior to drug administration as well as s/s of infection and bleeding B. Instruct pt in self-assessment of s/s of infection and bleeding C. Refer to sec. on bone marrow depression, chap. 4
III. *Alteration in skin integrity, related to*			
A. Alopecia	III. A. 1. More common with 5-day courses of treatment. Uncommon with 1-day courses 2. Diffuse thinning, loss of eyelashes and eyebrows	III. A. 1. Pt will verbalize feelings re hair loss, and identify strategies to cope with change in body image	III. A. 1. Assess pt for s/s of hair loss 2. Discuss with pt impact of hair loss, and strategies to minimize distress; i.e, wig, scarf, cap (begin before therapy is initiated) 3. Refer to sec. on alopecia, chap. 4
B. Changes in nails and skin	B. 1. Nail loss and brittle cracking of nails may occur 2. Photosensitivity/photophobia may occur 3. Maculopapular rash sometimes occurs on the extremities and trunk (rarely serious) 4. Chemical phlebitis may occur during continuous infusions related to high pH of drug	B. 1. Pt will verbalize feelings re changes in nails and skin and will identify strategies to cope with changes in body image	B. 1. Assess pt for changes in nails and skin 2. Discuss with pt impact of changes and strategies to minimize distress (e.g., wearing nail polish for women or long sleeve tops) 3. Instruct pt in importance of staying out of sun or wearing sunscreen if sun exposure is unavoidable 4. Assess skin for rash or other changes. Report changes to MD (pt may need antihistamines or steroids) 5. Consider implanted venous access device, and discuss with pt and physician

| IV. *Sensory perceptual alterations* | IV. A. Occasional cerebellar ataxia (reversible when drug is discontinued)
B. Somnolence
C. Ocular changes: conjunctivitis, increased lacrimation, photophobia, oculomotor dysfunction, blurred vision
D. Occasional euphoria | IV. A. Early neurological changes will be identified
B. Pt will identify strategies for coping with neurological changes | IV. A. Assess cerebellar function prior to each treatment
B. Teach pt safety precautions as needed
C. Assess pt for ocular changes. Report changes
D. Refer to sec. on neurotoxicity, chap. 4 |

DRUG

Flutamide (Eulexin)

Class: Antiandrogen

MECHANISM OF ACTION

Antiandrogen which exerts its effect by inhibiting androgen uptake or by inhibiting nuclear binding of androgen in target tissues or both.

METABOLISM

Rapidly and completely absorbed. Excreted mainly via urine. Biologically active metabolite reaches maximum plasma levels in approximately 2 hours. Plasma half-life is 6 hours. Largely plasma bound.

DOSAGE/RANGE

250 mg every 8 hours

DRUG PREPARATION

None (provided in 125-mg tablets)

DRUG ADMINISTRATION

PO

SPECIAL CONSIDERATIONS

None

Flutamide (Eulexin)

Nursing Diagnosis	Defining Characteristics	Expected Outcomes	Nursing Interventions
I. *Alteration in comfort*	I. A. Hot flashes occur commonly	I. A. 1. Pt will be without hot flashes B. Discomfort will be identified and treated early	I. A. Inform pt that hot flashes may occur B. Encourage pt to report symptoms early
II. *Sexual dysfunction*	II. A. Causes decreased libido and impotence in about a third of pts B. Gynecomastia occurs in about 10% of pts	II. A. 1. Pt and significant other will verbalize understanding of changes in sexuality and body image that may occur	II. A. As appropriate, explore with pt and significant other issues of reproductive and sexuality patterns and the impact that chemotherapy may have on them B. Discuss strategies to preserve sexuality and reproductive health C. See sec. on gonadal dysfunction, chap. 4
III. *Altered nutrition: less than body requirements related to*			
A. Diarrhea	III. A. Occurs in about 10% of pts	III. A. 1. Pt will have minimal diarrhea	III. A. 1. Encourage pt to report onset of diarrhea 2. Administer or teach pt to self-administer antidiarrheals 3. Guaiac stools 4. Refer to sec. on diarrhea, chap. 4
B. Nausea and vomiting	B. Occurs in about 10% of pts	B. 1. Pt will be without nausea and vomiting 2. Nausea and vomiting, should they occur, will be minimal	B. 1. Inform pt of possibility of nausea and vomiting. Obtain prescription for antiemetic if necessary 2. Encourage small, frequent feedings of cool, bland foods 3. Refer to sec. on nausea and vomiting, chap. 4

DRUG

Hexamethylmelamine (HXM, Altretamine)

Class: Alkylating agent

MECHANISM OF ACTION

The exact mechanism of action is unknown. May inhibit incorporation of thymidine and uridine into DNA and RNA, respectively. Hexamethylmelamine is felt not to act as an alkylating agent *in vitro*, but it may be activated to an alkylating agent in the body *in vivo*. Also may act as an antimetabolite with activity in S-phase.

METABOLISM

Well absorbed orally although bioavailability is variable. Peak plasma concentration in 1 hour. Metabolized extensively in the liver, with majority excreted in the urine. Some of the drug is excreted as respiratory CO_2. Half-life of the parent compound 4.7–10.2 hours.

DOSAGE/RANGE

4–12 mg/kg/day (divided in 3 or 4 doses) $\times$ 21–90 days
or
240 mg/m^2 (6 mg/kg)–320 mg/m^2 (8 mg/kg) daily $\times$ 21 days, repeated every 6 weeks

DRUG PREPARATION

Available in 50-mg and 100-mg capsules from the National Cancer Institute (NCI).

DRUG ADMINISTRATION

Oral

SPECIAL CONSIDERATIONS

Nausea and vomiting can be minimized if patient takes dose 2 hours after meal and at bedtime.

Vitamin B$_6$ may be administered concurrently to decrease neurological complications.

Nadir 3 to 4 weeks after treatment.

Hexamethylmelamine

Nursing Diagnosis	Defining Characteristics	Expected Outcomes	Nursing Interventions
I. Infection and bleeding, related to bone marrow depression	I. A. Mild bone marrow depression B. Nadir 21–28 days after beginning treatment C. Rapid recovery within 1 week of drug discontinuance	I. A. Pt will be without s/s of infection or bleeding B. Early s/s of infection or bleeding will be identified	I. A. Monitor CBC, platelet count prior to drug administration, as well as s/s of infection and bleeding B. Instruct pt in self-assessment of s/s of infection and bleeding C. Refer to sec. on bone marrow depression, chap. 4
II. Altered nutrition: less than body requirements related to			
A. Nausea and vomiting	II. A. 1. Nausea occurs in 50%–70% of pts and is dose-dependent 2. Tolerance may develop, usually after at least 3 weeks	II. A. 1. Pt will be without nausea and vomiting 2. Nausea and vomiting, if they occur, will be minimal	II. A. 1. Premediate with antiemetics and continue throughout therapy as needed (tolerance may develop after 3 weeks). Teach pt self-administration 2. If nausea occurs, encourage small, frequent feedings of cool, bland foods 3. Divide daily dose into 4 parts and give 1–2 hours pc and at bedtime 4. Refer to sec. on nausea and vomiting, chap. 4
B. Diarrhea and abdominal cramps	B. Gastrointestinal effects often dose-limiting	B. 1. Pt will have minimal diarrhea 2. Pt will develop strategies to minimize discomfort from cramps	B. 1. Encourage pt to report onset of diarrhea 2. Administer or instruct pt in self-administration of antidiarrheal medication 3. Refer to sec. on diarrhea, chap. 4 4. Discuss possible strategies to decrease distress from cramping: heat, position change
C. Anorexia	C. Anorexia has been noted as a side effect in clinical trials	C. Pt will maintain baseline weight ± 5%	C. 1. Encourage small, frequent feedings of favorite foods, especially high-calorie, high-protein foods 2. Encourage use of spices 3. Weekly weights

(continued)

Hexamethylmelamine (continued)

Nursing Diagnosis	Defining Characteristics	Expected Outcomes	Nursing Interventions
III. *Sensory/perceptual alterations related to*			
A. Peripheral neuropathies	III. A. 1. Rarely occur, 5% incidence 2. *Sensory and motor:* paresthesia, hypersthesia, hyperreflexia, and numbness may occur and are reversible with drug discontinuance	III. A. 1. Pt will report alterations in sensation, perception	III. A. 1. Instruct pt that these may occur, and to report s/s of sensory/perceptual alterations, if these occur 2. Discuss with physician initiating *pyridoxine* 100 mg TID when hexamethylmelamine is begun to prevent or minimize these side effects 3. If these changes occur, discuss drug discontinuance with MD
B. CNS effects	B. 1. Agitation, confusion, hallucinations, depression and Parkinson-like symptoms may occur, and usually resolve after discontinuance of therapy 2. More common with continuous (>3 mos) therapy than with pulse-dosing regimens	B. Neurological s/s will be minimized	B. 1. Coinsider that hexamethylmelamine may exacerbate the neurotoxicity of other chemotherapy agents; e.g. vinca alkaloids 2. Refer to sec. on neurotoxicity, chap. 4
IV. *Alteration in skin integrity*	IV. Skin rashes, pruritus, eczematous skin lesions may occur but are rare	IV. A. Skin will remain intact B. Early s/s of alterations in skin integrity will be identified	IV. A. Assess for changes in skin color, texture, and integrity B. Teach pt self-assessment of skin, and to report these changes C. Assess type of discomfort that exists, and develop strategy to provide symptom relief

DRUG

Hydroxyurea (Hydrea)

Class: Miscellaneous/Antimetabolite

MECHANISM OF ACTION

Antimetabolite that prevents conversion of ribonucleotides to deoxyribonucleotides by inhibiting the converting enzyme ribonucleoside diphosphate reductase. DNA synthesis is thus inhibited. Cell cycle phase specific—S phase. May also sensitize cells to the effects of radiation therapy, although the process is not clearly understood.

METABOLISM

Rapidly absorbed from gastrointestinal tract. Peak plasma level reached in 2 hours, with plasma half-life of 3–4 hours. About half the drug is metabolized in the liver, half excreted in urine as urea and unchanged drug. Some of the drug is eliminated as respiratory CO_2. Crosses blood–brain barrier.

DOSAGE/RANGE

500–3000 mg orally daily (dose reduced in renal dysfunction)

25 mg/kg orally as a continuous dose

100 mg/kg IV daily $\times$ 3 days

DRUG PREPARATION

None. Available in 500 mg capsules.

DRUG ADMINISTRATION

Oral

SPECIAL CONSIDERATIONS

Hydroxyurea has a side effect of dramatically lowering the WBC in a relatively short period of time (24–48 hours). In leukemia patients endangered by the potential complication of leukostasis, this is the desired effect.

May need to pretreat with allopurinal to protect patient from tumor lysis syndrome.

Dermatologic radiation recall phenomena may occur.

In combination with radiation therapy, mucosal reactions in the radiation field may be severe.

Hydroxyurea

Nursing Diagnosis	Defining Characteristics	Expected Outcomes	Nursing Interventions
I. Infection and bleeding related to bone marrow depression	I. A. Leukopenia more common than thrombocytopenia B. WBC may start dropping in 24–48 hours. Nadir seen in 10 days with recovery within 10–30 days C. Severity of leukopenia is dose related	I. A. Pt will be without s/s of infection or bleeding B. Early s/s of infection or bleeding will be identified	I. A. Monitor CBC, platelet count prior to drug administration, as well as s/s of infection or bleeding B. Instruct pt in self-assessment of s/s of infection or bleeding C. Drug dosage may be titrated for higher or lower than normal blood values D. See sec. on bone marrow depression, chap. 4
II. Altered nutrition: less than body requirements related to			
A. Anorexia	II. A. Mild to moderate	II. A. Pt will maintain baseline weight ±5%	II. A. 1. Encourage small, frequent feedings of favorite foods, especially high-calorie, high-protein foods 2. Encourage use of spices 3. Weekly weights
B. Stomatitis	B. Uncommon	B. Oral mucous membranes will remain intact without infection	B. 1. Teach pt oral assessment and mouth care 2. Encourage pt to report early stomatitis 3. Teach pt oral hygiene 4. See sec. on stomatitis/mucositis, chap. 4
C. Diarrhea	C. Uncommon	C. Pt will have minimal diarrhea	C. 1. Encourage pt to report onset of diarrhea 2. Administer or teach pt to self-administer antidiarrheal medications 3. See sec. on diarrhea, chap. 4
D. Hepatic dysfunction	D. Hepatitis is rare, but may occur; there are also disturbances in liver function studies	D. Hepatic dysfunction will be identified early	D. 1. Monitor SGOT, SGPT, LDH, alkaline phosphatase and bilirubin periodically during treatment 2. Notify MD of any elevations

III. *Alteration in skin integrity, related to*

A. Alopecia	III. A. Uncommon though may be slight to diffuse thinning	III. A. Pt will verbalize feelings re hair loss, and identify strategies to cope with changes in body image	III. A. 1. Assess pt for s/s of hair loss 2. Discuss with pt impact of hair loss and strategies to minimize distress; i.e., wig, scarf, cap (begin before therapy is initiated) 3. See sec. on alopecia, chap. 4
B. Dermatitis	B. 1. Dermatitis is uncommon, usually mild and reversible 2. Symptoms may include facial erythema, rash, pruritus 3. Rarely, post–irradiation therapy erythema (recall) may occur	B. 1. Skin will remain intact 2. Early skin impairment will be identified	B. 1. Assess skin integrity 2. If dermatitis severe, discuss drug discontinuance with MD 3. Topical medications as appropriate 4. Radiation recall occurs when hydroxyurea is administered during or after irradiation therapy and may occur weeks or months after therapy
IV. *Alteration in renal function related to chemotherapy (rare)*	IV. Reversible renal tubular dysfunction evidenced by elevated BUN, creatinine, and uric acid levels	IV. Pt will be without renal dysfunction	IV. A. Monitor BUN and creatinine prior to drug dose as half of drug is excreted unchanged in urine B. Provide or instruct pt in hydration of *at least* 2–3 L of fluid/day during and for at least 48 hours after therapy C. Monitor I/O D. Weekly weights E. Refer to sec. on nephrotoxicity, chap. 4

(continued)

Hydroxyurea *(continued)*

Nursing Diagnosis	Defining Characteristics	Expected Outcomes	Nursing Interventions
V. *Potential for sexual/ reproductive dysfunction*	V. A. Gonadal function and fertility are affected (may be permanent or transient) B. Reported to be excreted in breast milk	V. A. Pt and significant other will understand need for contraception B. Pt and significant other will identify strategies to cope with sexual and reproductive dysfunction	V. A. As appropriate, explore with pt and significant other issues of reproductive and sexuality patterns and impact chemotherapy will have B. Discuss strategies to preserve sexuality and reproductive health (i.e., contraception, sperm banking) C. See sec. on gonadal dysfunction, chap. 4
VI. *Sensory/perceptual alterations*	VI. A. S/s may include disorientation, drowsiness, headache, vertigo B. Symptoms usually do not last more than 24 hours	VI. A. Mental status changes and other disturbances will be identified early	VI. A. Obtain baseline mental status—neurological function B. Assess status changes during chemotherapy C. Encourage pt to report any changes

DRUG

Idarubicin (DMDR, 4 Demethoxydaunorubicin)

Class: Investigational (antitumor antibiotic)

MECHANISM OF ACTION

Cell cycle phase specific for S phase.

Analog of daunorubicin. Has a marked inhibitory effect on RNA synthesis.

METABOLISM

Excreted primarily in the bile and urine, with approximately 25% of the intravenous dose accounted for over 5 days.

The halflife of this agent is 6–9.4 hours.

DOSAGE/RANGE

Drug is undergoing clinical trials; consult individual protocol for specific dosages.

DRUG PREPARATION

Available as a red powder. The drug is reconstituted with Normal Saline injection.

DRUG ADMINISTRATION

Drug is a vesicant. Administer IV push over 10 to 15 minutes into the side arm of a freely running IV.

SPECIAL CONSIDERATIONS

Vesicant.

Discolored urine (pink to red) may occur up to 48 hours after administration.

Cardiomyopathy is less common and less severe than with doxorubicin and daunorubicin.

Drug is light sensitive.

Idarubicin

Nursing Diagnosis	Defining Characteristics	Expected Outcomes	Nursing Interventions
I. *Infection and bleeding, related to bone marrow depression*	I. A. Hematologic toxicity is dose limiting B. Leukopenia nadir 10–20 days with recovery in 1–2 weeks C. Thrombocytopenia usually follows leukopenia and is mild D. BM toxicity is not cumulative	I. A. Pt will be without s/s of infection or bleeding B. Early s/s of infection or bleeding will be identified	I. A. Monitor CBC, platelet count prior to drug administration as well as s/s of infection or bleeding B. Instruct pt in self-assessment of s/s of infection or bleeding C. Dose modifications often necessary (35%–50%) if compromised bone marrow function D. See sec. on bone marrow depression, chap. 4
II. *Altered nutrition: less than body requirements related to* A. Nausea and vomiting	II. A. Usually mild to moderate, though nausea and vomiting are seen to some degree in most patients	II. A. 1. Pt will be without nausea and vomiting 2. Nausea and vomiting, if they occur, will be minimal	II. A. 1. Premediate with antiemetics and continue prophylactically × 24 hrs to *prevent* nausea and vomiting at least first treatment 2. Encourage small, frequent feedings of cool, bland foods and liquids 3. Refer to sec. on nausea and vomiting, chap. 4
B. Anorexia	B. Commonly occurs	B. Pt will maintain baseline weight ±5%	B. 1. Encourage small, frequent feedings of favorite foods, especially high-calorie, high-protein foods 2. Encourage use of spices 3. Weekly weights
C. Stomatitis	C. Mild	C. Oral mucous membranes will remain intact without infection	C. 1. Teach pt oral assessment and mouth care 2. Encourage pt to report early stomatitis 3. Teach pt oral hygiene 4. See sec. on stomatitis, chap. 4

II. D. Diarrhea	II. D. Infrequent and mild	II. D. Pt will have minimal diarrhea	II. D. 1. Encourage pt to report onset of diarrhea 2. Administer or teach pt to self-administer antidiarrheal medications 3. See sec. on diarrhea, chap. 4
E. Hepatitic dysfunction	E. Hepatitis is rare but may occur 2. There are also disturbances in liver function studies	E. Hepatic dysfunction will be identified early	E. 1. Monitor SGOT, SGPT, LDH, alkaline phosphatase, and bilirubin periodically during treatment 2. Notify MD of any elevations

III. *Alteration in skin integrity, related to*

A. Alopecia	III. A. 1. Occurs in about 30% of pts after oral drug and can be partial after IV drug 2. Begins after 3 + weeks and hair may grow back while on therapy 3. May be slight to diffuse thinning	III. A. Pt will verbalize feelings re hair loss and identify strategies to cope with change in body image	III. A. 1. Assess pt for s/s of hair loss 2. Discuss with pt impact of hair loss and strategies to minimize distress; i.e., wigs, scarf, cap (begin before therapy is initiated) 3. See sec. on alopecia, chap. 4
B. Skin changes: darkening of nail beds, skin ulcer/necrosis, sensitivity to sunlight, skin itching at irradiated areas	B. Skin changes seen as hyperpigmentation of nail beds, sensitivity to sunlight, radiation recall, and potential necrosis with extravasation	B. 1. Skin will remain intact 2. Early skin impairment will be identified	B. 1. Assess skin for integrity 2. If severe, discuss drug discontinuance with MD 3. Assess pt for changes in skin, nails 4. Discuss with pt impact of changes and strategies to minimize distress; i.e., wearing nail polish (women), long sleeved tops

(continued)

Idarubicin (continued)

Nursing Diagnosis	Defining Characteristics	Expected Outcomes	Nursing Interventions
			III. B. 5. Administer according to policies for vesicant drugs
			a. Careful technique is used during venipuncture. See sec. on intravenous administration, chap. 7
			b. Administer vesicant through freely flowing IV, constantly monitoring IV site and pt response
			c. Nurse should be THOROUGHLY familiar with institutional policy and procedure for administration of a vesicant agent
			d. If vesicant drug is administered as a continuous infusion, drug must be given through a patent central line
			e. If extravasation is suspected:
			1) stop drug administered
			2) aspirate any residual drug and blood from IV tubing, IV catheter/needle, and IV site if possible
			3) instill antidote into area of apparent infiltration, IF ANTIDOTE EXISTS, as per MD orders and institutional policy and procedure
			4) apply cold or topical medication as per MD order and institutional policy and procedure
			f. Assess site regularly for pain, progression of erythema, induration, and for evidence of necrosis

III. B. 5. g. When in doubt about whether drug is infiltrating, TREAT AS AN INFILTRATION

h. Teach pt to assess site and notify MD if condition worsens

i. Arrange next clinic visit for assessment of site depending on drug, amount infiltrated, extent of potential injury, and pt variables

j. Document in pt's record as per institutional policy and procedure. See sec. on reactions, chap. 6

IV. *Alteration in cardiac output, related to cumulative doses of Idarubicin*	IV. A. Cardiac toxicity is similar characteristically but less severe than that seen with daunorubicin and doxorubicin B. CHF due to cardiomyopathy seen after large cumulative doses	IV. Early s/s of cardiomyopathy will be identified	IV. A. Assess pt for s/s of cardiomyopathy B. Obtain baseline cardiac functions (EKG changes uncommon) C. Discuss GBPS with MD D. Assess quality and regularity of heartbeat E. Instruct pt to report dyspnea, shortness of breath F. Teach pt the potential of irreversible CHF with cumulative dosages G. Refer to sec. on cardiotoxicity, chap. 4

DRUG

Ifosfamide (IFEX)

Class: Alkalating agent

MECHANISM OF ACTION

Analogue of cyclophosphamide and is cell cycle phase nonspecific. Destroys DNA throughout the cell cycle by binding to protein and DNA cross-linking with DNA, and causing chain scission as well as inhibition of DNA synthesis. Ifosfamide has been shown to be effective in tumors previously resistant to cyclophosphamide. Activated by microsomes in the liver.

METABOLISM

Only about 50% of the drug is metabolized with much of the drug excreted in the urine almost completely unchanged. Half-life is 13.8 hours for high dose versus 3–10 hours for lower doses.

DOSAGE/RANGE

IV bolus/push: 50 mg/kg/day
  or 2 g/m^2/day × 5 days
  or 2400 mg/m^2/day × 3 days
Continuous infusion: 1200 mg/m^2/day × 5 days
Single dose: 5000 mg/m^2
Dose-limiting toxicity has been renal and bladder dysfunction.

DRUG PREPARATION

Available as a powder and should be reconstituted with sterile water for injection.
Solution is chemically stable for 7 days but discard after 8 hours due to lack of bacteriostatic preservative of the solution.
May be diluted further in either D$_5$W or normal saline.

DRUG ADMINISTRATION

IV bolus—administer over 30 minutes.
Continuous infusion—administer intravenously for 5 days. Mesna should be administered with ifosfamide: it is begun simultaneously with the drug and repeated at 4 and 8 hours after the ifosfamide. (See drug sheet on mesna.) Mesna, ascorbic acid, and Mucomyst have been utilized to protect the bladder. Pre- and posthydration (1500–2000 cc/day) or continuous bladder irrigations are recommended to prevent hemorrhagic cystitis.

SPECIAL CONSIDERATIONS

Metabolic toxicity is increased by simultaneous administration of barbiturates.
Activity and toxicity of the drug may be altered by allopurinol, chloroquine, phenothiazides, potassium iodide, chloramphenicol, imipramine, vitamin A, corticosteroids, and succinylcholine.
Nausea and vomiting (moderate to severe) beginning 3–6 hours after administration is seen in approximately 50% of patients.
Renal function—BUN, serum creatinine, and creatinine clearance must be determined prior to treatment.
Leukopenia is mild to moderate, with rare thrombocytopenia and anemia.
Therapy requires the concomitant administration of a uroprotector such as mesna and pre- and posthydration; may also require catheterization and constant bladder irrigation, and/or ascorbic acid.
Test urine for occult blood.

Ifosfamide

Nursing Diagnosis	Defining Characteristics	Expected Outcomes	Nursing Interventions
I. *Altered urinary elimination*			
A. Hemorrhagic cystitis	I. A. 1. Symptoms of bladder irritation 2. Hemorrhagic cystitis with hematuria, dysuria, urinary frequency 3. Preventable with uroprotection and hydration	I. A. 1. Pt will be without hemorrhagic cystitis 2. Hemorrhagic cystitis, if it occurs, will be detected early	I. A. 1. Assess presence of RBC in urine prior to successive doses, especially if symptoms are present, as well as BUN and creatinine 2. Administer drug with concomitant uroprotector, e.g., mesna 3. Encourage *prehydration:* PO intake of 2–3 L/day prior to chemotherapy; *posthydration:* increase po fluids to 2–3 L for 2 days after chemotherapy 4. If possible, administer drug in morning to minimize drug accumulation in bladder during sleep 5. Instruct pt to empty bladder every 2–3 hours, before bedtime, and during night when awake 6. Monitor urinary output and total body balance
B. Renal toxicity	B. 1. Symptoms of renal toxicity 2. ↑ BUN, ↑ serum creatinine, ↓ urine creatinine clearance (usually reversible) 3. Acute tubular necrosis, pyelonephritis, glomerular dysfunction 4. Metabolic acidosis	B. Renal dysfunction will be identified early	B. 1. Assess urinary elimination pattern prior to each drug dose 2. If rigorous regimen is adhered to, minimal renal toxicity will result 3. Monitor BUN and creatinine

(continued)

Ifosfamide (continued)

Nursing Diagnosis	Defining Characteristics	Expected Outcomes	Nursing Interventions
II. Altered nutrition: less than body requirements			
A. Nausea and vomiting	II. A. 1. Nausea and vomiting occur in 58% of pts 2. Dose and schedule dependent with ↑ severity with higher dose and rapid injection 3. Occurs within a few hours of drug administration and may last 3 days	II. A. 1. Pt will be without nausea and vomiting 2. Nausea and vomiting, if they occur, will be minimal	II. A. 1. Premedicate with antiemetics and continue prophylactically to *prevent* nausea and vomiting for 24 hours at least first treatment 2. Encourage small, frequent feedings of cool, bland foods and liquids 3. Refer to sec. on nausea and vomiting, chap. 4
B. Hepatotoxicity	B. 1. Elevations of serum transaminate and alkaline phosphatase may occur 2. Usually transient and resolve spontaneously 3. No apparent sequelae	B. Early hepatotoxicity will be identified	B. Monitor LFTs (liver function tests) during treament
III. *Infection and bleeding, related to bone marrow depression*	III. A. Leukopenia is mild to moderate B. Thrombocytopenia and anemia are rare C. Dosage adjustment may be necessary when ifosfamide is combined with other chemotherapy agents D. Pts at risk for BMD: pts with impaired renal function, and ↓ bone marrow reserve (bone marrow metastases, prior XRT)	III. A. Pt will be without s/s of infection or bleeding B. Early s/s of infection or bleeding will be identified	III. A. Monitor CBC, platelet count prior to drug administration, as well as s/s of infection or bleeding B. Instruct pt in self-assessment of s/s of infection or bleeding C. Dose reduction may be necessary when given in combination with other agents causing BMD D. Refer to sec. on bone marrow depression, chap. 4

IV. Alteration in skin integrity, related to

A. Alopecia	IV. A. A. Incidence 83%, with 50% experiencing severe hair loss in 2–4 weeks	IV. A. A. Pt will verbalize feelings re hair loss and identify strategies to cope with change in body image	IV. A. 1. Discuss with pt anticipated impact of hair loss; suggest wig, as appropriate, prior to actual hair loss 2. Explore with pt response to hair loss, and alternative strategies to minimize distress 3. See sec. on alopecia, chap. 4 B. Carefully monitor injection site during drug administration, infusion for s/s of phlebitis, irritation, vein patency
B. Sterile phlebitis at injection site; irritation with extravasation	B. 1. Drug is not activated until it reaches hepatic microsomes, so drug doesn't cause tissue damage (is not a vesicant). Incidence <2%	B. 1. Skin injury will be prevented 2. Early injury will be identified	
C. Skin changes	C. 1. Skin hyperpigmentation, dermatitis, nail ridging may occur	C. 1. Early skin impairment will be identified 2. Pt will verbalize feelings re changes in nail or skin color or texture and identify strategies to cope with change in body image	C. 1. Assess skin integrity 2. Assess impact of skin changes on body image 3. Discuss strategies to minimize distress

(continued)

Ifosfamide (*continued*)

Nursing Diagnosis	Defining Characteristics	Expected Outcomes	Nursing Interventions
V. *Sensory/perceptual alterations: confusion, activity intolerance, fatigue*	V. A. Intact drug passes easily into CNS, however *active* metabolites do not B. Lethargy and confusion may be seen with high doses, lasting 1–8 hours, usually spontaneously reversible C. CNS side effects occur in about 12% of pts treated including somnolence, confusion, depressive psychosis, hallucinations D. Less frequent S/E dizziness, disorientation, cranial nerve dysfunction, seizures E. Incidence of CNS side effects may be higher in pts with compromised renal function, as well as in pts receiving high dose	V. A. Neurologic alterations will be identified early B. Pt and family will manage distress safely	V. A. Identify pts at risk (↓ renal function) and observe closely B. Assess neurological and mental status prior to and during drug administration and on follow-up C. Instruct pt to report any alterations in behavior, sensation, perception D. Develop a plan of care with pt and family if side effects develop to manage distress and promote safety
VI. *Potential for sexual dysfunction*	VI. A. Drug is carcinogenic, mutagenic, and teratogenic B. Drug is excreted in breast milk	VI. A. Pt and significant other will understand need for contraception B. Pt and significant other will identify strategies to cope with sexual dysfunction	VI. A. As appropriate, explore with pt and significant other issues of reproductive and sexual patterns, and impact chemotherapy will have B. Discuss strategies to preserve sexuality, and reproductive health (i.e., sperm banking, contraception) C. See sec. on gonadal dysfunction, chap. 4

DRUG

L-asparaginase (EISPAR)

Class: Miscellaneous agents (Enzyme)

MECHANISM OF ACTION

Hydrolysis of serum asparagine occurs which deprives leukemia cells of the required amino acid. Normal cells are spared because they generally have the ability to synthesize their own asparagine.

Cell cycle specific for G_1 postmitotic phase.

Some leukemic cells are unable to synthesize asparagine. These cells must obtain asparagine from an exogenous source, the patient's serum. Administration of the enzyme L-asparaginase causes hydrolysis of asparagine to aspartate, resulting in rapid depletion of the asparagine concentration in the patient's serum.

METABOLISM

Metabolism of L-asparaginase is independent of renal and hepatic function. The drug is not recovered in the urine and does not appear to cross the blood–brain barrier.

DOSAGE/RANGE

IM or IV varies with protocol

DRUG PREPARATION

IV Injection: Reconstitute with sterile water for injection or sodium chloride injection (without preservative) and use within 8 hours of restoration.

IV Infusion: Dilute with sodium chloride injection or 5% dextrose injection and use within 8 hours, only if clear; if gelatinous particles develop, filter through a 5.0-micron filter.

The lyophilized powder must be stored under refrigeration. The reconstituted solution must also be stored under refrigeration if it is not used immediately. The solution must be discarded within 8 hours after preparation.

DRUG ADMINISTRATION

Use in a hospital setting. Make preparations to treat anaphylaxis at each administration of the drug.

SPECIAL CONSIDERATIONS

Potential reduction in antineoplastic effect of methotrexate when given in combination.

Anaphylaxis is associated with the administration of this drug.

Intravenous administration of L-asparaginase concurrently with or immediately before prednisone and vincristine administration may be associated with increased toxicity.

L-asparaginase

Nursing Diagnosis	Defining Characteristics	Expected Outcomes	Nursing Interventions

I. *Potential for injury, related to hypersensitivity or anaphylaxis reactions*	I. A. Occurs in 20%–35% of pts
	B. Increased incidence after several doses administered but may occur with first dose
	C. Occurs less often with IM route of administration
	D. May be life threatening reaction, but usually mild
	  1. Urticarial eruptions
	  2. Fever (100°–101°F) seen in half of pts
	  3. Chills
	  4. Facial redness
	  5. Hypotension
	  6. Shortness of breath
	  7. Hives
	  8. Diaphoresis
		I. Early s/s of hypersensitivity or anaphylactic reactions will be identified	I. A. Teach pt of the potential of a hypersensitivity or anaphylaxis reaction and to immediately report any unusual symptoms
			B. Obtain baseline vital signs and note pt's mental status
			C. Skin testing, prior to administering full dose, is recommended by manufacturer
			D. Assess pt for at least 30 mins after the drug is given for s/s of a reaction. See sec. on reactions, chap. 6
			E. 1. Administer therapy according to MD orders
			  2. Review standing orders for management of pt in anaphylaxis and identify location of anaphylaxis kit containing epinephrine 1:1000, hydrocortisone sodium succinate (Solucortef), diphenhydramine HCl (Benadryl), Aminophylline, and others
			  3. Observe for following s/s during infusion usually occurring within first 15 mins of start of infusion:
			  Subjective
			  generalized itching
			  nausea
			  chest tightness
			  crampy abdominal pain
			  difficulty speaking
			  anxiety
			  agitation
			  sense of impending doom
			  uneasiness
			  desire to urinate/defecate
			  dizziness
			  chills

I. E. 3. *Objective*
flushed appearance (angioedema of face, neck, eyelids, hands, feet)
localized or generalized urticaria
respiratory distress ± wheezing
hypotension
cyanosis
4. If reaction occurs, stop infusion and notify MD
5. Place pt in supine position to promote perfusion of visceral organs
6. Monitor vital signs until stable
7. Provide emotional reassurance to pt and family
8. Maintain patent airway, and have CPR equipment ready if needed
9. Document incident
10. Discuss with MD desensitization versus drug discontinuance for further dosing
F. *Escherichia coli* preparation of L-asparaginase and *Erwinia carotovora* preparation are non–cross resistant so if an anaphylaxis reaction occurs with one, the other preparation may be used

II. *Altered nutrition: less than body requirements related to*
A. Nausea and vomiting

II. A. 1. 50%–60% of pts experience mild to severe nausea and vomiting starting within 4–6 hrs after treatment

II. A. 1. Pt will be without nausea and vomiting
2. Nausea and vomiting, if they occur, will be minimal

II. A. 1. Premedicate with antiemetics and continue prophylactically × 24 hrs to *prevent* nausea and vomiting
2. Encourage small, frequent feedings of cool, bland foods and liquids
3. Refer to sec. on nausea and vomiting, chap. 4

(continued)

L-asparaginase (*continued*)

Nursing Diagnosis	Defining Characteristics	Expected Outcomes	Nursing Interventions
II. B. Anorexia	II. B. Commonly occurs	II. B. Pt will maintain baseline weight ±5%	II. B. 1. Encourage small, frequent feedings of favorite foods, especially high-calorie, high-protein foods 2. Encourage use of spices 3. Weekly weights
C. Hyperglycemia	C. 1. Transient reaction caused by effects on the pancreas 2. ↓ insulin synthesis 3. Pancreatitis in 5% of pts	C. 1. Pt will be without s/s of hypergly-cemia or pancreatitis 2. Early s/s of hyperglycemia or pancreatitis will be identified	C. 1. Teach pt of the potential of hyperglycemia and pancreatitis and to report any unusual symptoms; i.e., increased thirst, urination, and appetite 2. Monitor serum glucose, amylase and lipase levels periodically during treatment 3. Report any laboratory elevations to MD 4. Treat hyperglycemia issues with diet or insulin as ordered by MD 5. Treat pancreatitis per MD orders
III. *Hepatic dysfunction or thromboembolic potential*	III. A. Two-thirds of pts have elevated LFTs starting within first 2 weeks of treatment; i.e., SGOT, bilirubin, and alkaline phosphatase B. Hepatically derived clotting factors may be depressed resulting in excessive bleeding or blood clotting. Relatively uncommon	III. A. Hepatic dysfunction will be identified early	III. A. Monitor SGOT, bilirubin, alkaline phosphatase, albumin, and clotting factors—PT, PTT, librinogen B. Teach pt of the potential of excessive bleeding or blood clotting and to report any unusual symptoms C. Assess pt for s/s of bleeding or thrombosis

Nursing Diagnosis	Defining Characteristics	Expected Outcomes	Nursing Interventions
IV. *Mental status alteration*	IV. A. 25% of pts experience some changes in mental status—commonly lethargy, drowsiness, and somnolence, rarely coma B. Predominately seen in adults C. Malaise ("Blahs") occur in most pts and generally gets worse with subsequent doses D. Drug does not cross blood–brain barrier	IV. A. Pt will be without changes in mental status, e.g., depression	IV. A. Teach pt of the potential of CNS toxicity and to report any unusual symptoms B. Obtain baseline neurologic and mental function C. Assess pt for any neurologic abnormalities and report changes to MD D. Discuss with pt the impact of malaise of his/her general sense of well-being and strategies to minimize the distress
V. *Alteration in mobility, related to soreness at injection site*	V. A. Pt may complain of sore muscle at injection site	V. A. Pt will not complain of altered mobility due to sore muscles	V. A. Rotate injection sites to decrease potential for soreness B. Utilize standard nursing practice for IM injections
VI. *Infection, bleeding, and fatigue, related to bone marrow depression*	VI. A. Bone marrow suppression is not common B. Mild anemia may occur C. Serious leukopenia and thrombocytopenia are rare	VI. A. Pt will be without s/s of infection, bleeding, or anemia B. Early s/s of infection, bleeding, or anemia will be identified	VI. A. Monitor CBC, platelet count prior to drug administration, as well as s/s of infection, bleeding, or anemia B. Instruct pt in self-assessment of s/s of infection, bleeding, or anemia C. Refer to sec. on bone marrow depression, chap. 4
VII. *Potential for sexual dysfunction*	VII. A. Drug is teratogenic	VII. A. Pt and significant other will understand need for contraception	VII. A. As appropriate, explore with pt and significant other issues of reproductive and sexual patterns, and impact chemotherapy will have B. Discuss strategies to preserve sexuality and reproductive health (i.e., sperm banking, contraception) C. See sec. on gonadal dysfunction, chap. 4

DRUG

Leucovorin calcium (Folinic acid, Citrovorum factor)

Class: Water soluble vitamin in the folate group (Folinic acid)

MECHANISM OF ACTION

Acts as an antidote for methotrexate and other folic acid antagonists. Circumvents the biochemical block of the enzyme inhibiters (e.g., dihydrofolate reductase [DHFR]) to permit DNA and RNA synthesis.

METABOLISM

Metabolized primarily in the liver. 50% of the single dose is excreted in 6 hours in the urine (80%–90% of dose) and stool (8% of dose).

DOSAGE/RANGE

Dose of drug and duration of rescue is dependent on serum methotrexate levels.

MTX Level	Leucovorin
$< 5.0(10)^{-7}M$	10 mg/m^2 every 6 hours
$5(10)^{-7}M$–$5(10)^{-6}M$	30–40 mg/m^2 every 6 hours
$> 5(10)^{-6}M$	100 mg/m^2 every 3–6 hours

DRUG PREPARATION

Drug is supplied in ampules or vials.

Reconstitute vials with sterile water for injection.

Dilute reconstituted vials or ampules further with D$_5$W or Normal Saline.

DRUG ADMINISTRATION

Administered 24 hours after first methotrexate dose is begun. Dose every 6 hours for up to 12 doses.

First dose is given IV: others can be administered orally or IM.

IV doses are given via bolus over 15 minutes.

Doses must be given *exactly on time* in order to rescue normal cells from methotrexate toxicity.

SPECIAL CONSIDERATIONS

It is imperative that the patient receive the leucovorin on schedule to avoid fatal methotrexate toxicity. Notify the physician if the patient is unable to take the dose orally, as it must then be given IV.

Usually free of side effects but allergic reaction and local pain may occur.

Leucovorin calcium

Nursing Diagnosis	Defining Characteristics	Expected Outcomes	Nursing Interventions
I. *Potential for injury related to*			
A. Allergic reaction	I. A. Allergic sensitization has been reported: facial flushing, itching	I. A. 1. Pt will be without an allergic reaction 2. If allergic reaction occurs, it will be minimized	I. A. 1. Monitor pt for s/s of allergic reaction 2. Diphenhydramine is effective for relieving symptoms of allergic reaction
B. Drug interaction	B. Leucovorin in large amounts may counteract the antiepileptic effects of phenobarbital, phenytoin, and pyrimidone	B. Pt will maintain baseline neurological status	B. 1. Monitor pt for symptoms of increased seizure activity (if on antiepileptic drugs) 2. Monitor antiepileptic drug levels
II. *Altered nutrition, less than body requirements related to nausea and vomiting*	II. Oral leucovorin rarely causes nausea or vomiting	II. A. 1. Pt will be without nausea and vomiting	II. A. Administer oral leucovorin with antacids or milk

DRUG

Leuprolide acetate (Lupron)

Class: Antihormone

MECHANISM OF ACTION

Is a luteinizing hormone-releasing hormone (LHRH) analogue which suppresses the secretion of follicle stimulating hormone (FSH) and luteinizing hormone (LH) from the pituitary gland. The decrease in LH causes the Leydig cells to reduce testosterone production to castrate levels.

METABOLISM

Metabolism and elimination characteristics of leuprolide in humans have not yet been fully elucidated. Several enzymes in the hypothalamus and anterior pituitary may be responsible for the metabolism of endogenous gonadotropin-releasing hormones and leuprolide may be metabolized in a similar way.

DOSAGE/RANGE

For palliative treatment of prostate cancer:
  1 mg/day subcutaneous
(up to 20 mg/day have been used, but without clear clinical advantages)

DRUG PREPARATION

Use syringes provided by manufacturer.

Solution should be inspected for particulate matter, discoloration.

Store solution at room temperature.

DRUG ADMINISTRATION

Give SQ.

SPECIAL CONSIDERATIONS

Patient should be instructed in proper administration techniques, in signs and symptoms of infection at site, and sites should be rotated.

Initially, drug causes increased LH secretion resulting in increased testosterone secretion and tumor flare. Usually disappears after 2 weeks.

Leuprolide acetate

Nursing Diagnosis	Defining Characteristics	Expected Outcomes	Nursing Interventions
I. *Altered nutrition: less than body requirements related to*			
A. Anorexia	I. A. Causes decreased appetite	I. A. Pt will maintain baseline weight ±5%	I. A. 1. Encourage small, frequent feedings of favorite foods, especially high-calorie, high-protein foods 2. Encourage use of spices 3. Monitor weight weekly
B. Nausea and vomiting	B. May occur	B. 1. Pt will be without nausea and vomiting 2. Nausea and vomiting, should they occur, will be minimal	B. 1. Inform pt of possibility of nausea and vomiting 2. Obtain order or prescription for antiemetic if necessary 3. Encourage small feedings of cool, bland foods 4. Refer to sec. on nausea and vomiting, chap. 4
II. *Alteration in comfort*	II. A. Headache, dizziness, hot flashes may occur B. Tumor "flare" may also occur initially (bone and tumor pain, transient increase in tumor size) C. Breast tenderness has been reported	II. A. Pt will be without headache, hot flashes, pain B. Discomfort will be identified and treated early	II. A. Inform pt that symptoms may occur, that "flare" reaction will subside after the initial two weeks of therapy B. Encourage pt to report symptoms early; administer analgesics as needed
III. *Potential for sexual dysfunction*	III. A. Frequently causes decreased libido and erectile impotence	III. A. Pt and significant other will verbalize understanding of changes in sexuality that may occur B. Pt and significant other will identify strategies to cope with sexual dysfunction	III. A. As appropriate, explore with pt and significant other issues of reproductive and sexual patterns and impact chemotherapy may have on them B. Discuss strategies to preserve sexuality and reproductive health C. See sec. on gonadal dysfunction, chap. 4

DRUG

Lomustine (CCNU, CeeNU)

Class: Alkylating agent (Nitrosourea)

MECHANISM OF ACTION

Nitrosourea alkylates DNA with a reactive chloroethyl carbonium ion, producing strand breaks and cross-links which inhibit RNA and DNA synthesis. Interferes with enzymes and histadine utilization. Is cell cycle phase nonspecific.

METABOLISM

Completely absorbed from gastrointestinal tract. Metabolized rapidly, partly proteinbound. Undergoes hepatic recirculation. Lipid soluble: crosses blood–brain barrier. 75% excreted in urine within 4 days.

DOSAGE/RANGE

100–300 mg/m^2 orally every 6 weeks

DRUG PREPARATION

(Oral): Available in 10-mg, 30-mg, and 100-mg capsules.

DRUG ADMINISTRATION

Administer on an empty stomach at bedtime.

SPECIAL CONSIDERATIONS

Give orally, on empty stomach.

Consumption of alcohol should be avoided for a short period after taking CCNU.

Absorbed 30 to 60 minutes after administration. Therefore, vomiting usually does not affect efficacy.

Lomustine (CCNU, CeeNU)

Nursing Diagnosis	Defining Characteristics	Expected Outcomes	Nursing Interventions
I. *Infection and bleeding related to myelosuppression*	I. A. Nadir: platelets: 26–34 days, lasting 6–10 days WBC: 41–46 days, lasting 9–14 days B. Delayed and cumulative bone marrow depression with successive dosing—recovery 6–8 weeks C. Bone marrow depression is dose-limiting toxicity	I. A. Pt will be without infection or bleeding B. Early s/s of infection and bleeding will be identified	I. A. Drug should be administered every 6–8 weeks due to delayed nadir and recovery B. Monitor CBC, platelets prior to drug administration (WBC >4000/mm^3 and platelets >100,000/mm^3) C. Dispense only *one* dose at a time D. See sec. on bone marrow depression, chap. 4
II. *Alteration in nutrition: less than body requirements related to*			
A. Nausea and vomiting	II. A. Onset 2–6 hours after taking dose; may be severe	II. A. Nausea and vomiting will be minimized or prevented	II. A. 1. Administer drug on an empty stomach at bedtime 2. Premedicate with antiemetic and sedative or hypnotic to promote sleep 3. Discourage food or fluid intake for 2 hours after drug administration 4. Refer to sec. on nausea and vomiting, chap. 4
B. Anorexia	B. May last for several days	B. Pt will maintain weight ± 5% of baseline	B. 1. Encourage small, frequent feedings of favorite foods 2. Encourage high-calorie, high-protein foods 3. Weekly weights
C. Diarrhea	C. Occurs infrequently	C. Pt will have minimal diarrhea	C. 1. Encourage pt to report onset of diarrhea 2. Administer or teach pt to self-administer antidiarrheal medication 3. See sec. on diarrhea, chap. 4

(continued)

Lomustine (CCNU, CeeNU) (continued)

Nursing Diagnosis	Defining Characteristics	Expected Outcomes	Nursing Interventions
II. D. Stomatitis	II. D. Occurs infrequently	II. D. Oral mucous membranes will remain intact and without infection	II. D. 1. Teach pt oral assessment and mouth care 2. Encourage pt to report early stomatitis 3. See sec. on stomatitis/mucositis, chap. 4
E. Hepatic dysfunction	E. Transient reversible elevations in liver function studies may occur	E. Hepatic dysfunction will be identified early	E. 1. Monitor SGOT, SGPT, LDH, alkaline phosphatase, and bilirubin—notify MD of elevations
III. Activity intolerance	III. A. Neurologic dysfunction may occur rarely: confusion, lethargy, disorientation, ataxia	III. A. Neurologic dysfunction will be identified early	III. A. Perform neurologic assessment as part of prechemotherapy assessment B. Assess orientation and level of consciousness, gait, activity tolerance
IV. Altered urinary elimination	IV. A. After prolonged therapy with high cumulative doses, tubular atrophy, glomerular sclerosis, and interstitial nephritis have occurred, leading to renal failure	IV. A. Early renal dysfunction will be identified	IV. A. Monitor BUN, creatinine prior to dosing, especially in pts receiving prolonged or high cumulative dose therapy B. If abnormalities are noted, a creatinine clearance should be determined
V. Sensory/perceptual alterations (visual)	V. A. Ocular damage may occur rarely: optic neuritis, retinopathy, blurred vision	V. A. Visual disturbances will be identified early	V. A. Assess vision during prechemotherapy assessment B. Encourage pt to report any visual changes
VI. Potential for sexual dysfunction related to mutagenic and teratogenic qualities of CCNU	VI. A. Drug is teratogenic, mutagenic, and carcinogenic	VI. A. Pt and significant other will understand the need for contraception	VI. A. As appropriate, discuss birth control measures B. See sec. on gonadal dysfunction, chap. 4
VII. Body image disturbance related to alopecia (rare)	VII. A. Alopecia is rare but may occur	VII. A. Pt will verbalize feelings re hair loss and strategies to cope with change in body image	VII. A. Assess pt for hair loss B. Discuss with pt impact of hair loss and obtaining wig or alternative C. See sec. on alopecia, chap. 4

DRUG

Mechlorethamine hydrochloride (nitrogen mustard, mustargen, HN_2)

Class: Alkylating agent

MECHANISM OF ACTION

Produces interstrand and intrastrand cross-linkages in DNA, causing miscoding, breakage, and failures of replication. Is cell cycle phase nonspecific.

METABOLISM

Undergoes chemical transformation after injection with less than 0.01% excreted unchanged in urine. Drug is rapidly inactivated by body fluids. 50% of the inactive metabolites are excreted in the urine within 24 hours.

DOSAGE/RANGE

IV: 0.4 mg/kg *or* 12–16 mg/m^2 IV as single agent 6 mg/m^2 IV days 1 and 8 of 28-day cycle with MOPP regimen

Topical: (dilute 10 mg in 60 mL sterile water; apply with rubber gloves)

Intracavitary (pleural, peritoneal, pericardial): 0.2–0.4 mg/kg

DRUG PREPARATION

Add sterile water or NS to each vial. Wear eye and hand protection when mixing.

Administer via sidearm or rapidly running IV.

Drug must be used within 15 minutes of reconstitution.

DRUG ADMINISTRATION

Intravenous. This drug is a *potent vesicant*. Give through a freely running IV to avoid extravasation which can lead to ulceration, pain, and necrosis. Check hospital's policy and procedure for administration of a vesicant.

SPECIAL CONSIDERATIONS

Drug is a *vesicant*. Give through a running IV to avoid extravasation. *Antidote* is sodium thiosulfate (dilute 4 ml sodium thiosulfate injection USP (10%) with 6 ml sterile water or injection, USP and inject subcutaneously in area of infiltration).

Nadir is 6 to 8 days after treatment.

Side effects occur in the reproductive system, such as amenorrhea and azospermia.

Severe nausea and vomiting.

Systemic toxic effects may occur with intracavitary drug administration.

Mechlorethamine hydrochloride

Nursing Diagnosis	Defining Characteristics	Expected Outcomes	Nursing Interventions
I. Altered nutrition: less than body requirements related to			
A. Nausea and vomiting	I. A. 1. Occurs in ~ 100% of pts 2. Within 30 mins to 2 hrs of drug administration, and up to 8 hrs after 3. Can be severe	I. A. 1. Pt will be without nausea and vomiting 2. Nausea and vomiting, if they occur, will be minimal	I. A. 1. Premedicate with antiemetics and continue prophylactically 2. Antiemetic and sedative may need to be started evening before if pt develops anticipatory nausea and vomiting 3. Lorazepam/metoclopramide/ dexamethasone has been used successfully to prevent or minimize nausea and vomiting 4. Encourage small, frequent feedings of cool, bland foods, dry toast, crackers 5. Monitor I/O to detect fluid volume deficit 6. Notify MD for more aggressive antiemetic if vomitus ≥750 cc 7. Refer to sec. on nausea and vomiting, chap. 4
B. Anorexia, Taste distortion (metallic taste)	B. 1. Taste alterations contribute to the anorexia that pts experience	B. 1. Pt will maintain baseline weight ± 5%	B. 1. Encourage small, frequent feedings of favorite foods, especially high-calorie, high-protein foods 2. Encourage use of spices 3. Weekly weights
C. Diarrhea	C. 1. May occur up to several days after drug administration	C. 1. Pt will have minimal diarrhea	C. 1. Encourage pt to report onset of diarrhea 2. Administer or teach pt to self-administer antidiarrheal medication 3. Diet modifications 4. Refer to sec. on diarrhea, chap. 4

I. D. Stomatitis	I. D. Occurs rarely	I. D. Oral mucous membrane will remain intact without infection	I. D. 1. Teach pt oral assessment and mouth care 2. Perform oral assessment prior to drug administration 3. Encourage pt to report early stomatitis 4. See sec. on stomatitis/mucositis, chap. 4
II. Infection and bleeding, related to bone marrow depression	II. A. Potent myelo-suppressant B. Nadir 6–8 days with recovery in 4 weeks C. Pts at risk for profound BMD are those with previous extensive XRT, previous chemotherapy, or with compromised bone marrow function D. Lymphocyte depression occurs within 24 hours of drug dose	II. A. Pt will be without s/s of infection or bleeding B. Early s/s of infection or bleeding will be identified	II. A. Monitor CBC, platelet count prior to drug administration, assess for s/s of infection or bleeding B. Instruct pt in self-assessment of s/s of infection or bleeding C. Refer to sec. on bone marrow depression, chap. 4
III. Impaired skin integrity related to A. Alopecia	III. A. 1. Usually occurs as diffuse thinning	III. A. 1. Pt will verbalize feelings re hair loss, and identify strategies to cope with changes in body image	III. A. 1. Discuss with pt anticipated impact of hair loss—suggest wig as appropriate prior to actual hair loss 2. Explore with pt response to actual hair loss, and plan strategies to minimize distress; i.e., wig, scarf, cap 3. Refer to sec. on alopecia, chap. 4

(continued)

Mechlorethamine hydrochloride *(continued)*

Nursing Diagnosis	Defining Characteristics	Expected Outcomes	Nursing Interventions

III. B. Extravasation	III. B. 1. Drug is a *potent vesicant*, causing tissue necrosis and sloughing if extravasation occurs
	
	2. Thrombosis or thrombophlebitis may occur despite all precautions and venous access device may be required
		III. B. 1. Extravasation will not occur
		
		2. If extravasation occurs, tissue damage will be minimal
			III. B. 1. Careful technique is used during venipuncture. See sec. on intravenous administration, chap. 7
			
			2. Administer vesicant through freely flowing IV, constantly monitoring IV site and pt response
			
			3. Nurse should be THOROUGHLY familiar with institutional policy and procedure for administration of a vesicant agent
			
			4. If extravasation is suspected:
			  a. Stop drug administered
			  b. Aspirate any residual drug and blood from IV tubing, IV catheter/needle, and IV site if possible
			  c. Instill antidote into area of apparent infiltration, Sodium Thiosulfate (⅙ M), as per MD orders and institutional policy and procedure
			  d. Apply cold or topical medication as per MD order and institutional policy and procedure
			
			5. Assess site regularly for pain, progression of erythema, induration, and for evidence of necrosis
			
			6. When in doubt about whether drug is infiltrating, TREAT AS AN INFILTRATION
			
			7. Teach pt to assess site and notify MD if condition worsens.

III. B. 8. Arrange next clinic visit for assessment of site depending on drug, amount infiltrated, extent of potential injury, and pt variables

9. Document in pt's record as per institutional policy and procedure. See sec. on reactions, ch. 6

10. *Consider* venous access device if peripheral veins are difficult to access

11. Warm packs may decrease discomfort of phlebitis

12. Have standing orders, and sodium thiosulfate injection, USP (10%) close by in the event of actual infiltration of drug: dilute sodium thiosulfate with sterile water for injection and inject subcutaneously in area of infiltration

C. Skin eruptions

C. 1. Maculopapular rash (rare)

C. 1. Skin discomfort will be minimized and skin will remain intact

C. 1. This is not an indication to stop the drug

2. Discuss with MD symptomatic management

D. Delayed cutaneous hypersensitivity

D. 1. Is seen with topical application

D. 1. Skin will be monitored for delayed cutaneous hypersensitivity

D. 1. This is not an indication to stop the drug

2. Discuss with MD symptomatic management

IV. *Alteration in comfort related to chills, fever, diarrhea*

IV. A. May occur immediately after drug administration

B. Also weakness, drowsiness, headache may occur

IV. A. 1. Pt will verbalize discomfort

IV. A. Assess pt for these symptoms during hour following treatment

B. Instruct pt to report these symptoms and teach self-management at home if outpt

C. Provide symptomatic management per MD with acetaminophen, antidiarrheal medication

(continued)

Mechlorethamine hydrochloride *(continued)*

Nursing Diagnosis	Defining Characteristics	Expected Outcomes	Nursing Interventions
V. *Potential for sexual dysfunction*	V. A. Drug is teratogenic, carcinogenic B. Amenorrhea occurs in female C. Impaired spermatogenesis occurs in male D. If administered to pregnant pt, spontaneous abortion or fetal abnormalities may occur	V. A. Pt and significant other will understand need for contraception B. Pt and significant other will identify strategies to cope with sexual dysfunction	V. A. As appropriate, explore with pt and significant other issues of reproductive and sexual patterns, and anticipated impact chemotherapy will have B. Discuss strategies to preserve sexuality and reproductive health (sperm banking, contraception, etc.) C. Refer to sec. on gonadal dysfunction, chap. 4
VI. *Sensory/perceptual alterations related to* A. Tinnitus, deafness	VI. A. 1. Tinnitus, deafness and other signs of eighth cranial nerve damage occur *rarely*, especially with high drug doses or regional perfusion techniques	VI. A. Hearing problems will be identified early	VI. A. 1. Assess hearing ability, presence of tinnitus prior to drug doses 2. If high doses of drug are given, or regional perfusion used, schedule pt for periodic audiometry 3. Instruct pt to report s/s of hearing loss
B. Temporary aphasia and paresis	B. 1. Occurs very rarely	B. Sensory and perceptual changes will be identified early	B. 1. Refer to sec. on neurotoxicity, chap. 4
VII. *Potential for injury, related to severe allergic reactions or anaphylaxis*	VII. A. Occurs rarely	VII. A. Allergic reaction or anaphylaxis will be detected early B. Airway will remain patent C. Systolic BP will remain within 20 mm Hg of baseline	VII. A. Review standing orders for management of pt in anaphylaxis and identify location of anaphylaxis kit containing epinephrine 1:1000, hydrocortisone sodium succinate (Solucortef), diphenhydramine HCl (Benadryl), Aminophylline and others B. Prior to drug administration, obtain baseline vital signs and record mental status

VII. C. Observe for following s/s during infusion usually occuring within first 15 minutes of start of infusion:

Subjective

generalized itching

nausea

chest tightness

crampy abdominal pain

difficulty speaking

anxiety

agitation

sense of impending doom

uneasiness

desire to urinate or defecate

dizziness

chills

Objective

flushed appearance (angioedema of face, neck, eyelids, hands, feet)

localized or generalized urticaria

respiratory distress ± wheezing

hypotension

cyanosis

D. Stop infusion and notify MD

E. Place pt in supine position to promote perfusion of visceral organs

F. Monitor vital signs until stable

G. Provide emotional reassurance to pt and family

H. Maintain patent airway, and have CPR equipment ready if needed

I. Document incident

J. Discuss with MD desensitization versus drug discontinuance for further dosing

DRUG

Melphalan (Alkeran, l-PAM, Phenylalanine Mustard, l-sarcolysin)

Class: Alkylating agent

MECHANISM OF ACTION

Prevents cell replication by causing breaks and cross-linkages in DNA strands with subsequent miscoding and breakage. Is cell cycle phase nonspecific. Drug is derivative of nitrogen mustard.

METABOLISM

Variable bioavailability after oral administration, especially if taken with food. Therefore, dose is titrated to WBC count. 20%–50% of drug is excreted in feces over 6 days, 50% excreted in urine within 24 hours. After IV administration, parent compound disappears from plasma with a half-life of about 2 hours.

DOSAGE/RANGE

6 mg/m^2 orally daily $\times$ 5 days every 6 weeks for myeloma *or* 0.1 mg/kg orally $\times$ 2–3 weeks, then maintenance of 2–4 mg daily when bone marrow has recovered

8 mg/m^2 IV daily $\times$ 5 days (experimental)

DRUG PREPARATION

Oral—Available in 2-mg tablets.

IV—dilute reconstituted vial in D$_5$W. Administer over 30–45 minutes.

DRUG ADMINISTRATION

Serious hypersensitivity reactions reported with IV.

Take oral preparation on an empty stomach.

IV infusion should be given in 100–150 ml of D$_5$W or NS over 15–30 minutes.

SPECIAL CONSIDERATIONS

Nadir 14 to 21 days after treatment.

Increased risk of nephrotoxicity when given with cyclosporine.

Melphalan

Nursing Diagnosis	Defining Characteristics	Expected Outcomes	Nursing Interventions
I. Infection and bleeding, related to bone marrow depression	I. A. Bone marrow depression may be pronounced B. Leukopenia and thrombocytopenia 14–21 days after intermittent dosing schedules C. May be delayed in onset, and cumulative with nadir extended to 5–6 weeks D. Combined immunosuppression from disease (i.e., multiple myeloma) and drug may prolong vulnerability to infection E. Thrombocytopenia may be persistent	I. A. Pt will be without s/s of infection or bleeding B. Early s/s of infection or bleeding will be identified early	I. A. Monitor CBC, platelets prior to drug administration, and assess for s/s of infection or bleeding B. Hold drug if WBC <3000/mm³ or platelet count <100,000/mm³ and discuss with MD C. Teach pt self-assessment techniques, and self-care measures to minimize risk of infection and bleeding D. Refer to sec. on bone marrow depression, chap. 4
II. Altered nutrition: less than body requirements related to			
A. Nausea and vomiting	II. A. 1. Mild at low, continuous dosing; severe following high doses	II. A. 1. Pt will be without nausea and vomiting 2. Nausea and vomiting, if they occur, will be minimal	II. A. 1. Administer drug (oral) on empty stomach 2. Premedicate with antiemetic (oral) one hour before oral dose 3. Use aggressive antiemetic regimen for IV Alkeran 4. Refer to sec. on nausea and vomiting, chap. 4
B. Anorexia	B. 1. Occurs rarely	B. 1. Pt will maintain baseline weight ±5%	B. 1. Encourage small, frequent feedings of favorite foods, especially high-calorie, high-protein foods 2. Encourage use of spices 3. Weekly weights

(continued)

Melphalan (continued)

Nursing Diagnosis	Defining Characteristics	Expected Outcomes	Nursing Interventions
II. C. Stomatitis	II. C. 1. Infrequent occurrence (rare)	II. C. 1. Oral mucous membrane will remain intact without infection	II. C. 1. Teach pt oral assessment 2. Assess oral mucosa prior to drug administration 3. Encourage pt to report (early) stomatitis 4. Refer to sec. on stomatitis, chap. 4
III. *Impaired skin integrity, related to alopecia, maculopapular rash, urticaria*	III. A. Alopecia is minimal if it occurs at all B. Maculopapular rash and urticaria are infrequent	III. A. Pt will develop strategy to manage distress associated with skin side effects	III. A. Assess skin integrity and presence of rash, urticaria, alopecia prior to dosing B. Assess impact of these alterations on pt and develop plan to manage symptom distress
IV. *Potential for impaired gas exchange, related to pulmonary toxicity*	IV. A. Rare, but may occur, especially with continued chronic dosing B. Bronchopulmonary dysplasia and pulmonary fibrosis	IV. A. Early s/s of pulmonary toxicity will be identified	IV. A. Assess pulmonary status for s/s of pulmonary dysfunction B. Assess lung sounds prior to dosing C. Instruct pt to report cough or dyspnea D. Discuss pulmonary function studies to be performed periodically with MD
V. *Potential for injury related to* A. Second malignancy	V. A. 1. Acute myelogenous and myelomonocytic leukemias may occur after continuous long-term dosing 2. Especially in pts with ovarian cancer and multiple myeloma 3. Heralded by preleukemic pancytopenia of several weeks duration 4. Chromosomal abnormalities characteristic of acute leukemia	V. A. 1. Malignancy, if it occurs, will be identified early	V. A. 1. Pts receiving prolonged continuous therapy should be closely followed during and after treatment

V. B. Drug infiltration when given IV	V. B. 1. Painful burning can occur	V. B. 1. Drug infiltration will not occur	V. B. 1. Drug administration is meticulous. Refer to sec. on IV administration, chap. 7
C. Anaphylaxis and hypersensitivity reactions	C. 1. Severe hypersensitivity reactions can occur with IV administration, including diaphoresis, hypotension, and cardiac arrest	C. 1. Hypersensitivity reactions will be detected early 2. Airway will be patent 3. BP will remain within 20 mm Hg of baseline 4. Anaphylaxis, if it occurs, will be detected early	C. 1. Review standing orders for management of pt in anaphylaxis and identify location of anaphylaxis kit containing epinephrine 1:1000, hydrocortisone sodium succinate (Solucortef), diphenhydramine HCl (Benadryl), Aminophylline, and others 2. Prior to drug administration, obtain baseline vital signs and record mental status 3. Administer drug slowly, diluted as per MD order 4. Observe for following s/s, usually occurring within first 15 minutes of infusion *Subjective* Generalized itching Nausea Chest tightness Crampy abdominal pain Difficulty speaking Anxiety Agitation Sense of impending doom Uneasiness Desire to urinate/defecate Dizziness Chills

(continued)

Melphalan *(continued)*

Nursing Diagnosis	Defining Characteristics	Expected Outcomes	Nursing Interventions
			V. C. 4. *Objective* Flushed appearance (angioedema of face, neck, eyelids, hands, feet) Localized or generalized urticaria Respiratory distress ± wheezing Hypotension Cyanosis
			5. For generalized allergic reaction stop infusion and notify MD
			6. Place pt in supine position to promote perfusion of visceral organs
			7. Monitor vital signs
			8. Provide emotional reassurance to pt and family
			9. Maintain patent airway, and have CPR equipment ready if needed
			10. Document incident
			11. Discuss with MD desensitization versus drug discontinuance for further dosing
VI. *Potential for sexual dysfunction*	VI. A. Potentially mutagenic and teratogenic	VI. A. Pt and significant other will understand potential sexual dysfunction	VI. A. Encourage pt to verbalize goals re family, and discuss options, such as sperm banking
			B. As appropriate, discuss or refer for counseling re birth control measures during therapy
			C. Refer to sec. on gonadal dysfunction, chap. 4

DRUG

6-Mercaptopurine (Purinethol, 6-MP)

Class: Antimetabolite

MECHANISM OF ACTION

One of two thiopurine antimetabolites (with 6-TG) which are converted to monophosphate nucleotides and inhibit de novo purine synthesis. The nucleotides are also incorporated into DNA. Cell cycle phase specific (S phase).

METABOLISM

Metabolized by the enzyme xanthine oxidase in the kidney and liver. Because xanthine oxidase is inhibited by allopurinol, concurrent use of the latter necessitates a dose reduction of 6-MP to $\frac{1}{4}$ the normal dose. 50% of the drug is excreted in the urine. Plasma half-life: 20–40 minutes.

DOSAGE/RANGE

100 mg/m^2 orally daily $\times$ 5 days

Children: 70 mg/m^2 daily for induction then 40 mg/m^2 daily for maintenance

IV use is investigational

DRUG PREPARATION

Oral: None. Available in 50 mg tablets.

IV: reconstitute 500-mg vial with sterile water for concentration of 10 mg/ml.

Store IV solution at room temperature: discard after 8 hours.

DRUG ADMINISTRATION

IV use is investigational; consult protocol.

SPECIAL CONSIDERATIONS

Elevated serum glucose levels and elevated serum uric acid levels could be related to the effects of medication.

Patients receiving allopurinol concurrently may require dosage reduction due to xanthine oxidase inhibition.

When given with nondepolarizing muscle relaxants there is decreased neuromuscular blockage.

When given with warfarin there is a decreased hypothrombinemic effect.

Reduce dose in cases of hepatic or renal dysfunction.

6-Mercaptopurine

Nursing Diagnosis	Defining Characteristics	Expected Outcomes	Nursing Interventions
I. *Altered nutrition: less than body requirements related to*			
A. Nausea and vomiting	I. A. 1. Uncommon; mild when they do occur	I. A. 1. Pt will be without nausea and vomiting	I. A. 1. Consider premedicating with antiemetics for first dose
		2. Nausea and vomiting, if they do occur, will be minimal	2. Encourage small, frequent feedings of cool, bland foods and liquids
			3. Assess for symptoms of fluid/electrolyte imbalance if pt's vomiting is significant
			4. Monitor I/O, daily weights, check lab results
			4. Refer to sec. on nausea and vomiting, chap. 4
B. Anorexia	B. 1. Infrequent; mild	B. 1. Pt will maintain baseline weight ± 5%	B. 1. Encourage small, frequent feedings of favorite foods, especially high-calorie, high-protein foods
			2. Encourage use of spices
C. Stomatitis	C. 1. Uncommon; but appears as white patchy areas similar to thrush	C. 1. Oral mucous membranes will remain intact and with infection	C. 1. Teach oral assessment and mouth care regimen
			2. Encourage pt to report early stomatitis
			3. Provide pain relief measures, if indicated
			4. Refer to sec. on stomatitis, chap. 4
D. Diarrhea	D. 1. Occurs occasionally; mild	D. 1. Pt will have minimal diarrhea	D. 1. Encourage pt to report onset of diarrhea
			2. Administer or teach pt to self-administer antidiarrheal medication
			3. Guaiac all stools
			4. If diarrhea is protracted, ensure adequate hydration, monitor I/O and electrolytes, and teach hygiene to pt
			4. Refer to sec. on diarrhea, chap. 4

I. E. Hepatotoxicity	I. E. 1. Reversible cholestatic jaundice may develop after 2–5 mos of treatment 2. Hepatic necrosis may develop	I. E. 1. Early hepatoxicity will be identified	I. E. 1. Monitor SGOT, SGPT, LDH, alkaline phosphatase, and bilirubin periodically during treatment 2. Notify MD of any elevations 3. Hepatic toxicity may be an indication for discontinuing treatment
II. *Potential for infection and bleeding, related to bone marrow depression*	II. A. Nadir varies from 5 days to 6 weeks after treatment B. Leukopenia more prominent than thrombocytopenia C. Blood counts may continue to fall after therapy is stopped	II. A. Pt will be without s/s of infection or bleeding B. Early s/s of infection or bleeding will be identified	II. A. Monitor CBC, platelet count prior to drug administration, as well as s/s of infection or bleeding B. Instruct in self-assessment of s/s of infection or bleeding C. Refer to sec. on bone marrow depression, chap. 4
III. *Potential for impaired skin integrity*	III. A. Skin eruptions, rash may occur	III. A. Distress related to alterations in skin condition will be minimized	III. A. Advise pt these changes may occur B. Instruct pt in symptomatic care if distress related to skin reactions occurs

DRUG

Mesna (Mesnex)

  Class: Sulfydryl

MECHANISM OF ACTION

Used to prevent ifosfamide-induced hemorrhagic cystitis. Drug is rapidly metabolized by the metabolite dimesna. In the kidney dimesna is reduced to mesna which binds to the urotoxic ifosfamide metabolites acrolein and 4-hydroxy-ifosfamide, resulting in their detoxification.

METABOLISM

Rapidly metabolized, remains in the intravascular compartment and is rapidly eliminated by the kidneys. The drug is eliminated in 24 hours as mesna (32%) and dimesna (33%). Majority of the dose is eliminated within 4 hours.

DOSAGE/RANGE

Recommended clinical dose 240 mg/m^2 IV bolus
15 minutes before ifosfamide
4 hours after ifosfamide
8 hours after ifosfamide
  Mesna dose is 20% of ifosfamide dose.

DRUG PREPARATION

Dilute mesna with D$_5$W, D$_5$/NS, or Normal Saline to create a designated final concentration.

DRUG ADMINISTRATION

Diluted solution is stable for 24 hours at room temperature.

Refrigerate and use reconstituted solution within 6 hours.

SPECIAL CONSIDERATIONS

At clinical doses, mild nausea and vomiting and diarrhea are the only side effects expected.

Mesna

Nursing Diagnosis	Defining Characteristics	Expected Outcomes	Nursing Interventions
I. *Potential for injury related to maintenance of bladder mucosal integrity*	I. A. Mesna uniquely concentrates in the bladder and has a very low degree of toxicity, making it the uroprotector of choice against ifosfomide-related urotoxicity	I. A. Pt will be free of bladder irritation and hemorrhagic cystitis	I. A. Daily U/A B. Assess for hematuria per hospital policy and procedure C. Hydrate vigorously

DRUG

Methotrexate (Amethopterin, Mexate, Folex)

Class: Antimetabolite, folic acid antagonist

MECHANISM OF ACTION

Blocks the enzyme dihydrofolate reductase (DHFR) which inhibits the conversion of folic acid to tetrahydrofolic acid, resulting in an inhibition of the key precursors of DNA, RNA, and cellular proteins. May synchronize malignant cells in the S phase: at high plasma levels, passive entry of the drug into tumor cells can potentially overcome drug resistance.

METABOLISM

Bound to serum albumin, concurrent use of drugs that displace methotrexate from serum albumin should be avoided. Salicylates, sulfonamides, dilantin, some antibacterials including tetracycline, chloramphenicol, paraminobenzoic acid, and alcohol should be avoided, as they will delay excretion. Drug is absorbed from gastrointestinal tract and peaks in 1 hour. Plasma half-life = 2 hours; 50%–100% of dose is excreted into the systemic circulation, with peak concentration 3–12 hours after administration.

DOSAGE/RANGE

IV: Low: 10–50 mg/m^2
    Med: 100–500 mg/m^2
    High: 500 mg/m^2 and above with leucovorin rescue

IT: 10–15 mg/m^2

IM: 25 mg/m^2

DRUG PREPARATION

5-, 50-, 100- and 200-mg vials are available already reconstituted.

Powder is available in vials without preservative for IT and high-dose administration (reconstitute with preservative-free NS).

DRUG ADMINISTRATION

5–149 mg: slow IVP

150–499 mg: IV drip over 20 minutes

500–1500 mg: infusion, per protocol with leucovorin rescue

SPECIAL CONSIDERATIONS

High doses cross the blood–brain barrier: reconstitute with preservative-free NS.

With high doses (1–7.5 gm/m^2) urine should be alkalinized both before and after administration, as the drug is a weak acid and can crystallize in the kidneys at an acid pH. Alkalinize with bicarbonate, add to pre- and posthydration. High doses should only be given under the direction of a qualified oncologist at an institution that can provide rapid serum methotrexate level readings.

Leucovorin rescue must be given *on time* per orders to prevent excessive toxicity and to achieve maximum therapeutic response (see leucovorin calcium table).

Avoid folic acid and its derivatives during methotrexate therapy.

Kidney function must be adequate to excrete drug and avoid excessive toxicity. Check BUN and creatinine before each dose.

Methotrexate

Nursing Diagnosis	Defining Characteristics	Expected Outcomes	Nursing Interventions
I. *Altered nutrition: less than body requirements related to*			
A. Nausea and vomiting	I. A. 1. Nausea and vomiting are uncommon with low dose; more common (39%) with high dose 2. May occur during drug administration and last 24–72 hours	I. A. 1. Pt will be without nausea and vomiting 2. Nausea and vomiting, should they occur, will be minimal	I. A. 1. Premedicate with antiemetics if giving high-dose methotrexate—continue prophylactically for 24 hrs (at least) to *prevent* nausea and vomiting 2. Encourage small, frequent feedings of cool, bland foods and liquids 3. Assess for symptoms of fluid and electrolyte imbalance—monitor I/O, daily weights if administered inpatient 4. See sec. on nausea and vomiting, chap. 4
B. Stomatitis	B. 1. Common: indication for interruption of therapy 2. Occurs in 3–5 days with high dose, 3–4 weeks with low dose 3. Appears initially at corners of mouth	B. 1. Oral mucous membranes will remain intact and without infection	B. 1. Assess oral cavity every day 2. Teach pt oral assessment and mouth care regimens 3. Encourage pt to report early stomatitis 4. Provide pain relief measures, if indicated 5. See sec. on stomatitis, chap. 4 6. Explore pt compliance to rescue; discuss ↑ rescue dose
C. Diarrhea	C. 1. Common: is an indication for interruption of therapy, as enteritis and intestinal perforation may occur 2. Melena, hematemesis may occur	C. 1. Pt will have minimal diarrhea	C. 1. Assess pt for diarrhea—guiac all stools 2. Encourage pt to report onset of diarrhea 3. Administer or teach pt to self-administer antidiarrheal medications 4. See sec. on diarrhea, chap. 4

(continued)

Methotrexate (continued)

Nursing Diagnosis	Defining Characteristics	Expected Outcomes	Nursing Interventions
I. D. Hepatotoxicity	I. D. 1. Usually subclinical and reversible, but can lead to cirrhosis 2. Increased risk of hepatotoxicity when given with other hepatotoxic agents, like alcohol 3. Transient increase in LFTs with high dose 1–10 days after treatment—may become jaundiced	I. D. 1. Early hepatoxicity will be identified	I. D. 1. Monitor LFTs prior to drug dose, especially with high dose methotrexate 2. Assess pt prior to and during treatment for s/s of hepatoxicity
E. Anorexia	E. Mild	E. 1. Pt will maintain baseline weight ± 5%	E. 1. Encourage small, frequent feedings of favorite foods, especially high-calorie, high-protein foods 2. Encourage use of spices 3. Q day weights
II. *Potential for infection and bleeding, related to bone marrow depression*	II. A. Nadir seen 10–14 days after drug administration B. Bone marrow depression occurs in about 10% of pts	II. A. Pt will be without s/s of infection or bleeding B. S/s of infection or bleeding will be identified early	II. A. Monitor CBC, platelet count prior to drug administration as well as s/s of infection or bleeding B. Instruct pt in self-assessment of s/s of infection or bleeding C. Administer leucovorin calcium as ordered D. See care plan for leucovorin calcium

III. *Potential for altered urinary elimination related to renal toxicity*	III. A. As an organic acid, methotrexate is insoluble in acid urine B. At doses greater than 1 gm/m² (i.e., high dose), drug may precipitate in renal tubules, causing acute tubular necrosis (ATN)	III. A. Pt will maintain normal patterns of urinary elimination B. Renal toxicity will be avoided	III. A. Prehydrate pt with alkaline solution for several hours prior to drug administration B. Maintain high urine output with a urine pH of greater than 7.0 (hydration fluid may need further alkalinization); dipstick each void C. Record I/O D. Monitor BUN and serum creatinine before, during, and after drug administration. Increases in these values may require methotrexate dose reductions or leucovorin dose increases
IV. *Potential for impaired gas exchange, related to pulmonary toxicity*	IV. A. Pneumothorax (high dose): rare, occurs within first 48 hours after drug administration in pts with pulmonary metastasis B. Allergic pneumonitis (high dose): rare but accompanied by eosinophilia, patchy pulmonary infiltrates, fever, cough, shortness of breath. Occurs 1–5 months after initiation of treatment C. Pneumonitis (low dose) symptoms usually disappear within a week, with or without use of steroids—interstitial pneumonitis may be a fatal complication	IV. A. Early s/s of pulmonary toxicity will be identified	IV. A. Assess for s/s of pulmonary dysfunction before each dose and between doses (see "Defining Characteristics") B. Discuss pulmonary function studies to be performed periodically with MD C. Assess lung sounds prior to drug administration D. Instruct pt to report cough or dyspnea

(continued)

Methotrexate *(continued)*

Nursing Diagnosis	Defining Characteristics	Expected Outcomes	Nursing Interventions
V. *Potential for alteration in skin integrity*	V. A. Alopecia and dermatitis are uncommon B. Pruritis, urticaria may occur C. Photosensitivity, sunburnlike rash 1–5 days after treatment; also, can develop radiation recall reaction	V. A. Pt will verbalize feelings about potential changes in body image and will identify strategies to cope with them B. Pt will identify strategies to minimize, avoid, or treat body image changes	V. A. Assess pt for s/s of hair loss B. Discuss with pt impact of hair loss, and strategies to minimize distress C. See sec. on alopecia, chap. 4 D. Instruct pt to avoid sun if possible, to stay covered or wear sunscreen if sun exposure is unavoidable
VI. *Potential for sensory and perceptual alterations*	VI. A. CNS effects: dizziness, malaise, blurred vision B. IT administration may increase CSF pressure C. Brain XRT followed by IV MTX may also cause neurological changes	VI. A. Early s/s of neurological toxicity will be identified	VI. A. Monitor for CNS effects of drug: dizziness, blurred vision, malaise B. Monitor for symptoms of increased CSF pressure: seizures, paresis, headache, nausea and vomiting, brain atrophy, fever C. If IV methotrexate follows brain XRT, monitor for symptoms of increased CSF pressure
VII. *Potential for alterations in comfort*	VII. A. Sometimes causes back pain during administration	VII. A. Pt will report comfort throughout drug administration	VII. A. Monitor pt for back and flank pain. Slow down infusion rate if it occurs B. Administer analgesics if pain occurs (must avoid ASA-containing products, as they displace methotrexate from serum albumin)

DRUG

Methyl-CCNU (semustine, MeCCNU, methyl lomustine)

Class: Alkylating agent (nitrosourea); investigational agent

MECHANISM OF ACTION

Alkylation and carbamoylation by semustine metabolites interfere with the synthesis and function of DNA, RNA, and proteins. Also inhibits DNA repair. Semustine is lipid soluble and easily enters the brain. Is cell cycle phase nonspecific.

METABOLISM

From 10%–20% of the drug is excreted in the urine.

DOSAGE/RANGE

150–200 mg/m^2 PO once every 6 to 10 weeks

DRUG PREPARATION

Oral—available in 10-mg, 50-mg and 100-mg capsules

DRUG ADMINISTRATION

Administer at bedtime on an empty stomach or 3–4 hours after a meal to minimize nausea and monitoring.

SPECIAL CONSIDERATIONS

Dose reduction necessary if patient has liver impairment.

Dispense one dose of semustine at a time.

Bone marrow recovery should occur prior to administration:

WBC >4000/mm^3 and
platelets >100,000/mm^3

Methyl-CCNU (semustine, MeCCNU)

Nursing Diagnosis	Defining Characteristics	Expected Outcomes	Nursing Interventions
I. Potential for infection and bleeding related to myelosuppression	I. A. Nadir: platelets: 4 weeks, but may be delayed to 8 weeks with recovery 4–10 weeks later WBC: occurs later than platelet B. Cumulative bone marrow suppression with subsequent dosing may occur: 2nd or 3rd drug dose may be reduced 25%–50% C. Persistent thrombocytopenia may occur	I. A. 1. Pt will be without infection or bleeding 2. Early s/s of infection and bleeding will be identified	I. A. 1. Monitor WBC platelets prior to drug administration (see Special Considerations) B. WBC >4000/mm³ and platelets >100,000/mm³ C. Dispense only one drug dose at a time D. Do not administer more often than once every 6 weeks E. Dose reduce if bone marrow or liver impairment F. Refer to sec. on bone marrow depression, chap. 4
II. Alteration in nutrition: less than body requirements related to			
A. Nausea and vomiting	II. A. Onset 4–6 hours after drug dosing and may be severe	II. A. Nausea and vomiting will be minimized or prevented	II. A. 1. Premedicate with antiemetic and sedative or hypnotic 2. Administer at night on empty stomach 3. Discourage food or fluid for 6 hours after drug dose 4. Refer to sec. on nausea and vomiting, chap. 4
B. Anorexia	B. Occurs rarely	B. Pt will maintain baseline weight ±5%	B. 1. Encourage favorite foods, especially those that are high-calorie, high-protein 2. Encourage small, frequent feedings
C. Stomatitis	C. Occurs rarely	C. Oral mucous membranes will remain intact without infection	C. 1. Inspect oral mucosa prior to dosing 2. Teach pt oral exam, mouth care pc and hs 3. Refer to sec. on stomatitis/mucositis, chap. 4

Nursing Diagnosis	Signs and Symptoms	Outcome Goals/Evaluation	Interventions
II. D. Hepatic dysfunction	II. D. Delayed hepatocullular damage may occur *rarely*	II. D. Hepatic dysfunction will be identified early	II. D. 1. Monitor SGOT, LDH, alkaline phosphatase, bilirubin 2. Notify MD of elevations, and discuss prior to administering subsequent drug dose
III. *Activity intolerance*	III. A. Neurologic dysfunction may occur *rarely*, including disorientation, lethargy, ataxia	III. A. Neurologic dysfunction will be identified early	III. A. Perform neurologic assessment as part of prechemotherapy assessment B. Assess orientation and level of consciousness, gait, activity tolerance
IV. *Sensory/perceptual alterations (visual)*	IV. A. Ocular damage may occur *rarely*, including optic neuritis, retinopathy, blurred vision	IV. A. Visual disturbances will be identified early	IV. A. Assess vision during prechemotherapy assessment B. Encourage pt to report any visual changes
V. *Altered urinary elimination*	V. A. Renal dysfunction infrequent but may occur late in treatment B. Tubular atrophy and glomerular sclerosis, ultimately renal failure	V. A. Early renal dysfunction will be identified	V. A. Monitor BUN, creatinine prior to dosing, especially in pts receiving prolonged or high cumulative doses B. If abnormalities are noted, determine renal creatinine clearance
VI. *Potential for sexual dysfunction, related to mutagenic and teratogenic qualities of MeCCNU*	VI. A. Drug is teratogenic and mutagenic	VI. A. Pt and significant other will understand need for contraception	VI. A. As appropriate, discuss birth control measures B. See sec. on gonadal dysfunction, chap. 4
VII. *Body image disturbance, related to alopecia*	VII. A. Alopecia infrequent	VII. A. Pt will verbalize feelings re hair loss and strategies to cope with change in body image	VII. A. Assess pt for hair loss B. Discuss with pt impact of hair loss and obtaining wig or alternative head cover C. See sec. on alopecia, chap. 4

(continued)

Methyl-CCNU (semustine, MeCCNU)

Nursing Diagnosis	Defining Characteristics	Expected Outcomes	Nursing Interventions
VIII. *Impaired gas exchange, related to pulmonary fibrosis*	VIII. A. Pulmonary fibrosis occurs rarely	VIII. A. Early pulmonary fibrosis/dysfunction will be identified	VIII. A. Assess pts at risk, those with 1. Preexisting lung disease 2. High cumulative doses B. Monitor pulmonary function studies periodically for pulmonary dysfunction

DRUG

Mitoguazone dihydrochloride (methyl-GAG, methyl-G)

Class: Investigational

MECHANISM OF ACTION

Methyl-GAG interferes with protein synthesis by inhibiting specific enzyme products. This process ultimately inhibits DNA synthesis. There are also theories that it may bind directly to DNA and act as a mitochrondrial poison. The exact mechanism of action is not clearly understood. Is cell cycle nonspecific.

METABOLISM

Methyl-GAG is administered by intravenous infusion or by deep intramuscular injection. There is a prolonged retention of methyl-GAG with an associated delay in excretion. 60% of drug dose is excreted intact in urine with < 20% being excreted in feces. At 72 hours postinfusion only 14% of the drug dose is excreted in urine. The remainder of the drug is slowly excreted over at least the next two weeks. The mean half-life is 136–224 hours.

DOSAGE/RANGE

Currently methyl-GAG is given in doses 260–800 mg/m^2. IV weekly, or 3–4 mg/kg deep intramuscular injection weekly. Clinical trials with methyl-GAG have been underway since the 1960s, but the optimal dosing schedule has yet to be determined. It is clear that schedules of administering it every 10–14 days offer less toxicity.

DRUG PREPARATION

Methyl-GAG is available as a lyophilized power in 30-ml vials of 1 gm of drug each. The drug is supplied by the National Cancer Institute. Each 30-ml vial is reconstituted with 9.3 ml of sodium chloride injection. This solution is chemically stable for 48 hours at room temperature or re-frigerated, but as it lacks bacteriostatic preservatives, the solution should be discarded after 8 hours. The reconstituted solution may be further diluted in 500 ml D$_5$W or NS.

DRUG ADMINISTRATION

Methyl-GAG intravenous infusions should be administered over 30–45 minutes. Intravenous push administration may cause orthostatic hypotension and thus is not recommended. This drug may also be administered by deep intramuscular injection. The total volume of drug per each injection site should not exceed 7.5 ml.

SPECIAL CONSIDERATIONS

Irritant.

Administered by intravenous infusion or deep injection.

Reports of rare occurences of hypotension and bronchospasm during infusion.

Toxicities somewhat unpredictable. Seem to be cumulative rather than dose related (may be due to rate of excretion).

Majority of patients experience facial flushing (may involve whole body) and warmth halfway into infusion, which resolve completely with 15 minutes after infusions. This issue can be decreased by decreasing the rate of infusion.

Dose-limiting toxicities include: muscle weakness, malaise, myopathies, GI mucositis, and hypoglycemia.

Mucositis may represent toxicity from drug accumulation.

Anorexia and weight loss have been noted in clinical trials.

Mitoguazone dihydrochloride (methyl-GAG)

Nursing Diagnosis	Defining Characteristics	Expected Outcomes	Nursing Interventions
I. *Potential for injury related to hypersensitivity reactions*	I. A. Almost all pts experience some hypersensitivity reactions, usually facial flushing and numbness, but may involve entire body. Bronchospasm occurs in 4% of pts B. Especially seen with IM injections C. Starts 5–15 mins after injection D. Hypotension may occur, especially with rapid infusions E. Dizziness and bronchospasm rarely occur F. Usually responds to steroids, epinephrine, or antihistamines	I. Early s/s of hypersensitivity reactions will be identified	I. A. Review standing orders for management of pt in anaphylaxis and identify location of anaphylaxis kit containing epinephrine 1:1000, hydrocortisone sodium succinate (Solucortef), diphenhydramine HCl (Benadryl), Aminophylline, and others B. 1. Prior to drug administration, obtain baseline vital signs and record mental status 2. Assess pt for at least 30 mins after the drug is given for s/s of a reaction 3. Teach pt about the potential for hypersensitivity reactions and to report any unusual symptoms C. Observe for following s/s during infusion, usually occuring within first 15 mins of start of infusion: *Subjective* generalized itching nausea chest tightness crampy abdominal pain difficulty speaking anxiety agitation sense of impending doom uneasiness desire to urinate or defecate dizziness chills

		I. C. *Objective*	flushed appearance (angioedema of face, neck, eyelids, hands, feet) localized or generalized urticaria respiratory distress ± wheezing hypotension cyanosis
			D. If reaction occurs, stop infusion and notify MD
			E. Place pt in supine position to promote perfusion of visceral organs
			F. Monitor vital signs until stable
			G. Provide emotional reassurance to pt and family
			H. Maintain patent airway, and have CPR equipment ready if needed
			I. Document incident
			J. Discuss with MD desensitation versus drug discontinuance for further dosing
II. *Potential for infection and bleeding related to bone marrow depression*	II. A. Dose-related, occurring in 13% of pts. Profound with daily dosing; rare with intermittent dosing	II. A. Pt will be without s/s of infection or bleeding	II. A. Monitor CBC, platelet count prior to drug administration, as well as s/s of infection or bleeding
	B. Leukopenia is more common than thrombocytopenia	B. Early s/s of infection or bleeding will be identified	B. Instruct pt in self-assessment of s/s of infection or bleeding
	C. Thrombocytopenia is mild to moderate		C. Dose reduction may be necessary in setting of compromised bone marrow function
			D. See sec. on bone marrow depression, chap. 4

(continued)

Mitoguazone dihydrochloride (methyl-GAG) (continued)

Nursing Diagnosis	Defining Characteristics	Expected Outcomes	Nursing Interventions
III. *Altered nutrition: less than body requirements related to*			
A. Nausea and vomiting (rare)	III. A. 1. Nausea is more common than vomiting 2. Rarely an unclear reaction occurs resulting in prolonged vomiting 3. Nausea usually limited to first 24 hrs after therapy	III. A. 1. Pt will be without nausea and vomiting 2. Nausea and vomiting, if they occur, will be minimal	III. A. 1. Premedicate with antiemetics and continue prophylactically × 24 hrs to prevent nausea and vomiting at least for first treatment 2. Encourage small, frequent feedings of cool, bland foods and liquids 3. See sec. on nausea and vomiting, chap. 4
B. Mucositis	B. 1. May be severe and dose-limiting 2. May progress from stomatitis to ulcerative mucositis with bloody diarrhea in 24% of pts 3. S/s start 7–14 days after administration 4. S/s may include inflammation or ulceration of any mucosal membrane, anorexia, weight loss, abdominal pain, diarrhea 5. Occurs in 20% of pts and may represent drug accumulation	B. 1. Mucous membranes will remain intact without infection 2. Pt will maintain baseline weight ± 5% 3. Pt will have minimal diarrhea	B. 1. Teach pt oral assessment 2. Encourage pt to report onset of mucositis, diarrhea 3. Teach pt oral hygiene 4. Encourage small, frequent feedings of favorite foods, especially high-calorie, high-protein foods 5. Encourage use of spices 6. Weekly weights 7. Administer or teach pt to self-administer antidiarrheal medications 8. See sec. on stomatitis/mucositis, chap. 4

III. C. Hypoglycemia	III. C. 1. Rare and delayed reaction, more common with daily dosing than intermittent dosing 2. S/s include muscle weakness, lethargy, confusion, flushing, restlessness, numbness, malaise	III. C. 1. Pt will be without s/s of hypoglycemia 2. Early s/s of hypoglycemia will be identified	III. C. 1. Teach pt about the potential for hypoglycemia and to report any unusual symptoms; i.e., mental status changes, muscle weakness, palpitations 2. Monitor serum glucose levels 3. Report any laboratory abnormalities to MD 4. Treat hypoglycemia with diet or medication as ordered by MD

IV. *Impaired skin integrity related to*

A. Alopecia	IV. A. 1. Uncommon; may be slight to diffuse thinning	IV. A. 1. Pt will verbalize feelings regarding hair loss and identify strategies to cope with change in body image	IV. A. 1. Assess pt for s/s of hair loss 2. Discuss with pt impact of hair loss, and strategies to minimize distress; i.e., wigs, scarf, cap (begin before therapy initiated) 3. See sec. on alopecia, chap. 4
B. Changes in skin	B. 1. May be inflammatory reactions on hands, feet, lower extremities 2. S/s may include erythema, edema, pain, dermatitis, ulcers, vasculitis 3. Subcutaneous nodules may form at injection site 4. Chemical thrombophlebitis and cellulitis occur	B. 1. Pt will verbalize feelings regarding skin changes and identify strategies to cope with changes in body image	B. 1. Assess pt for inflammatory skin reactions or formation of subcutaneous nodules at injection sites 2. Discuss with pt impact of changes and strategies to minimize distress; i.e., wearing nonirritating socks, cotton gloves, long pants 3. Rotate injection sites 4. Warm soaks to nodules as appropriate 5. Administer corticosteroids as ordered

(continued)

Mitoguazone dihydrochloride (methyl-GAG) *(continued)*

Nursing Diagnosis	Defining Characteristics	Expected Outcomes	Nursing Interventions
V. *Potential for injury related to myopathy and peripheral neuropathies*	V. A. 24% of pts experience myopathy syndrome—may be quite severe, necessitating narcotic analgesia. Reversible when treatment is held B. Peripheral neuropathies are rare	V. A. Early s/s of myopathy and peripheral neuropathies will be identified B. Pt will not experience injuries as a result of skeletal or neurological changes	V. A. Teach pt about the potential for myopathy or peripheral neuropathies and to report any unusual symptoms; i.e., muscle weakness and wasting, numbness B. Obtain baseline physical. Assess muscular and neurological function C. Dose decrease or rescheduling of dose administration may be necessary

DRUG

Mitomycin (Mitomycin C, Mutamycin)

Class: Antitumor antibiotic

MECHANISM OF ACTION

Drug acts as alkylating agent and inhibits DNA synthesis by cross-linking of DNA. Alkylating and cross-linking mitomycin metabolites interfere with structure and function of DNA.

METABOLISM

Drug is rapidly cleared by the liver. May need to modify dose in presence of liver abnormalities. 10% of drug is excreted unchanged.

DOSAGE/RANGE

2 mg/m^2 IV every day times five days

15–20 mg/m^2 IV every 6–8 weeks

Bladder instillations 20–60 mg (1 mg/ml)

DRUG PREPARATION

Depending on vial size, dilute with sterile water to obtain concentration of 0.5 mg/mL.

DRUG ADMINISTRATION

IV. This drug is a potent vesicant. Give through the sidearm of a running IV so as to avoid extravasation which can lead to ulceration, pain, and necrosis. Check individual hospital policy for administration of a vesicant.

SPECIAL CONSIDERATIONS

Drug is a potent vesicant. Give through running IV to avoid extravasation.

Intertitial pneumotitis.

Mitomycin

Nursing Diagnosis	Defining Characteristics	Expected Outcomes	Nursing Interventions
I. *Altered nutrition: less than body requirements related to*			
A. Nausea and vomiting	I. A. 1. Mild to moderate nausea and vomiting occur within 1–2 hours, lasting up to 3 days	I. A. 1. Pt will be without nausea and vomiting 2. Nausea and vomiting, if they occur, will be minimal	I. A. 1. Premedicate with antiemetics and continue prophylactically × 24 hrs to prevent nausea and vomiting at least for first treatment 2. Encourage small, frequent feedings of cool, bland foods and liquids 3. See sec. on nausea and vomiting, chap. 4
B. Stomatitis	B. 1. Mucocutaneous toxicity	B. Oral mucous membrane will remain intact without infection	B. 1. Teach pt oral assessment and oral hygiene regimen 2. Encourage pt to report early stomatitis 3. See sec. on stomatitis, chap. 4
II. *Potential for infection related to myelosuppression*	II. A. Myelosuppression is the dose-limiting toxicity. Toxicity is delayed and cumulative B. Initial nadir occurs at approximately 4–6 weeks C. Usually by the third course, 50% drug modifications are necessary	II. A. Pt will be without infection B. Early s/s of infection will be identified	II. A. Monitor WBC, Hct, platelets prior to drug administration B. Monitor pts for s/s of infection: teach pt self-assessment C. Drug dosage should be reduced or held for lower-than-normal blood values D. See sec. on bone marrow depression, chap. 4
III. *Potential for alteration in comfort related to fever*	III. A. Fever with malaise in almost all pts is related to length and duration of drug schedule	III. A. Pt will remain comfortable during therapy	III. A. Assess pt for symptoms during the treatment. Discuss with MD B. Premedicate with prescribed medication C. Evaluate the effectiveness of the symptomatic relief prescribed and administered D. Monitor the quantity of cumulative dose

IV. *Potential for impaired skin integrity related to*

A. Extravasation

IV. A. 1. Extravasation of drug can cause severe tissue necrosis, erythema, burning, tissue sloughing	IV. A. 1. Extravasation will be prevented or treated appropriately, if it does occur	IV. A. 1. Careful technique is used during venipuncture. See sec. on intravenous administration, chap. 7
	2. Skin and underlying tissue damage will be minimized	2. Administer vesicant through freely flowing IV, constantly monitoring IV site and pt response
		3. Nurse should be THOROUGHLY familiar with institutional policy and procedure for administration of a vesicant agent
		4. If vesicant drug is administered as a continuous infusion, drug must be given through a patent central line
		5. If extravasation is suspected:
		a. Stop drug administered
		b. Aspirate any residual drug and blood from IV tubing, IV catheter/needle, and IV site if possible
		c. Instill antidote into area of apparent infiltration, IF ANTIDOTE EXISTS, as per MD orders and institutional policy and procedure
		d. Apply cold or topical medication as per MD order and instutional policy and procedure
		6. Assess site regularly for pain, progression of erythema, induration, and for evidence of necrosis
		7. When in doubt about whether drug is infiltrating, TREAT AS AN INFILTRATION

(continued)

Mitomycin *(continued)*

Nursing Diagnosis	Defining Characteristics	Expected Outcomes	Nursing Interventions
			IV. A. 8. Teach pt to assess site and notify MD if condition worsens
			9. Arrange next clinic visit for assessment of site depending on drug, amount infiltrated, extent of potential injury, and pt variables
			10. Document in pt's record as per institutional policy and procedure. See sec. on reactions, ch. 6
B. Alopecia	B. 1. Alopecia has been reported	B. 1. Pt will verbalize feelings re hair loss and identify strategies to cope with changes in body image	B. 1. Discuss with pt impact of hair loss
			2. Suggest wig as appropriate prior to actual hair loss
			3. Explore with pt response to actual hair loss and plan strategies to minimize distress; i.e., wig, scarf, cap
			4. See sec. on alopecia, chap. 4
C. Skin reactions	C. 1. Discoloration of fingernails; usually dark half-circles	C. 1. Skin discomfort will be minimized and skin will remain intact	C. 1. Discuss with pt feelings about skin changes
		2. Pt will verbalize feelings re skin changes	2. Reinforce pt teaching on the action and side effects of mitomycin
			3. Offer emotional support

| V. Potential for injury related to Hemolytic Uremic Syndrome | V. A. (2%) Pts may experience significant increase in creatinine unrelated to total dose or duration of therapy
B. Hold drug for creatinine >1.7 mg/dl
C. Thrombotic microangiopathy may occur with anemia, thrombocytopenia
D. Blood transfusions may exacerbate condition
E. Often fatal | V. A. Alterations in renal function will be identified early | V. A. Monitor renal function, hematocrit, platelets prior to each drug dose; hold dose if serum creatinine is >1.7 mg/dl
B. If renal failure occurs, hemofiltration or dialysis may be necessary
C. Discuss risks and benefits with MD and pt if renal insufficiency is present and blood transfusion(s) are required |

DRUG

Mitotane (o,P'-DDD; Lysodren)

Class: Antihormone

MECHANISM OF ACTION

Adrenocortical suppressant with direct cytotoxic effect on mitochondria of adrenal cortical cells. Forces a drop in steroid secretion and alters the peripheral metabolism of steroids.

METABOLISM

34%–45% of oral dose is absorbed from the gastrointestinal tract. Metabolized partly in the liver and kidneys to a water-soluble metabolite that is then excreted in the bile and urine. Small amount of drug passes into the CSF.

DOSAGE/RANGE

Dose ranges from 2–16 gm/day orally.

Usual doses 2–10 gm/day.

Treatment usually begins with low doses (2 gm/day) and gradually increases.

Daily dose is divided into 3–4 doses.

DRUG PREPARATION

None

DRUG ADMINISTRATION

Oral

SPECIAL CONSIDERATIONS

Hypersensitivity reactions are rare, but have occurred.

Mitotane

Nursing Diagnosis	Defining Characteristics	Expected Outcomes	Nursing Interventions
I. *Altered nutrition, less than body requirements related to*			
A. Nausea and vomiting	I. A. 1. Occurs in 75% of pts, and may be dose-limiting toxicity 2. Anorexia may also occur	I. A. 1. Pt will be without nausea and vomiting 2. Nausea or vomiting, should they occur, will be treated early	I. A. 1. Nausea and vomiting may be reduced by beginning therapy with a low dose and increasing it as tolerated 2. Premedicate with antiemetics to prevent nausea and vomiting; continue as needed 3. Encourage small, frequent feedings of cool, bland foods and liquids 4. Inform pt that nausea and vomiting can occur; encourage pt to report onset 5. See sec. on nausea and vomiting, chap. 4
B. Diarrhea	B. Occurs in 20% of pts	B. 1. Pt will have minimal diarrhea	B. 1. Encourage pt to report onset of diarrhea 2. Administer or teach administration of antidiarrheal medication 3. If diarrhea is protracted, ensure adequate hydration, monitor I/O and electrolytes, teach perineal hygiene 4. See sec. on diarrhea, chap. 4
II. *Potential for injury, related to neurological toxicity*	II. A. Lethargy and somnolence most common: resolve with discontinuation of therapy B. Dizziness, vertigo occur in about 15% of pts C. Other CNS manifestations are depression, vertigo, muscle tremors, confusion, headache	II. A. Pt will maintain baseline cognitive function B. Pt will report onset of cognitive changes	II. A. Teach the pt and family about possible neurological toxicity: assess safety of planned activities (i.e., pt should avoid activities that require alertness) B. Encourage pt and family to report onset of symptoms, as they may necessitate discontinuing therapy

(continued)

Mitotane (continued)

Nursing Diagnosis	Defining Characteristics	Expected Outcomes	Nursing Interventions
III. *Potential for impaired skin integrity*	III. A. Skin irritation or rash occurs in about 15% of pts B. Sometimes resolves during treatment	III. A. Skin will remain intact B. Early signs of skin impairment will be identified	III. A. Inform pt that rash is expected and will resolve when treatment is finished B. Assess skin for integrity—recommend measures to decrease irritation, if indicated

DRUG

Mitoxantrone (Novantrone)

Class: New class of antineoplastics—anthracenediones. Antitumor antibiotic

MECHANISM OF ACTION

Inhibits both DNA and RNA synthesis regardless of the phase of cell division. Intercalates between base pairs thus distorting DNA structure. DNA-dependent RNA synthesis and protein synthesis are also inhibited.

METABOLISM

Excreted in both the bile and urine for 24–36 hours as virtually unchanged drug. Mean half-life is 5.8 hours. Peak levels achieved immediately. FDA approved for acute nonlymphocytic leukemia in adults.

DOSAGE/RANGE

10–14 mg/m^2 daily for 1 to 3 days

10–24 mg/m^2/day (clinical trials use—see specific protocol)

DRUG PREPARATION

Available as dark blue solution.

May be diluted in D$_5$W, NS or D$_5$NS.

Solution is chemically stable at room temperature for at least 48 hours.

Intact vials should be stored at room temperature. If refrigerated, a precipitate may form. This precipitate can be redissolved when vial is warmed to room temperature.

DRUG ADMINISTRATION

IV push over 3 minutes through the arm of a freely running infusion. IV bolus over 5–30 minutes.

SPECIAL CONSIDERATIONS

Nonvesicant. There have been rare reports of tissue necrosis after drug infiltration.

Incompatible with admixtures containing heparin.

Patient may experience blue-green urine for 24 hours after drug administration.

Mitoxantrone (Novantrone)

Nursing Diagnosis	Defining Characteristics	Expected Outcomes	Nursing Interventions
I. *Potential for injury related to*			
A. Infection	I. A. 1. Potent bone marrow depression: nadir 9–10 days 2. Granulocytopenia is usually the dose-limiting toxicity 3. Toxicity may be cumulative	I. A. 1. Pt will be without infection 2. Early s/s of infection and bleeding will be identified	I. A. 1. Monitor WBC, Hct, platelets prior to drug administration 2. Drug dosage should be reduced or held for lower-than-normal blood values 3. Instruct pt in self-assessment of s/s of infection 4. See sec. on bone marrow depression, chap. 4
B. Bleeding	B. 1. Thrombocytopenia uncommon, but can be severe when it occurs	B. 1. Pt will be without s/s of bleeding 2. Bleeding, if it occurs, will be identified and treated early	B. 1. Instruct pt in self-assessment of s/s of bleeding
C. Allergic reactions	C. 1. Hypersensitivity has been reported occasionally 2. Hypotension 3. Urticaria 4. Dyspnea 5. Rashes	C. 1. Allergic reactions will be detected early	C. 1. Prior to drug administration, obtain baseline vital signs 2. Observe for s/s of allergic reaction 3. Subjective s/s: generalized itching, dizziness 4. Objective s/s: flushed appearance (angioedema of face, neck, eyelids, hands, feet), localized or generalized urticaria 5. Document incident 6. Discuss with MD densensitization for future dose, versus drug discontinuance

II. *Nutrition alteration, less than body requirements related to*

	Assessment	Expected Outcomes	Interventions
A. Nausea and vomiting	II. A. 1. Typically not severe 2. Occurs in 30% of pts	II. A. 1. Pt will be without nausea and vomiting 2. Nausea and vomiting, if they occur, will be minimal	II. A. 1. Premedicate with antiemetic and continue prophylactically × 24 hrs to prevent nausea and vomiting, at least for first treatment 2. Encourage small, frequent feedings of cool, bland food and liquids 3. Refer to sec. on nausea and vomiting, chap. 4
B. Mucositis	B. 1. More common with prolonged dosing 2. Occurs in 5% of pts 3. Usually within 1 week of therapy	B. 1. Oral mucous membranes will remain intact and without infection	B. 1. Teach pt oral assessment and oral hygiene regimen 2. Encourage pt to report early stomatitis 3. See sec. on stomatitis, chap. 4

III. *Potential for impaired skin integrity related to*

	Assessment	Expected Outcomes	Interventions
A. Alopecia	III. A. 1. Mild to moderate 2. Occurs in 20% of pts	III. A. 1. Pt will verbalize feelings regarding hair loss 2. Pt will identify strategies to cope with changes in body image	III. A. 1. Discuss with pt impact of hair loss 2. Suggest wig as appropriate prior to actual hair loss 3. Explore with pt response to actual hair loss and plan strategies to minimize distress, i.e., wig, scarf, cap 4. Refer to sec. on alopecia, chap. 4
B. Extravasation	B. 1. Not a vesicant 2. Stains skin blue without ulcers 3. Rare reports of tissue necrosis following extravasation	B. 1. Skin discomfort will be minimized 2. Skin will remain intact 3. Pt will verbalize feelings re skin changes	B. 1. Careful technique is used during venipuncture. See sec. on IV administration, chap. 7 2. Administer drug through freely flowing IV, constantly monitoring IV site and pt response

(continued)

Mitoxantrone (Novantrone) (continued)

Nursing Diagnosis	Defining Characteristics	Expected Outcomes	Nursing Interventions
			III. B. 3. Teach pt to assess site and notify provider if condition worsens 4. Arrange next clinic visit for assessment of site depending on drug, amount infiltrated, extent of potential injury, and pt variables 5. Document in pt's record as per institutional policy and procedure. See sec. on reactions, ch. 6
IV. *Potential for alteration in cardiac output*	IV. A. CHF B. Decreased left ventricular ejection fraction occurs in about 3% of pts C. Increased cardiotoxicity with cumulative dose greater than 180 mg/m^2 D. Cumulative lifetime dose must be reduced if pt has had previous anthracycline therapy	IV. A. Early s/s of cardiomyopathy will be identified	IV. A. Assess for s/s of cardiomyopathy B. Assess quality and regularity of heartbeat C. Baseline EKG D. Instruct pt to report dyspnea, shortness of breath, swelling of extremities, orthopnea E. Discuss frequency of GBPs with MD
V. *Alternation in metabolic pattern*	V. A. In leukemia pts, rapid tumor lysis may occur with resultant hyperuricemia	V. A. Hyperuricemia will be identified early	V. A. Hydrate pt B. Alkalinize urine C. Administer allopurinal as per MD order D. Evaluate the effects of allopurinal by monitoring uric acid levels E. Monitor blood values of electrolytes, BUN, and creatinine

Nursing diagnosis			
VI. *Potential for anxiety*	VI. A. Urine will be green/blue × 24 hours B. Sclera may become discolored blue	VI. A. Pt will verbalize understanding of physiological changes expected with treatment	VI. A. Explain to pt changes that may occur with therapy, and that they are only temporary
VII. *Potential for sexual dysfunction*	VII. A. Drug is mutagenic and teratogenic	VII. A. Pt and significant other will understand the need for contraception	VII. A. As appropriate, explore with pt and significant other issues of reproductive and sexuality patterns and impact chemotherapy may have B. Discuss strategies to preserve sexual and reproductive health (i.e., sperm banking, contraception) C. See sec. on gonadal dysfunction, chap. 4

DRUG

Pentostatin (2'-deoxycofomycin, DCF)

Class: Investigational agent; antitumor antibiotic

MECHANISM OF ACTION

Cell cycle phase nonspecific. A potent inhibitor of adenosine deaminase. Interferes with DNA replication and disrupts RNA processing. It has potent lymphocytotoxic properties. The major mechanism of action is not yet clearly understood.

METABOLISM

The majority of pentostatin is excreted from the body via the urine, as unchanged drug. The mean half-life is 4.9–6.2 hours.

Clinical trials have shown a relationship between pentostatin's complete excretion and the patient's renal function. Patients with creatinine clearance ≤ 50 mL/min should NOT receive this agent.

DOSAGE/RANGE

Drug is undergoing clinical trials, consult individual protocol for specific dosages.

DRUG PREPARATION

This drug is supplied by the National Cancer Institute.

Available as a white powder.

Reconstitute with sodium chloride injection.

This solution is chemically stable at room temperature for at least 72 hours, but since it lacks bacteriostatic preservatives, discard the solution after 8 hours.

DRUG ADMINISTRATION

Drug is a vesicant. Administer IV push over 5 minutes through the side arm of a freely running IV.

SPECIAL CONSIDERATIONS

Drug is a vesicant.

Dose-limiting toxicities involve renal and neurotoxicities.

Requires adequate renal function.

Pentostatin

Nursing Diagnosis	Defining Characteristics	Expected Outcomes	Nursing Interventions
I. Potential for infection and bleeding related to bone marrow depression	I. A. Severe/profound leukopenia and thrombocytopenia B. Mild anemia	I. A. Patient will be without s/s of infection or bleeding B. Early s/s of infection or bleeding will be identified	I. A. Monitor CBC, platelet count prior to drug administration as well as s/s of infection or bleeding B. Instruct pt in self-assessment of s/s of infection or bleeding C. Dose reduction often necessary (35%–50%), if compromised bone marrow function D. Transfuse with platelets, red cells per MD orders E. Refer to sec. on bone marrow depression, chap. 4
II. Potential for altered urinary elimination related to nephrotoxicity	II. A. Renal insufficiency—mild; reversible—increased BUN, and creatinine common B. May include hyperuricemia if hydration, allopurinol are inadequate or if tumor lysis is acute	II. A. Pt will be without s/s of nephrotoxicity	II. A. Monitor BUN and creatinine prior to drug dose as drug is excreted in urine B. Provide, or instruct pt in hydration of at least 3 liters of fluid/day C. Monitor I/Os D. Hold drug if renal functions are elevated E. Refer to sec. on nephrotoxicity, chap. 4
III. Altered nutrition: less than body requirements related to			
A. Nausea and vomiting	III. A. 1. Nausea and vomiting may be mild to severe and seen in at least ⅔ of pts	III. A. 1. Pt will be without nausea and vomiting 2. Nausea and vomiting, if they occur, will be minimal	III. A. 1. Premedicate with antiemetics and continue prophylactically × 24 hrs to prevent nausea and vomiting 2. Encourage small, frequent feedings of cool, bland foods and liquids 3. Refer to sec. on nausea and vomiting, chap. 4
B. Hepatic dysfunction	B. 1. Hepatitis is rare but may occur; also disturbances in liver functions, i.e., mild SGOT	B. 1. Hepatic dysfunction will be identified early	B. 1. Monitor LFTs, especially SGOT 2. Notify MD of any elevations 3. Refer to sec. on hepotoxicity, chap. 4

(continued)

Pentostatin (continued)

Nursing Diagnosis	Defining Characteristics	Expected Outcomes	Nursing Interventions
IV. *Potential for mental status changes*	IV. A. Neurotoxicity varies from lethargy and somnolence to coma B. Occurs in 60% of cases C. Begins several days after pentostatin infusion and may last for up to 3 weeks	IV. A. Neurotoxicity will be identified early	IV. A. Teach pt about the potential for neurological reactions and to report any unusual symptoms B. Obtain baseline neurological and mental function C. Assess pt for any neurological abnormalities and report changes to MD D. Concomitant psychotropic drugs may exacerbate the s/s E. Refer to sec. on neurotoxicity, chap. 4
V. *Potential for impaired gas exchange related to pulmonary toxicity*	V. A. Infiltrates and nodules may occur in pts with prior history of receiving bleomycin, or lung irradiation	V. A. Early s/s of pulmonary toxicity will be identified	V. A. Obtain baseline pulmonary function B. Assess for s/s of pulmonary dysfunction, i.e., lung sounds C. Discuss with MD pulmonary function studies to be performed periodically D. Instruct pt to report cough or dyspnea E. Refer to sec. on pulmonary toxicity, chap. 4
VI. *Potential for sensory/perceptual alterations*	VI. A. Severe yet reversible conjunctivitis B. Responds to steroid eye drops	VI. A. Conjunctivitis will be prevented (or at least identified early)	VI. A. Obtain baseline opthalmic assessment B. Teach pt of the potential of opthalmic reactions and to report any unusual symptoms C. Administer steroid eye drops during drug administration
VII. A. *Alteration in skin integrity related to extravasation potential*	VII. A. Pentostatin is a potent vesicant B. Vesicant drugs cause erythema, burning, tissue necrosis, tissue sloughing	VII. A. Extravasation, if it occurs, is detected early with early intervention B. Skin and underlying tissue damage is minimized	VII. A. Careful technique is used during venipuncture. See sec. on intravenous administration, chap. 7 B. Administer vesicant through freely flowing IV, constantly monitoring IV site and pt response

VII. C. Nurse should be THOROUGHLY familiar with institutional policy and procedure for administration of a vesicant agent

D. If vesicant drug is administered as a continuous infusion, drug must be given through a patent central line

E. If extravasation is suspected:

1. Stop drug administered

2. Aspirate any residual drug and blood from IV tubing, IV catheter/needle, and IV site if possible

3. Instill antidote into area of apparent infiltration, IF ANTIDOTE EXISTS, as per MD orders and institutional policy and procedure

4. Apply cold or topical medication as per MD order and institutional policy and procedure

F. Assess site regularly for pain, progression of erythema, induration, and for evidence of necrosis

G. When in doubt about whether drug is infiltrating, TREAT AS AN INFILTRATION

H. Teach pt to assess site and notify MD if condition worsens.

I. Arrange next clinic visit for assessment of site depending on drug, amount infiltrated, extent of potential injury, and pt variables

J. Document in pt's record as per institutional policy and procedure. See sec. on reactions, ch. 6

DRUG

Plicamycin (mithramycin, Mithracin)

Class: Antibiotic. Isolated from *Streptomyces plicatus*

MECHANISM OF ACTION

In the presence of magnesium ions the drug binds with guanine bases of DNA and inhibits DNA-directed RNA synthesis. Cell cycle specific for S phase.

METABOLISM

Metabolism is not clearly understood. About half of the drug is excreted within 18–24 hours. Crosses blood–brain barrier and concentrations of drug in CSF equals blood concentration 4–6 hours after administration.

DOSAGE/RANGE

Dose for Testicular Cancer: 25–30 mcg/kg IV alternating days until toxicity occurs

Hypercalcemia: 25 mcg/kg IV times one dose

DRUG PREPARATION

For each 2.5-mg vial add sterile water to obtain concentration of 500 mcg/ml.

DRUG ADMINISTRATION

IV drug is an irritant; avoid extravasation. Administer over 4–6 hours to minimize nausea and vomiting.

SPECIAL CONSIDERATIONS

Alternate day therapy greatly reduces the incidences and severity of stomatitis, hemorrhage, and facial flushing and swelling.

Do not administer to patient with a coagulation disorder or impaired bone marrow function because of the risk of hemorrhagic diathesis.

Crosses the blood–brain barrier.

Metallic taste with administration.

Plicamycin

Nursing Diagnosis	Defining Characteristics	Expected Outcomes	Nursing Interventions
I. *Altered nutrition, less than body requirements related to*			
A. Nausea and vomiting	I. A. 1. Severe nausea and vomiting begins 6+ hours after dose and may last 24 hours (at therapeutic doses)	I. A. 1. Pt will be without nausea and vomiting 2. Nausea and vomiting, if they occur, will be minimal	I. A. 1. Premedicate with antiemetics and continue prophylactically to *prevent* nausea and vomiting, at least for first treatment 2. Encourage small, frequent feedings of cool, bland foods and liquids 3. See sec. on nausea and vomiting, chap. 4
B. Anorexia	B. 1. Commonly occurs	B. 1. Pt will maintain baseline weight ±5%	B. 1. Encourage small, frequent feedings of favorite foods, especially high-calorie, high-protein foods 2. Encourage use of spices 3. Weekly weights
C. Stomatitis	C. 1. Alternate day therapy greatly reduces the incidence and severity of stomatitis	C. 1. Oral mucous membranes will remain intact without infection	C. 1. Teach pt oral assessment and oral hygiene regimens 2. Encourage pt to report early stomatitis 3. Pain relief measures if needed. 4. See sec. on stomatitis, chap. 4
D. Potential for taste alterations	D. 1. Taste alterations can occur	D. 1. Pt will eat adequate calories, proteins, minerals	D. 1. Suggest increased use of spices as tolerated 2. Help pt and significant others develop menu based on past favorite foods 3. Dietary consultation as needed 4. Discuss dietary supplements of zinc and selenium

(continued)

Plicamycin (continued)

Nursing Diagnosis	Defining Characteristics	Expected Outcomes	Nursing Interventions
II. Potential for infection and bleeding, related to bone marrow depression	II. A. Leukopenia nadir 7–14 days with recovery by 1–2 weeks B. Less frequent thrombocytopenia, but ⅓ of pts develop a coagulopathy. Alternate-day instead of daily dosing reduces bleeding complications C. Mild anemia D. Potent immuno-suppressant	II. A. Pt will be without s/s of infection or bleeding B. Early s/s of infection or bleeding will be identified	II. A. Monitor CBC, platelet count prior to drug administration, as well as s/s of infection or bleeding B. Instruct pt in self-assessment of s/s of infection or bleeding C. Dose reduction often necessary (35%–50%) if compromised bone marrow function D. See sec. on bone marrow depression, chap. 4
III. *Potential for impaired skin integrity, related to*			
A. Alopecia	III. A. 1. Occurs in 30%–50% of pts, especially with IV dosing 2. Some degree of hair loss expected in all pts 3. Begins after 3+ weeks, and hair may grow back on therapy 4. May be slight to diffuse thinning	III. A. 1. Pt will verbalize feelings re hair loss, and identify strategies to cope with change in body image	III. A. 1. Assess pt for s/s of hair loss 2. Discuss with pt impact of hair loss, and strategies to minimize distress; i.e., wig, scarf, cap (begin before therapy initiated) 3. See sec. on alopecia, chap. 4

B. Changes in nails, skin	B. Hyperpigmentation of nails and skin, transverse ridging of nails ("band-ing") may occur	B. 1. Pt will verbalize feelings re changes in nail or skin color or texture, and identify strategies to cope with change in body image	B. 1. Assess pt for changes in skin, nails 2. Discuss with pt impact of changes and strategies to minimize distress; i.e., wearing nail polish (women), long sleeved tops
IV. *Potential for sexual dysfunction*	IV. A. Drug is mutagenic and teratogenic B. Testicular atrophy sometimes with reversible oligo- and azoospermia C. Amenorrhea often occurs in females D. Drug is excreted in breast milk	IV. A. Pt and significant other will understand need for contraception B. Pt and significant other will identify strategies to cope with sexual dysfunction	IV. A. As appropriate, explore with pt and significant other issues of reproductive and sexuality patterns, and impact chemotherapy will have B. Discuss strategies to preserve sexual and reproductive health (i.e., sperm banking, contraception) C. See sec. on gonadal dysfunction, chap. 4
V. *Alteration in metabolism*	V. A. Drug may decrease calcium and lead to hypocalcemia. Monitor for muscle stiffness, twitching B. In some cases when calcium is abnormally high (as in hypercalcemia from breast cancer), this drug may be used to decrease calcium level	V. A. Hypocalcemia will be identified and treated early	V. A. Monitor blood calcium levels B. Instruct pt about s/s of neuro/muscular involvement such as, muscle stiffness, weakness, or twitching C. Instruct pt about CNS manifestations of hypocalcemia: weakness, drowsiness, lethargy, irritability, headache, confusion, depression

DRUG

Procarbazine Hydrochlorozide (Natulanar, Matulane)

Class: Miscellaneous agent

MECHANISM OF ACTION

Uncertain, but appears to affect preformed DNA, RNA, and protein. It is a methylhydrazine derivative.

METABOLISM

Most of the drug is excreted in the urine. Procarbazine crosses the blood–brain barrier. Rapidly absorbed from the gastrointestinal tract, metabolized by the liver.

DOSAGE/RANGE

100 to 300 mg daily PO from 7 to 14 days every 4 weeks. Given in combination with other drugs.

DRUG PREPARATION

None

DRUG ADMINISTRATION

Oral. Available in 50 mg capsules.

SPECIAL CONSIDERATIONS

Procarbazine is synergistic with CNS depressants. Barbiturates, antihistamine, narcotic, and hypotensive agents or phenothiazine antiemetics should be used with caution.

Antabuse-like reaction may result if the patient consumes ETOH. Symptoms include headache, respiratory difficulties, nausea and vomiting, chest pain, hypotension, and mental status changes.

Exhibits weak MOA (monoamine oxidase) inhibitor activity. Foods containing high amounts of tyramine should be avoided: substances like beer, wine, cheese, brewer's yeast, chicken livers, and bananas. Consumption of foods high in tyramine in combination with procarbazine may lead to intracranial hemorrhage or hypertensive crisis.

When taken in combination with digoxin there is a decreased bioavailability of digoxin.

Procarbazine Hydrochlorozide

Nursing Diagnosis	Defining Characteristics	Expected Outcomes	Nursing Interventions
I. *Potential for infection and bleeding related to bone marrow depression (BMD)*	I. A. Major dose-limiting toxicity B. Thrombocytopenia occurs in ½ pts, evidenced by a delayed onset (28 d after treatment) and lasting 2–3 weeks C. Leukopenia seen in ⅔ of pts with nadirs occurring after initial thrombocytopenia D. Anemias may be due to BMD or hemolysis	I. A. Pt will be without s/s of infection or bleeding B. Early s/s of infection or bleeding will be identified	I. A. Monitor CBC, platelet count prior to drug administration, as well as s/s of infection, bleeding, and anemia B. Instruct pt in self-assessment of s/s of infection, bleeding, and anemia C. Dose reduction often necessary (35%–50%) if compromised bone marrow function D. Platelet and red cell transfusions per MD order E. Refer to sec. on BMD, chap. 4
II. *Altered nutrition less than body requirements related to*			
A. Nausea and vomiting	II. A. 1. Nausea and vomiting occur in 70% of pts and may be a dose-limiting toxicity	II. A. 1. Pt will be without nausea and vomiting 2. Nausea and vomiting, if they occur, will be minimal	II. A. 1. Premedicate with antiemetics and continue prophylactically × 24 hrs to *prevent* nausea and vomiting 2. Encourage small, frequent feedings of cool, bland foods and liquids 3. Minimize nausea and vomiting by dividing the total daily dosage into 3–4 doses. Also taking the pills at bedtime may decrease the sense of nausea 4. May administer nonphenothiazine antiemetics 5. Refer to sec. on nausea and vomiting, chap. 4
B. Diarrhea	B. 1. Uncommon but rarely may be protracted and thus would be an indication for dose reduction	B. 1. Pt will have minimal diarrhea	B. 1. Encourage pt to report onset of diarrhea 2. Administer, or teach pt to self-administer antidiarrheal medications 3. See sec. on diarrhea, chap. 4

(continued)

Procarbazine Hydrochlorozide

Nursing Diagnosis	Defining Characteristics	Expected Outcomes	Nursing Interventions
II. C. Stomatitis	II. C. 1. Rare	II. C. 1. Oral mucous membranes will remain intact without infection	II. C. 1. Teach pt oral assessment 2. Encourage pt to report early stomatitis 3. Teach pt oral hygiene regimen 4. See sec. on stomatitis, chap. 4
D. Anorexia	D. 1. Rare	D. 1. Pt will maintain baseline weight ± 5%	D. 1. Encourage small, frequent feedings of favorite foods, especially high-calorie, high-protein foods 2. Encourage use of spices 3. Weekly weights
III. *Potential for sensory/perceptual alterations* A. Neurotoxicity	III. A. 1. Symptoms occur in 10%–30% of pts. Seen as lethargy, depression, freq. nightmares, insomnia, nervousness, or hallucinations 2. Tremors, coma, convulsions less common 3. Symptoms usually disappear when drug is discontinued 4. Crosses into CSF	III. A. 1. Early s/s of neurotoxicity will be identified	III. A. 1. Teach pt the potential of neurotoxicity and provide early counseling about these effects 2. Assess pts for any symptoms of neurotoxicity 3. Discuss strategies with pt to preserve general sense of well-being 4. Obtain baseline neurological and motor function 5. CNS toxicity may be manifested as reactions to other drugs, e.g., barbiturates, narcotics, and phenothiazine antiemetics

Nursing Diagnosis	Assessment	Expected Outcomes	Interventions
III. B. *Peripheral neuropathy*	III. B. 1. 10% of pts exhibit paresthesias, decrease in deep tendon reflexes 2. Foot drop and ataxia occasionally reported 3. Reversible when drug discontinued	III. B. 1. Pt will be without s/s of peripheral neuropathy	III. B. 1. Obtain baseline neurological and motor function 2. Assess pt for any changes in motor function, e.g., picking up pencil, buttoning buttons
C. *Flulike syndrome*	C. 1. Commonly occurs: fever, chills, sweating, lethargy, myalgias, and arthralgias	C. 1. Pt will report early s/s of flulike syndrome	C. 1. Teach pt the potential for flulike syndromes and how to distinguish from actual infection 2. Instruct pt to report any changes in condition
IV. *Potential for impaired skin integrity related to rare dermatitis reactions*	IV. A. Rarely occurs as alopecia, pruritis, rash, hyperpigmentation	IV. A. Pt will verbalize feelings regarding changes in hair loss, skin color or skin integrity, and identify strategies to cope with change in body image	IV. A. Assess pt for changes in skin, nails, and hair loss B. Discuss with pt impact of changes and strategies to minimize distress, i.e., wearing nail polish (women), long sleeved tops, wigs, scarfs, caps
V. *Potential for sexual dysfunction*	V. A. Drug is teratogenic B. Causes azoospermia C. Cessation of menses, though, may be reversible	V. A. Pt and significant other will understand need for contraception B. Pt and significant other will identify strategies to cope with sexual dysfunction	V. A. As appropriate, explore with pt and significant other issues of reproductive and sexuality patterns, and impact chemotherapy may have B. Discuss strategies to preserve sexual and reproductive health (i.e., sperm banking, contraception) C. See sec. on gonadal dysfunction, chap. 4
VI. *Potential for injury related to second malignancy, leukemia*	VI. A. Prolonged therapy may cause leukemia (related to drug's carcinogenic properties)	VI. A. Malignancy, if it occurs, will be identified early	VI. A. If receiving prolonged therapy, pt should be screened periodically B. Educate pts on the potential of secondary malignancies

DRUG

Progestational agents: medroxyprogesterone acetate (Provera, Depo-Provera); megestrol acetate (Megace, Pallace)

Class: Hormone

MECHANISM OF ACTION

Unclear, but progestational agents compete for androgen and progestational receptor sites on the cell. Has potent antiestrogenic properties that disturb estrogen receptor cycle. Also increases synthesis of RNA by interacting with DNA.

METABOLISM

Rapidly absorbed from gastrointestinal tract. Metabolized in the liver. Excreted in the urine. Peak plasma levels reached in 1–3 hours; biological halflife: 3½ days.

DOSAGE/RANGE

Medroxyprogesterone acetate:
Provera   20–80 mg orally daily
Depo-Provera   400–800 mg IM every month
               100 mg IM three times weekly
               (high dose) 1000–1500 mg daily

Megestrol acetate (Megace, Pallace):
       40 mg orally QID (breast cancer)
       80 mg orally QID (endometrial cancer)

DRUG PREPARATION

IM preparation is ready to use; shake vial well before drawing up medication.

DRUG ADMINISTRATION

Give via deep IM injection.

SPECIAL CONSIDERATIONS

Patients may become sensitive to oil carrier (oil in which drug is mixed).

Small risk of hypersensitivity reaction.

Progestational Agents

Nursing Diagnosis	Defining Characteristics	Expected Outcomes	Nursing Interventions
I. *Potential for injury, related to*			
A. Fluid retention	I. A. 1. May occur	I. A. 1. Fluid balance will be maintained	I. A. 1. Inform pt of potential for fluid retention, of s/s to watch for and to report to nurse or MD 2. Assess pt for s/s of fluid overload
B. Thromboembolic complications	B. 1. Thromboembolic complications may occur	B. 1. Pt will avoid injury related to abnormal blood clotting	B. 1. Teach pts and family s/s of thromboembolic events: positive Homan's Sign, localized pain, tenderness, erythema, sudden CNS changes, shortness of breath, etc. 2. Instruct pt to notify nurse or MD if any of the above occur
C. Sterile abscess	C. 1. May occur with IM administration	C. 1. Pt will avoid injury related to abscess formation	C. 1. Give drug via deep IM injection: apply pressure to injection site after administering 2. Inspect used sites: rotate sites systematically
II. *Altered nutrition, less than body requirements related to nausea*	II. A. Occurs infrequently	II. A. Pt will be without nausea	II. A. Inform pt that nausea can occur: encourage pt to report nausea B. Encourage small, frequent feedings of cool, bland liquids and foods C. Refer to sec. on nausea and vomiting, chap. 4

DRUG

Streptozocin (Streptozotocin, Zanosar)

Class: Alkylating agent (nitrosourea)

MECHANISM OF ACTION

A weak alkylating agent (nitrosourea) that causes interstrand cross-linking in DNA (is cell cycle phase nonspecific). Appears to have some specificity for neoplastic pancreatic endocrine cells. Glucose attached to nitrosourea appears to diminish myelotoxicity.

METABOLISM

60%–70% of total dose and 10%–20% of parent drug appears in urine. Drug is rapidly eliminated from serum in 4 hours with major concentrations occuring in liver and kidneys.

DOSAGE/RANGE

500 mg/m^2 IV every day $\times$ 5 days repeat every 3–4 weeks
or 1500 mg/m^2 IV every week

DRUG PREPARATION

Add sterile water or NS to vial.

If powder or solution contacts skin, wash immediately with soap and water.

Solution is stable 48 hours at room temperature, 96 hours if refrigerated.

DRUG ADMINISTRATION

Administer via voutrol over 1 hour.

Has also been given as continuous infusion or continuous arterial infusion into the hepatic artery.

If local pain or burning occurs, slow infusion and apply cool packs above injection site.

Irritant; avoid extravasation.

Administer with 1–2 liters of hydration to prevent nephrotoxicity.

SPECIAL CONSIDERATIONS

Increased risk of nephrotoxicity if given with other potentially nephrototoxic drugs.

Renal function must be monitored closely.

Drug is an irritant. Give through the sidearm of a running IV.

Streptozocin

Nursing Diagnosis	Defining Characteristics	Expected Outcomes	Nursing Interventions
I. *Potential for altered urinary elimination*	I. A. 60% of pts experience renal dysfunction B. Usually transient proteinuria and azotemia but may progress to permanent renal failure, especially if other nephrotoxic drugs are given concurrently C. S/s include: proteinuria, increased BUN, hypophosphatemia, glycosuria, renal tubular acidosis, decreased creatinine clearance D. Hypophosphatemia is probably earliest sign of renal dysfunction	I. A. Early renal dysfunction will be identified B. Permanent renal failure will be prevented	I. A. Closely monitor BUN, creatinine, phosphorus, urine protein, and 24 hr creatinine clearance prior to each treatment, and BUN, creatinine, pH of urine, glucose/protein of urine every shift during therapy B. If creatinine clearance is <25 mL/min, dose should be reduced by 50%–75% C. Strictly monitor I/O during therapy D. Hydration per MD, but usually 2–3L/day E. Refer to sec. on nephrotoxicity, chap. 4

(continued)

Streptozocin *(continued)*

Nursing Diagnosis	Defining Characteristics	Expected Outcomes	Nursing Interventions
II. *Altered nutrition, less than body requirements related to*			
A. Nausea and vomiting	II. A. 1. Nausea and vomiting occur in up to 90% of pts, beginning 1–4 hrs after drug dose 2. Significantly reduced when drug is given as continuous infusion 3. Nausea and vomiting may worsen during 5-consecutive-day therapy 4. Increased severity with doses >500mg/m^2	II. A. 1. Pt will be without nausea and vomiting 2. Nausea and vomiting, if they occur, will be minimal	II. A. 1. Premedicate with antiemetics and continue prophylactically × 24 hrs; use aggressive antiemetics when drug is given IV over 1 hour 2. Encourage small, frequent feedings of cool, bland foods and liquids 3. If pt has emesis >250 in 8 hr discuss with MD more aggressive antiemetics 4. Monitor I/O closely and replace fluids 5. Refer to sec. on nausea and vomiting, chap. 4
B. Diarrhea	B. 1. 10% of pts experience diarrhea with abdominal cramping	B. 1. Pt will have minimal diarrhea	B. 1. Encourage pt to report onset of diarrhea 2. Administer or teach pt to self-administer antidiarrheal medications 3. Teach pt diet modifications 4. Refer to sec. on diarrhea, chap. 4

II. C. Alterations in glucose metabolism

II. C. 1. Appears that damage to pancreatic beta cells causes sudden release of insulin with resulting hypoglycemia in about 20% of pts
2. Hyperglycemia may occur in pts with insulinomas and decreased glucose tolerance. Increased fasting or post-pranidial blood levels may occur

II. C. 1. Hypoglycemia will be identified and corrected
2. Hyperglycemia will be identified and corrected

II. C. 1. Monitor serum glucose levels every day or more frequently as needed, check urine glucose
2. Assess for, and instruct pt to report following s/s of hypoglycemia:
   a. muscle weakness and lethargy
   b. perspiration
   c. flushed feeling
   d. restlessness
   e. headache
   f. confusion
   g. trembling
   h. epigastric hunger pains
3. If s/s of hypoglycemia are found, encourage pt to eat or drink high glucose food and juice and notify MD
4. Hypoglycemia can be prevented with nicotinamide
5. Assess for s/s of hyperglycemia in pt with insulinomas and instruct pt in self-assessment

D. Hepatic dysfunction

D. 1. Liver function studies may be elevated but normalize with time
2. Hepatotoxicity occurs in ~50% of pts
3. Liver enzymes increase 2–3 weeks after therapy
4. Albumin decreases
5. Symptoms rarely occur
6. Painless jaundice may occur

D. 1. Early hepatotoxicity will be identified

D. 1. Monitor LFTs (liver function tests) prior to each treatment (alkaline phosphatase, SGOT, SGPT, albumin)
2. Assess for s/s of hepatic dysfunction: jaundice, yellowing of skin; sclera, orange-colored urine; white or clay-colored stools; itchy skin

(continued)

Streptozocin (*continued*)

Nursing Diagnosis	Defining Characteristics	Expected Outcomes	Nursing Interventions
III. *Potential for infection and bleeding related to bone marrow depression (BMD)*	III. A. BMD occurs in about 9–20% of pts B. Nadir 1–2 wks after administration C. Occasionally, severe leukopenia and thrombocytopenia occur D. Mild anemia may occur	III. A. Pt will be without s/s of infection or bleeding B. Early s/s of infection or bleeding will be identified	III. A. Monitor CBC, platelets prior to drug administration, as well as assess for s/s of infection or bleeding B. Instruct pt in self-assessment of s/s of infection or bleeding C. Refer to sec. on BMD, chap. 4
IV. *Potential for injury related to secondary malignancies*	IV. A. Drug is carcinogenic—secondary malignancies are well described	IV. A. Malignancy, if it occurs, will be identified early	IV. A. Pts receiving prolonged therapy should be screened periodically

DRUG

Tamoxifen citrate (Nolvadex)

Class: Antiestrogen

MECHANISM OF ACTION

Nonsteroidal antiestrogen which binds to estrogen receptors, forming an abnormal complex that migrates to the cell nucleus and inhibits DNA synthesis.

METABOLISM

Well absorbed from gastrointestinal tract and metabolized by liver. Undergoes enterohepatic circulation, prolonging blood levels. Excreted in feces. Elimination half-life is 7 days.

DOSAGE/RANGE

20–80 mg orally daily (most often, 20 mg BID)

DRUG PREPARATION

None. Available in 10 mg tablets.

DRUG ADMINISTRATION

Oral

SPECIAL CONSIDERATIONS

Measurement of estrogen receptors in tumor may be important in predicting tumor response and should be performed at same time as biopsy and before antiestrogen treatment is started.

Avoid antacids within 2 hours of taking enteric-coated tablets.

A "flare" reaction with bony pain and hypercalcemia may occur. Such reactions are short-lived and usually result in a tumor response if therapy is continued.

Tamoxifen Citrate

Nursing Diagnosis	Defining Characteristics	Expected Outcomes	Nursing Interventions
I. Potential for sexual dysfunction	I. A. May cause menstrual irregularity, hot flashes, milk production in breasts, vaginal discharge and bleeding B. Symptoms occur in about 10% of pts and are usually not severe enough to discontinue therapy	I. A. Pt and significant other will identify strategies for coping with sexual dysfunction	I. A. As appropriate, explore with pt and significant other issues of reproductive and sexuality patterns and impact drug may have on them B. Discuss strategies to preserve sexual and reproductive health C. Refer to sec. on gonadal dysfunction, chap. 4
II. Potential for alteration in comfort	II. A. May cause "flare" reaction initially (bone and tumor pain, transient increase in tumor size) B. Nausea, vomiting, and anorexia may occur	II. A. Pt will identify s/s of "flare" reaction, and strategies to cope with it B. Pt will avoid nausea, vomiting, and anorexia C. Nausea, vomiting, and anorexia, should they occur, will be minimal	II. A. Inform pt of possibility of "flare" reaction, s/s to be aware of, and encourage pt to report any s/s B. Inform pt of possibility of nausea, vomiting, and anorexia C. Encourage small, frequent feedings of high-calorie, high-protein foods
III. Potential for sensory/perceptual alteration	III. A. Retinopathy has been reported with high doses B. Corneal changes (infrequent), decreased visual acuity, and blurred vision have occurred C. Headache, dizziness, and lightheadedness are rare	III. A. Visual disturbance and CNS symptoms will be identified early	III. A. Obtain visual assessment prior to starting therapy B. Encourage pt to report any visual changes C. Instruct pt to report headache, dizziness, lightheadedness

IV. *Potential for infection and bleeding related to bone marrow depression*	IV. A. Mild transient leukopenia and thrombocytopenia occur rarely	IV. A. Patient will be without s/s of infection or bleeding	IV. A. Monitor CBC, platelet counts prior to therapy and after therapy has begun B. Instruct pt in self-assessment of s/s of infection or bleeding C. See sec. on bone marrow depression, chap. 4
V. *Potential for skin integrity impairment*	V. A. Skin rash, alopecia, peripheral edema are rare	V. A. Skin integrity will be maintained	V. A. Assess pt for s/s of hair loss, edema, and skin rash B. Instruct pt to report any of these symptoms C. Discuss with pt the impact of skin changes
VI. *Potential for injury related to hypercalcemia*	VI. A. Hypercalcemia uncommon	VI. A. Serum calcium will remain within normal limits	VI. A. Obtain serum calcium levels prior to therapy and at regular intervals during therapy B. Instruct pt in s/s of hypercalcemia: nausea, vomiting, weakness, constipation, loss of muscle tone, malaise, decreased urine output

DRUG

6-Thioguanine (Thioguanine, Tabloid, 6-TG)

Class: Thiopurine antimetabolite

MECHANISM OF ACTION

Converts to monophosphate nucleotides and inhibits de novo purine synthesis. The nucleotides are also incorporated into DNA. Cell cycle phase specific (S phase).

Thioguanine interferes with nucleic acid biosynthesis resulting in sequential blockage of the synthesis and utilization of the purine nucleotides.

METABOLISM

Absorption is incomplete and variable orally. Is metabolized in the liver by deamination and methylation. Metabolites are excreted in the urine and feces. Plasma half-life: 80–90 minutes.

DOSAGE/RANGE

Children and Adults: 100 mg/m^2 orally every 12 hours for 5–10 days, usually in combination with cytarabine

100 mg/m^2 IV daily × 5 days

1–3 mg/kg orally daily

DRUG PREPARATION

Available in 40 mg tablets.

Reconstitute 100-mg vial in 15 ml NS.

DRUG ADMINISTRATION

Given via IV bolus.

SPECIAL CONSIDERATIONS

Oral dose to be given on empty stomach to facilitate complete absorption.

Dose is titrated to avoid excessive stomatitis and diarrhea.

6-Thioguanine can be used in full doses with allopurinol.

6-Thioguanine

Nursing Diagnosis	Defining Characteristics	Expected Outcomes	Nursing Interventions
I. *Altered nutrition, less than body requirements related to*			
A. Nausea and vomiting	I. A. 1. Nausea and vomiting occur uncommonly, especially in children, but are dose-related	I. A. 1. Pt will be without nausea and vomiting 2. Nausea and vomiting, should they occur, will be minimal	I. A. 1. Treat symptomatically with antiemeties 2. Encourage small, frequent feedings of cool, bland foods and liquids 3. If vomiting occurs, assess for fluid and electrolyte imbalance. Monitor I/O and daily weights if pt is hospitalized
B. Anorexia	B. 1. Rare	B. 1. Pt will maintain baseline weight ± 5%	B. 1. Encourage small frequent feedings of favorite foods, especially high-calorie, high-protein foods 2. Encourage use of spices 3. Weekly weights
C. Stomatitis	C. 1. Rare, but most common with high doses	C. 1. Oral mucous membranes will remain intact and without infection	C. 1. Teach oral assessment and oral hygiene regimen 2. Encourage pt to report early stomatitis 3. Provide pain relief measures, if indicated 4. See sec. on stomatitis, chap. 4
D. Hepatotoxicity	D. 1. Rare, but may be associated with hepatic veno-occlusive disease or jaundice	D. 1. Hepatotoxicity will be identified early	D. 1. Monitor LFTs prior to drug dose 2. Assess pt prior to and during treatment for s/s of hepatotoxicity

(continued)

6-Thioguanine *(continued)*

Nursing Diagnosis	Defining Characteristics	Expected Outcomes	Nursing Interventions
II. *Potential for infection and bleeding, related to bone marrow depression*	II. A. Bone marrow depression occurs 1–4 weeks after treatment B. Leukopenia and thrombocytopenia are most common C. Drug may have prolonged or delayed nadir	II. A. Pt will be without s/s of infection or bleeding B. Early s/s of infection or bleeding will be identified	II. A. Monitor CBC, platelet count prior to drug administration, as well as s/s of infection or bleeding B. Instruct pt in self-assessment of s/s of infection or bleeding C. Administer platelet, red cell transfusions per MD order D. Refer to sec. on bone marrow depression, chap. 4
III. *Potential for sensory/perceptual alterations*	III. A. Loss of vibratory sensation, unsteady gait may occur	III. A. Neurological toxicity will be identified early	III. A. Assess vibratory sensation, gait before each dose and between treatments B. Report changes to MD C. Encourage pt to report any changes

DRUG

Thiotepa (Triethylene Thiophosphoramide)

Class: Alkylating agent

MECHANISM OF ACTION

Selectively reacts with DNA phosphate groups to produce chromosome cross-linkage with blocking of nucleoprotein synthesis. Acts as a polyfunctional alkylating agent. Cell cycle phase nonspecific agent. Mimics radiation-induced injury.

METABOLISM

Rapidly cleared following IV administration; 60% of dose is eliminated in urine within 24–72 hours. Slow onset of action, slowly bound to tissues, extensively metabolized.

DOSAGE/RANGE

Intravenous:
8 mg/m^2 (0.2 mg/kg) IV every day × 5 days repeated every 3–4 weeks *or*
30–60 mg IV, IM, or SQ once a week, depending on WBC

Intracavitary:
bladder: 60 mg in 60 ml sterile water once a week for 3–4 weeks

DRUG PREPARATION

Add sterile water to vial of lyophilized powder.

Further dilute with NS or D$_5$W.

Do not use solution unless it is clear.

Refrigerate vial until use (reconstituted solution is stable for 5 days).

DRUG ADMINISTRATION

IV, IM; intracavitary; intratumor, intra-arterial.

SPECIAL CONSIDERATIONS

Hypersensitivity reactions have occurred with this drug.

Is an irritant, should be given via a sidearm of a running IV.

Increased neuromuscular blockage when given with nondepolarizing muscle relaxants.

Thiotepa

Nursing Diagnosis	Defining Characteristics	Expected Outcomes	Nursing Interventions
I. Potential for infection and bleeding related to bone marrow depression (BMD)	I. A. 1. Nadir is 5–30 days after drug administration B. Thrombocytopenia and leukopenia may occur C. Anemia may occur with prolonged use D. May be cumulative toxicity with recovery of bone marrow in 40–50 days E. Thrombocytopenia is dose-limiting	I. A. Pt will be without s/s of infection or bleeding B. Early s/s of infection or bleeding will be detected	I. A. Monitor CBC, platelet count prior to drug administration; monitor for s/s of infection or bleeding B. Instruct pt in self-assessment of s/s of infection or bleeding C. Administer red cell and platelet transfusions per MD orders D. Refer to sec. on BMD, chap. 4
II. *Altered nutrition, less than body requirements related to*			
A. Nausea and vomiting	II. A. 1. Nausea and vomiting occurs in 10%–15% of pts 2. Dose dependent 3. Occurs 6–12 hours after drug dose	II. A. 1. Pt will be without nausea and vomiting 2. Nausea and vomiting, if they occur, will be minimal	II. A. 1. Premedicate with antiemetics especially with parenteral dosing of high dose. Continue antiemetics at least 12 hours after drug is given 2. Encourage small, frequent feedings of cool, bland dry foods 3. Refer to sec. on nausea and vomiting, chap. 4
B. Anorexia	B. 1. Occurs occasionally	B. 1. Pt will maintain baseline weight ± 5%	B. 1. Encourage small frequent feedings of favorite foods, especially high-calorie, high-protein foods 2. Encourage use of spices 3. Weekly weights

Nursing diagnosis	Defining characteristics	Expected outcomes	Nursing interventions
III. *Sexual dysfunction*	III. A. Drug is mutagenic B. Sterility may be reversible and incomplete C. Amenorrhea often reverses in 6–8 mos	III. A. Pt and significant other will identify coping strategies to deal with sexual dysfunction	III. A. As appropriate, explore with pt and significant other issues of reproductive and sexuality patterns and anticipated impact chemotherapy may have B. Discuss strategies to preserve sexuality and reproductive health (i.e., sperm banking) C. Refer to sec. on gonadal dysfunction, chap. 4
IV. *Potential for injury related to* A. Allergic reaction	IV. A. 1. Allergic responses may occur rarely: hives, bronchospasm, skin rash (dermatitis)	IV. A. 1. Allergic responses will be detected early and treated	IV. A. 1. Assess for s/s of allergic response during drug administration 2. Stop drug if bronchospasm occurs and notify MD 3. Discuss symptomatic treatment with MD
B. Secondary malignancies	B. 1. Secondary malignancies may occur with a prolonged therapy	B. 1. Secondary malignancy, if it occurs, will be detected early	B. 1. Instruct pt receiving prolonged therapy in importance of regular health maintenance examinations during and after therapy by primary care provider and oncologist
V. *Alteration in comfort*	V. A. Dizziness, headache, fever, and local pain may occur	V. A. Distress will be minimal	V. A. Assess for alterations in comfort B. Treat symptomatically

DRUG

Trimetrexate

Class: Investigational Agent Antimetabolite

MECHANISM OF ACTION

Nonclassical folate antagonist; potent inhibitor of dihydrofolate reductase. May be able to overcome mechanism(s) of methotrexate resistance as drug reaches higher concentration within tumor cells. Also, inhibits growth of parasitic infective agents (causing pneumocystis carinii, toxoplasmosis) in patients with immunodeficiency or myelodysplastic disorders.

METABOLISM

Significant percentage of drug is protein bound. Metabolized by liver, 10%–20% of dose is excreted by kidneys in 24 hours.

DOSAGE/RANGE

12 mg/m^2 IV daily $\times$ 5 repeat every 3 weeks
8 mg/m^2 IV daily $\times$ 5 repeat every 3 weeks
Maximum tolerated dose: 15 mg/m^2 day $\times$ 5

Maximum tolerated dose: 13.1 mg/m^2 day $\times$ 5 for patient without prior therapy; 7.6 mg/m^2 day $\times$ 5 for patient with prior therapy

DRUG PREPARATION

Stable 24 hours at room temperature or refrigerated.

DRUG ADMINISTRATION

IV bolus over 5 minutes.

Can be given as an IV infusion.

Incompatible with chloride solutions.

SPECIAL CONSIDERATIONS

Increased toxicity is seen in patients with low protein (drug is highly protein bound) and hepatic dysfunction. Dose reduction indicated.

Leukopenia is dose-limiting toxicity first seen at dose of 1.6 mg/m^2.

Other side effects are nausea and vomiting, rash, mucositis, diarrhea, SGOT elevations, thrombocytopenia.

Trimetrexate

Nursing Diagnosis	Defining Characteristics	Expected Outcomes	Nursing Interventions
I. Infection and bleeding related to bone marrow depression	I. A. Leukopenia is a dose-limiting toxicity: seen at doses of 1.6 mg/m^2 and higher B. Thrombocytopenia also occurs commonly	I. A. Pt will be without s/s of infection or bleeding B. Early s/s of infection or bleeding will be identified	I. A. Monitor CBC, platelet count prior to drug administration, as well as s/s of infection or bleeding B. Instruct pt in self-assessment of s/s of infection or bleeding C. Administer red cell, platelet transfusions per MD order D. Refer to sec. on bone marrow depression, chap. 4
II. *Altered nutrition: less than body requirements related to*			
A. Nausea and vomiting	II. A. 1. Nausea and vomiting have been reported in clinical trials	II. A. 1. Pt will be without nausea and vomiting 2. Nausea and vomiting, if they occur, will be minimal	II. A. 1. Premedicate with antiemetics and continue prophylactically × 24 hrs to prevent nausea and vomiting, at least for the first treatment 2. Encourage small, frequent feedings of cool, bland foods and liquids 3. Assess for symptoms of fluids and electrolyte imbalance: monitor I/O, daily weights if administered inpatient 4. Refer to sec. on nausea and vomiting, chap. 4
B. Stomatitis	B. 1. Has been reported to cause stomatitis	B. 1. Oral mucous membranes will remain intact and without infection	B. 1. Teach pt oral assessment and oral hygiene regimens 2. Encourage pt to report early stomatitis 3. Provide pain relief measures if indicated (e.g., topical anesthetics) 4. See sec. on stomatitis/mucositis, chap. 4

(continued)

Trimetrexate (*continued*)

Nursing Diagnosis	Defining Characteristics	Expected Outcomes	Nursing Interventions
II. C. Diarrhea	II. C. 1. Documented during clinical trials	II. C. Pt will have minimal diarrhea	II. C. 1. Encourage pt to report onset of diarrhea 2. Administer or teach pt to self-administer antidiarrheal medication 3. Watch all stools 4. Ensure adequate hydration, monitor I/0 5. See sec. on diarrhea, chap. 4
III. *Potential for hepatotoxicity*	III. A. Evidenced in SGOT elevations B. Increased drug toxicity in pts with low protein and hepatic dysfunction. Dose reductions may be necessary	III. A. Early hepatotoxicity will be identified	III. A. Monitor LFTs prior to drug dose B. Assess pt prior to and during treatment for s/s of hepatotoxicity C. See sec. on hepatotoxicity, chap. 4

DRUG

Vinblastine (Velban)

Class: Plant alkaloid extracted from the periwinkle plant (*Vinca rosea*)

MECHANISM OF ACTION

Drug binds to microtubular proteins thus arresting mitosis during metaphase; may inhibit RNA, DNA, and protein synthesis. Active in S and M phases (cell cycle phase specific).

METABOLISM

About 10% of drug is excreted in feces. Vinblastine is partially metabolized by the liver. Minimal amount of the drug is excreted in urine and bile. Dose modification may be necessary in the presence of hepatic failure.

DOSAGE/RANGE

0.1 mg/kg; 6 mg/m^2 IV weekly: continuous infusion 1.4–1.8 mg/day × 5 days

DRUG PREPARATION

Available in 10-mg vials. Store in refrigerator until use.

DRUG ADMINISTRATION

Intravenous. This drug is a *vesicant*. Give through the sidearm of a running IV so as to avoid extravasation which can lead to ulceration, pain, and necrosis. Refer to individual hospital policy and procedure for administration of a vesicant.

SPECIAL CONSIDERATIONS

Drug is a *vesicant*. Give through a running IV to avoid *extravasation*.

Dose modification may be necessary in the presence of hepatic failure.

Decreased pharmacologic effects of phenytoin when given with this drug.

Increases cellular uptake of methotrexate by certain malignant cells when administered sequentially, but less so than vincristine.

Vinblastine (Velban)

Nursing Diagnosis	Defining Characteristics	Expected Outcomes	Nursing Interventions
I. *Potential for infection and bleeding related to bone marrow depression (BMD)*	I. A. May cause severe BMD B. Nadir 4–10 days C. Neutrophils greatly affected D. In pts with prior XRT or chemotherapy, thrombocytopenia may be severe	I. A. Pt will be without s/s of infection or bleeding B. Early s/s of infection or bleeding will be identified	I. A. Monitor CBC, platelet count prior to drug administration B. Assess for s/s of infection or bleeding C. Instruct pt in self-assessment of s/s of infection or bleeding D Dose reduction if hepatic dysfunction 50% if bilirubin > 1.5 mg/dl 75% if bilirubin > 3.0 mg/dl E. Administer red cell, platelet transfusions as ordered F. Refer to sec. on bone marrow depression, chap. 4
II. *Potential for sensory/perceptual alterations*	II. A. Occur less frequently than with vincristine B. Occur in pts receiving prolonged or high-dose therapy C. Symptoms: paresthesias, peripheral neuropathy, depression, headache, malaise, jaw pain, urinary retention, tachycardia, orthostatic hypotension seizures D. Rare ocular changes: diplopia, ptosis, photophobia, oculomotor dysfunction, optic neuropathy	II. A. Sensory/perceptual changes will be identified early B. Dysfunction will be minimized C. Discomfort will be minimized	II. A. Assess sensory/perceptual changes prior to each drug dose, especially if dose is high (> 10 mg) or pt is receiving prolonged therapy B. Notify MD of alterations C. Discuss with pt impact changes have had, and strategies to minimize dysfunction and decrease distress D. Refer to sec. on neurotoxicity, chap. 4

III. *Constipation, potential*	III. A. Constipation results from neurotoxicity (central) and is less common than with vincristine B. Risk factors: high dose (>20 mg) C. May lead to adynamic ileus, abdominal pain	III. A. Constipation will be prevented B. Early s/s of adynamic ileus will be identified	III. A. Assess bowel elimination pattern each drug dose, especially if dose >20 mg B. Teach pt to promote bowel evaluation by fluids, 3 L/day, high fiber, bulky foods, exercise, stool softeners C. Suggest laxative if unable to move bowels at least once a day D. Instruct pt to report abdominal pain
IV. *Altered nutrition: less than body requirements related to* A. Nausea and vomiting	IV. A. 1. Rarely occur	IV. A. 1. Pt will be without nausea and vomiting 2. Nausea and vomiting, if they occur, will be minimal	IV. A. 1. Premedicate with antiemetics and continue prophylactically × 24 hrs to prevent nausea and vomiting, at least for the first treatment 2. Encourage small, frequent feedings of cool, bland foods and liquids 3. Assess for symptoms of fluid and electrolyte imbalance: monitor I/O, daily weights if administered inpatient 4. Refer to sec. on nausea and vomiting, chap. 4
B. Stomatitis	B. 1. Occurs occasionally, but may be severe	B. 1. Oral mucous membranes will remain intact and without infection	B. 1. Teach pt oral assessment 2. Teach, reinforce teaching, re oral hygiene regimens 3. Encourage pt to report early stomatitis 4. Provide pain relief measures if indicated (e.g., topical anesthetics) See sec. on stomatitis/mucositis, chap. 4

(continued)

Vinblastine (Velban) (continued)

Nursing Diagnosis	Defining Characteristics	Expected Outcomes	Nursing Interventions
IV. C. Diarrhea	IV. C. 1. Occasional, infrequent, and mild	IV. C. 1. Pt will have minimal diarrhea	IV. C. 1. Encourage pt to report onset of diarrhea 2. Administer or teach pt to self-administer antidiarrheal medication 3. Diet modification 4. See sec. on diarrhea, chap. 4
V. Potential for impaired skin integrity related to			
A. Alopecia	V. A. 1. Reversible and mild 2. Occurs in 45%–50% of pts receiving drug	V. A. 1. Pt will verbalize feelings regarding hair loss 2. Pt will identify strategies to cope with changes in body image	V. A. 1. Discuss with pt impact of hair loss 2. Suggest wig as appropriate prior to actual hair loss 3. Explore with pt response to actual hair loss and plan strategies to minimize distress, i.e., wig, scarf, cap 4. Refer to sec. on alopecia, chap. 4
B. Extravasation	B. 1. Drug is a potent vesicant and can cause irritation and necrosis if infiltrated	B. 1. Extravasation will be avoided 2. Skin will heal completely if extravasation occurs	B. 1. Refer to sec. on reactions, chap. 6 for safe administration of vesicant 2. Careful technique is used during venipuncture. See sec. on intravenous administration, chap. 7 3. Administer vesicant through freely flowing IV, constantly monitoring IV site and pt response 4. Nurse should be THOROUGHLY familiar with institutional policy and procedure for administration of a vesicant agent 5. If vesicant drug is administered as a continuous infusion, drug must be given through a patent central line

V. B. 6. If extravasation is suspected:
  a. Stop drug administered
  b. Aspirate any residual drug and blood from IV tubing, IV catheter/needle, and IV site if possible
  c. If drug infiltration is suspected, manufacturer suggests the following after withdrawing any remaining drug from IV: local installation of hyaluronidase, apply moderate heat

7. Assess site regularly for pain, progression of erythema, induration, and for evidence of necrosis

8. When in doubt about whether drug is infiltrating, TREAT AS AN INFILTRATION

9. Teach pt to assess site and notify MD if condition worsens

10. Arrange next clinic visit for assessment of site depending on drug, amount infiltrated, extent of potential injury, and pt variables

11. Document in pt's record as per institutional policy and procedure. See sec. on reactions, ch. 6

(continued)

Vinblastine (Velban) *(continued)*

Nursing Diagnosis	Defining Characteristics	Expected Outcomes	Nursing Interventions
V. C. Rash	V. C. 1. Uncommon	V. C. 1. Pt will identify strategies to cope with rash	V. C. 1. Assess impact of rash on pt: body image, comfort, and treat symptomatically
VI. *Potential for sexual dysfunction*	VI. A. Drug is possibly teratogenic B. Likely to cause zoospermia in men	VI. A. Pt and significant other will identify strategies to cope with sexual dysfunction	VI. A. As appropriate, explore with pt and significant other issues of reproductive and sexuality patterns and anticipated impact chemotherapy may have B. Discuss strategies to preserve sexual health (e.g., sperm banking) C. Refer to sec. on gonadal dysfunction, chap. 4

DRUG

Vincristine (Oncovin)

Class: Plant alkaloid extracted from the periwinkle plant (*Vinca rosea*)

MECHANISM OF ACTION

Drug binds to microtubular proteins thus arresting mitosis during metaphase. Cell cycle phase specific in M and S phases.

METABOLISM

The primary route for excretion is via the liver with about 70% of the drug being excreted in feces and bile. These metabolites are a result of hepatic metabolism and biliary excretion. A small amount is excreted in the urine. Dose modification may be necessary in the presence of hepatic failure.

DOSAGE/RANGE

0.4–1.4 mg/m^2 weekly (initially limited to 2 mg per dose)

DRUG PREPARATION

Supplied in 1-mg, 2-mg, and 5-mg vials. Refrigerate vials until use.

DRUG ADMINISTRATION

Intravenous. This drug is a *vesicant*. Give through a running IV to avoid extravasation which can lead to ulceration, pain, and necrosis. Refer to hospital's policy and procedure for administration of a vesicant.

SPECIAL CONSIDERATIONS

Drug is a *vesicant*. Give through a running IV to avoid *extravasation*.

Dose modification may be necessary in the presence of hepatic failure.

Decreased bioavailability of digoxin when given with this drug.

Increased cellular uptake of methotrexate by some malignant cells when given sequentially.

Vincristine

Nursing Diagnosis	Defining Characteristics	Expected Outcomes	Nursing Interventions
I. *Potential for sensory/perceptual alterations, related to*			
A. Peripheral neuropathies	I. A. 1. Peripheral neuropathies occur as a result of toxicity to nerve fibers 2. Absent deep tension reflexes 3. Numbness, weakness, myalgias, cramping 4. Late severe motor difficulties 5. Reversal or discontinuance of therapy necessary 6. Increased risk in elderly	I. A. 1. Sensory and perceptual changes will be identified early 2. Dysfunction will be minimized 3. Discomfort will be minimized	I. A. 1. Assess sensory and perceptual changes prior to each drug dose, i.e., presence of numbness or tingling of fingertips or toes 2. Assess for loss of tendon reflexes: foot drop, slapping gait 3. Assess for motor difficulties: clumsiness of hands, difficulty climbing stairs (buttoning shirt, walking on heels) 4. Notify MD of alterations; discuss holding drug if loss of deep tendon reflexes occur 5. Discuss with pt impact alterations have had, and strategies to minimize dysfunction and decrease distress 6. Discuss with pt type of alteration: memory, sensory/perceptual changes, temporary and reversible when drug stopped 7. See sec. on neurotoxicity, chap. 4
B. Cranial nerve damage and other nerve involvement	B. 1. Cranial nerve dysfunction may occur (rare) 2. Jaw pain (trigeminal neuralagia) 3. Diplopia 4. Vocal cord paresis 5. Mental depression 6. Metallic taste	B. 1. Symptoms of nerve dysfunction will be identified early	B. 1. Assess pt for s/s of nerve dysfunction before each dose 2. Notify MD of any changes

I. C. Constipation	I. C. 1. Autonomic neuropathy may lead to constipation and paralytic ileus 2. A concurrent use of vincristine, narcotic analgesics, or cholinergic medication may increase risk of constipation	I. C. 1. Constipation will be prevented 2. Early s/s of paralytic ileus will be identified	I. C. 1. Assess bowel elimination pattern prior to each chemotherapy administration 2. Teach pt to include bulky and high fiber foods in diet, increase fluids to 3 L/day, and exercise moderately to promote elimination 3. Suggest stool softeners if needed 4. Teach pt to use laxative if unable to move bowels at least once every 2 days 5. Instruct pt to report abdominal pain

II. *Potential for impaired skin integrity related to*

A. Alopecia and subsequent body image disturbance	II. A. 1. Complete hair loss occurs in 12%–45% of pts 2. Both men and women are at risk for body image disturbance 3. Hair will grow back	II. A. 1. Pt will verbalize feelings about hair loss and identify strategies to cope with changes in body image	II. A. 1. Discuss with pt anticipated impact of hair loss; suggest wig or toupe as appropriate prior to actual hair loss 2. Explore with pt response to hair loss, if it occurs, and strategies to minimize distress, i.e., wig, scarf, cap 3. See sec. on alopecia, chap. 4
B. Dermatitis	B. 1. Uncommon	B. 1. Pt will identify coping strategies	B. 1. Assess impact on pt: body image, comfort 2. Discuss strategies to minimize distress
C. Extravasation	C. 1. Drug is potent vesicant causing irritation and necrosis if infiltrated	C. 1. Extravasation will be avoided 2. Skin will heal completely if drug is extravasated	C. 1. Careful technique is used during venipuncture. See sec. on intravenous administration, chap. 7 2. Administer vesicant through freely flowing IV, constantly monitoring IV site and pt response 3. Nurse should be THOROUGHLY familiar with institutional policy and procedure for administration of a vesicant agent

(continued)

Vincristine *(continued)*

Nursing Diagnosis	Defining Characteristics	Expected Outcomes	Nursing Interventions
			II. C. 4. If vesicant drug is administered as a continuous infusion, drug must be given through a patent central line
			5. If extravasation is suspected:
			a. Stop drug administered
			b. Aspirate any residual drug and blood from IV tubing, IV catheter/needle, and IV site if possible
			c. If drug infiltration is suspected, manufacturer suggests the following after withdrawing any remaining drug from tubing: local injection of hyaluronidase, apply moderate heat
			6. Assess site regularly for pain, progression of erythema, induration, and for evidence of necrosis
			7. When in doubt about whether drug is infiltrating, TREAT AS AN INFILTRATION
			8. Teach pt to assess site and notify MD if condition worsens
			9. Arrange next clinic visit for assessment of site depending on drug, amount infiltrated, extent of potential injury, and pt variables
			10. Document in pt's record as per institutional policy and procedure. See sec. on reactions, ch. 6

III. *Potential for infection and bleeding related to bone marrow depression*	III. A. Rare myelo-suppression, mild when it occurs B. May have depression of pt over time requiring transfusion C. Nadir 10–14 days after treatment begins	III. A. Monitor WBC, Hct, platelets prior to drug administration B. See reduction if hepatic dysfunction: 50% reduction if BR >1.5 mg/dl; 75% reduction if BR >3.0 mg/dl C. See sec. on bone marrow depression, chap. 4
	III. A. Pt will be without bleeding or infection B. Early s/s of bleeding or infection will be detected	
IV. *Potential for sexual dysfunction*	IV. A. Impotence may occur related to neurotoxicity	IV. A. As appropriate, explore with pt and significant other issues of reproductive and sexuality patterns and impact chemotherapy may have B. Discuss strategies to preserve sexual health, i.e., alternative expressions of sexuality C. Reassure pt that impotency, if it occurs, is usually temporary, and reversible after drug discontinuance D. Refer to sec. on gonadal dysfunction, chap. 4
	IV. A. Pt and significant other will identify strategies to cope with sexual dysfunction	

DRUG

Vindesine (Eldisine, Desacetylvinblastine)

Class: Synthetic derivative of vinblastine; synthetic vinca alkaloid

MECHANISM OF ACTION

Inhibits microtubule formation causing metaphase arrest during M phase and causes some cell death during S phase. Cell cycle phase specific.

METABOLISM

Short plasma half-life (probably binds to tissue). Prolonged elimination suggesting drug may accumulate with repeated dosing. Excreted primarily by bile.

DOSAGE/RANGE

3–4 mg/m^2 q 1–2 weeks
1–1.3 mg/m^2 day × 5–7 days repeated every 3 wks
1.5–2 mg/m^2 2 × week

DRUG PREPARATION

10-mg vial, lyophilized powder, reconstituted with provided diluent or Normal Saline. Solution is stable for 2 weeks refrigerated.

DRUG ADMINISTRATION

Vesicant precautions. Administer slowly as intravenous push through sidearm of freely running IV, also may be given as continuous infusion.

SPECIAL CONSIDERATIONS

Do not give with other vinca alkaloids, such as vincristine or vinblastine as there is potential for cumulative neurotoxicity.

Dose reduction may be necessary in patients with abnormal liver function or if patient has received maximal doses of other vinca alkaloids.

Vindesine

Nursing Diagnosis	Defining Characteristics	Expected Outcomes	Nursing Interventions
I. *Potential for infection and bleeding related to bone marrow depression*	I. A. Dose-limiting side effect B. Nadir 5–10 days C. Neutropenia mild to moderate C. Thrombocytopenia mild, rare (may increase on treatment)	I. A. Patient will be without s/s of infection or bleeding B. Early s/s of infection or bleeding will be identified	I. A. Monitor CBC, platelet count prior to drug administration as well as s/s of infection or bleeding B. Instruct pt in self-assessment of s/s of infection or bleeding C. Dose reduction often necessary (35%–50%), if compromised bone marrow function D. Refer to sec. on bone marrow depression, chap. 4
II. *Potential for sensory/perceptual alteration related to* A. Peripheral neuropathy, cranial nerve damage, other nerve involvement	II. A. 1. Neurotoxicity similar to vincristine 2. Cumulative toxicity, mild 3. Begins with distal paresthesias, proximal muscle weakness, loss of deep tendon reflexes 4. Abdominal cramping common; constipation and ileus less common 5. Hoarseness, jaw pain (severe and transient, may occur)	II. A. 1. Sensory/ perceptual changes will be identified early 2. Dysfunction will be minimized 3. Discomfort will be minimized	II. A. 1. Obtain visual assessment prior to starting therapy 2. Encourage pt to report any visual changes 3. Instruct pt to report headache, dizziness, lightheadedness 4. Refer to sec. on neurotoxicity, chap. 4

(continued)

Vindesine (continued)

Nursing Diagnosis	Defining Characteristics	Expected Outcomes	Nursing Interventions
II. B. Constipation	II. B. 1. Autonomic neuropathy may lead to constipation and paralytic ileus	II. B. 1. Constipation will be prevented 2. Early s/s of paralytic ileus will be identified	II. B. 1. Assess bowel elimination pattern prior to each chemotherapy administration 2. Teach pt to include bulky and high fiber foods in diet, increase fluids to 3 L/day, exercise moderately to promote elimination 3. Suggest stool softeners if needed 4. Teach pt to use laxative if unable to move bowels at least once every 2 days 5. Instruct pt to report abdominal pain
III. *Potential for impaired skin integrity related to*			
A. Alopecia with subsequent body image disturbance	III. A. 1. Affects 80%–90%, with 25%–50% experiencing total hair loss 2. Alopecia may be progressive 3. Both men and women at risk for body image disturbance 4. Hair will grow back 5. Scalp tourniquet may be helpful if not contra-indicated	III. A. 1. Pt will verbalize feelings regarding hair loss 2. Pt will identify strategies to cope with changes in body image	III. A. 1. Discuss with pt impact of hair loss 2. Suggest wig as appropriate prior to actual hair loss 3. Explore with pt response to actual hair loss and plan strategies to minimize distress, i.e., wig, scarf, cap 4. Refer to sec. on alopecia, chap. 4
B. Rash	B. 1. Uncommon	B. 1. Patient will identify coping strategies	B. 1. Assess impact of rash on pt: body image, comfort; treat symptomatically

| III. C. Extravasation | III. C. 1. Inapparent or obvious infiltrations can occur
2. Presentation delayed; pain, phlebitis, blister formation occurs; may progress to ulceration and necrosis
3. Management similar to vincristine extravasation | III. C. 1. Extravasation will be avoided
2. Skin will heal completely if extravasation occurs | III. C. 1. Careful technique is used during venipuncture. See sec. on intravenous administration, chap. 7
2. Administer vesicant through freely flowing IV, constantly monitoring IV site and pt response
3. Nurse should be THOROUGHLY familiar with institutional policy and procedure for administration of a vesicant agent
4. If vesicant drug is administered as a continuous infusion, drug must be given through a patent central line
5. If extravasation is suspected:
  a. Stop drug administered
  b. Aspirate any residual drug and blood from IV tubing, IV catheter/needle, and IV site if possible
  c. If drug infiltration is suspected, manufacturer suggests the following after withdrawing any remaining drug from IV: local installation of hyaluronidase, apply moderate heat
  d. Apply heat or cold or topical medication as per MD order and institutional policy and procedure
6. Assess site regularly for pain, progression of erythema, induration, and for evidence of necrosis
7. When in doubt about whether drug is infiltrating, TREAT AS AN INFILTRATION |

(continued)

Vindesine *(continued)*

Nursing Diagnosis	Defining Characteristics	Expected Outcomes	Nursing Interventions
			III. C. 8. Teach pt to assess site and notify MD if condition worsens 9. Arrange next clinic visit for assessment of site depending on drug, amount infiltrated, extent of potential injury, and pt variables 10. Document in pt's record as per institutional policy and procedure. See sec. on reactions, ch. 6
IV. Altered nutrition: less than body requirements *related to*			
A. Nausea and vomiting	IV. A. 1. Typically not severe 2. Occurs in 30% of pts	IV. A. 1. Pt will be without nausea and vomiting 2. Nausea and vomiting, if they occur, will be minimal	IV. A. 1. Premedicate with antiemetic and continue prophylactically × 24 hrs to prevent nausea and vomiting, at least for first treatment 2. Encourage small, frequent feedings of cool, bland food and liquids 3. Refer to sec. on nausea and vomiting, chap. 4
B. Diarrhea	B. 1. Uncommon, but rarely may be protracted and thus would be an indication for dose reduction	B. 1. Pt will have minimal diarrhea	B. 1. Encourage pt to report onset of diarrhea 2. Administer, or teach pt to self-administer antidiarrheal medications 3. See sec. on diarrhea, chap. 4
C. Stomatitis	C. 1. Rare	C. 1. Oral mucous membranes will remain intact without infection	C. 1. Teach pt oral assessment 2. Encourage pt to report early stomatitis 3. Teach pt oral hygiene 4. See sec. on stomatitis/mucositis, chap. 4
D. Anorexia	D. 1. Rare	D. 1. Pt will maintain baseline weight ±5%	D. 1. Encourage small, frequent feedings of favorite foods, especially high-calorie, high-protein foods 2. Encourage use of spices 3. Weekly weights

DRUG

VM-26 (teniposide)

> **Class:** Investigational agent. Plant alkaloid, a derivative of the mandrake plant (*Mandragora officinarum*)

MECHANISM OF ACTION

Cell cycle specific in late S phase, early G_2 phase, causing arrest of cell division in mitosis. Inhibits uptake of thymidine into DNA so DNA synthesis is impaired.

METABOLISM

Drug binds extensively to serum protein. Metabolized by the liver and excreted in bile and urine.

DOSAGE/RANGE

100 mg/m^2 weekly for 6–8 weeks
50 mg/m^2 2 × wk × 4

DRUG PREPARATION

Available investigationally in 10 mg/ml 5-ml ampules. Add desired NS for injection, or 5% dextrose in water.

DRUG ADMINISTRATION

Do not administer the solution if a precipitate is noted.

SPECIAL CONSIDERATIONS

Rapid infusion, less than 30 minutes, may cause hypotension.

Chemical phlebitis may occur if drug is not properly diluted, or if infused too rapidly.

Anaphylaxis occurs rarely.

VM-26 (teniposide)

Nursing Diagnosis	Defining Characteristics	Expected Outcomes	Nursing Interventions
I. *Potential for injury during drug administration related to*			
A. Hypotension	I. A. 1. Hypotension may occur during rapid infusion	I. A. 1. Hypotension will be prevented	I. A. 1. Monitor BP prior to drug administration, and periodically during infusion at least during first drug administration 2. Infuse over at least 30–60 mins
B. Anaphylaxis	B. 1. Rarely occurs; may be characterized by fever, dyspnea, lumbar pain, progressive hypotension 2. May respond to drug discontinuance and IV hydrocortisone	B. 1. Anaphylaxis, if it occurs, will be managed successfully	B. 1. Have anaphylaxis tray with corticosteroids, antihistamines, epinephrine nearby when chemotherapy is administered 2. Monitor pt closely during infusion 3. Review standing orders for management of allergic reactions (hypersensitivity and anaphylaxis) per institutional policy and procedure 4. Prior to drug administration obtain baseline vital signs and record mental status 5. OBSERVE for following s/s, usually occuring within the first 15 minutes of infusion *Subjective* generalized itching nausea chest tightness crampy abdominal pain agitation anxiety sense of impending doom wheeziness desire to urinate or defecate dizziness chills

I. B.   5. *Objective*

flushed appearance (angioedema of the face, neck, eyelids, hands, feet)

localized or generalized urticaria

respiratory distress ± wheezing

hypotension

cyanosis

6. For generalized allergic response, stop infusion and notify MD

7. Place pt in supine position to promote perfusion of visceral organs

8. Monitor vital signs

9. Provide emotional reassurance to pt and family

10. Maintain patent airway, and have equipment ready for CPR if needed

11. Document incident

12. Discuss with MD desensitization versus drug discontinuance for further dose

13. Refer to sec. on reactions, chap. 6

(continued)

VM-26 (teniposide) (continued)

Nursing Diagnosis	Defining Characteristics	Expected Outcomes	Nursing Interventions
II. *Potential for infection and bleeding related to bone marrow depression*	II. A. Dose-limiting toxicity B. Leukopenia, but thrombocytopenia may also occur C. Nadir 3–14 days (~7 days) D. Dose reductions indicated for pts heavily pretreated with radiation or chemotherapy	II. A. Pt will be without s/s of infection or bleeding B. Early s/s of infection or bleeding will be identified	II. A. Monitor platelet count prior to drug administration, assess for s/s of infection or bleeding. Assess nadir counts B. Instruct pt in self-assessment techniques for infection, bleeding C. Dose reduction may be necessary based on nadir counts, history of previous XRT/chemotherapy, altered hepatic function D. Transfuse with red cells, platelets per MD order E. Refer to sec. on bone marrow depression, chap. 4
III. *Altered nutrition: less than body requirements related to* A. Nausea and vomiting	III. A. 1. May occur, but it is usually mild	III. A. 1. Pt will be without nausea and vomiting	III. A. 1. Premedicate with antiemetic and continue prophylactically × 24 hrs to prevent nausea and vomiting, at least for first treatment 2. Encourage small, frequent feedings of cool, bland food and liquids 3. See sec. on nausea and vomiting, chap. 4
B. Hepatic dysfunction	B. 1. Mild elevation of liver function tests may occur	B. 1. Hepatic dysfunction will be identified early	B. 1. Monitor SGOT, SGPT, LDH, alkaline phosphastase and bilirubin prior to drug administration 2. Notify MD of any elevations 3. See sec. on hepatotoxocity, chap. 4

Nursing Diagnosis	Defining Characteristics	Expected Outcomes	Nursing Interventions
IV. Potential for impaired skin integrity related to A. Alopecia	IV. A. 1. Occurs uncommonly (9%–30%) and is reversible	IV. A. 1. Pt will verbalize feelings regarding hair loss 2. Pt will identify strategies to cope with changes in body image	IV. A. 1. Discuss with pt impact of hair loss 2. Suggest wig as appropriate prior to actual hair loss 3. Explore with pt response to actual hair loss and plan strategies to minimize distress, i.e., wig, scarf, cap 4. Refer to sec. on alopecia, chap. 4
B. Irritation	B. 1. Phlebitis or perivascular irritation may occur if drug is too concentrated or is infused too rapidly	B. 1. Phlebitis, irritation will be minimal	B. 1. Use careful venipuncture technique and administer drug over 30–60 mins diluted to at least 5 volumes as per manufacturer's specifications 2. Refer to sec. on intravenous administration, chap. 7
V. Potential for alteration in cardiac output	V. A. Rarely palpitations may occur	V. A. Early cardiac rhythm abnormalities will be identified	V. A. Monitor HR, noting rhythm, when administering drug B. Notify MD of any irregularity C. EKG to identify irregular rhythm D. See sec. on cardiotoxicity, chap. 4
VI. Potential for sensory/perceptual alterations related to neurological toxicity	VI. A. Peripheral neuropathies may occur, and are mild	VI. A. Peripheral neuropathy will be identified early B. Pt will verbalize feelings re discomfort, dysfunction related to neuropathy, and identify alternative coping strategies	VI. A. Assess motor and sensory function prior to therapy B. Encourage pt to verbalize feelings re discomfort and sensory loss if these occur C. Assist pt to discuss alternative coping strategies D. Refer to sec. on neurotoxicity, chap. 4

BIBLIOGRAPHY

Agarwal R (1980) Deoxycoformycin toxicity in mice after long-term treatment. *Cancer Chemotherapy and Pharmacology,* 5(2): 83–87

Annual report to the FDA. CBDCA (NSC #241-240) (1985) Washington, DC, Government Printing Office

Beck S, Yasko JM (1984) *A Guideline for Oral Care.* Illinois, Sage Products

Becker T (1981) *Cancer Chemotherapy: A Manual for Nurses.* Boston, Little, Brown, & Co

Brager BL, Yasko JM (1984) *Care of the Client Receiving Chemotherapy.* Reston, Va, Reston Publishing Co

Cadman ED, Ignoffo RJ, Stagg RJ (1985) *Leucovorin: Uses With Methotrexate, Sequential Methrotrexate and 5-Fluorouracil, and With 5-Fluorouracil.* Wayne, NJ, Lederle Laboratories

Calvert AH, Harland JJ, Newell DR, et al (1985) Phase 1 studies with carboplatin at the Royal Marsden Hospital. *Cancer Treatment Review,* 12 (suppl A): 54

Canetta R, Franks C, Smaldone L, et al (1987) Clinical status of carboplatin. *Oncology,* July, 61–69

Carella AM, Santini G, Hartinengo M, et al (1985) 4-demethoxydaunorubicin (DMDR) in refractory or relapsed acute leukemia: a pilot study. *Cancer* 55(7): 1452

Carter SK, Canetta R, Roxencweig M (1985) Carboplatin: future directions. *Cancer Treatment Review,* 12 (suppl A): 145

Chabner BA, Myers CE (1985) Clinical pharmacology of cancer chemotherapy, in DeVita VT, Hellman S, Rosenberg SA (eds): *Cancer: Principles and Practice of Oncology* (ed 2). Philadelphia, Lippincott Co

Daghestani AN, et al (1985). Phase 1–2 clinical and pharmacological study of 4-demethoxydaunorubicin (DMDR) in adult patients with acute leukemia. *Cancer Research* 45(3): 1408–1412

Doria MI, Shepart KV, Lerin B, et al (1986) Liver pathology following hepatic arterial infusion chemotherapy: hepatic toxicity with FUDR. *Cancer* 58: 855–861

Dorr RT (1989) *MESNEXtm (mesna) Injection Dosing and Administration Guide—Rationale and Guidelines for Dosing and Administration.* Evansville, Ind, Bristol-Myers Company

Dorr RT, Fritz W (1980) *Cancer Chemotherapy Handbook.* New York, Elsevier Press

Eisenhower EA, Zee BC, Pater JL, Walsh WR (1988) Trimetrexate: predictors of severe or life-threatening toxic effects. *Journal of the National Cancer Institute.* 80(16): 1318–1322

Fischer DS, Knobf MT (1989) *The Cancer Chemotherapy Handbook* (ed 3). Chicago, Yearbook Medical Publishers

Forastiere AA, Natale RB, Takasugi BJ, et al (1987) A Phase I–II trial of carboplatin and 5-fluorouracil combination chemotherapy in advanced carcinoma of the head and neck. *Journal of Clinical Oncology* 5(2): 191 (February)

Foster BJ, Clagett-Carr K, Leyland-Jones B, Hoth D (1985) Results of NCI sponsored phase I trials with carboplatin. *Cancer Treatment Review,* 12 (suppl A): 43

Goodman M (1988) Concepts of hormonal manipulation in the treatment of cancer. *Oncology Nursing Forum* 15(5): 639–647

———— (1987) Management of nausea and vomiting induced by outpatient cisplatin therapy. *Seminars in Oncology Nursing* 3(1) (Suppl 1, Feb): 23–35

Govani LE, Hayes JE (1982) *Drugs and Nursing Implications.* Norwalk, Conn: Appleton-Century-Crofts

Grem JL, Ellenberg SS, King SA, Shoemaker DD (1989) Correlates of severe or life-threatening toxic effects from trimetrexate. *Journal of the National Cancer Institute* 80(16): 1313–1318

Grever MR, Siaw MFE, Jacob WF, et al (1981) The biochemical and clinical consequences of 2'-deoxycoformycin in refractory lymphoproliferative malignancies. *Blood* 57(3): 406–417

Grever MR, Malspers L, Balcerzak S, et al (1982) 2'-deoxycoformycin: A phase I clinical-pharmacokinetic investigation. *AACR Proceedings* 23(533): 36

Grochow LB, Noe DA, Dole GB, et al (1989) Phase I trial of trimetrexate gluconate on a five-day bolus schedule: clinical pharmacology and pharmacodynamics. *Journal of the National Cancer Institute* 81(2): 124–130

Groenwald SL, Frogge MH, Goodman M, Yarbro CH (1990) *Cancer Nursing Principles and Practice* (ed 2). Boston, Jones and Bartlett Publishers

Harris JR, Hellman S, Canellos GP, Fisher B (1985) Cancer of the breast, in DeVita VT, Hellman S, Rosenberg S (eds): *Cancer: Principles and Practice of Oncology* (ed 2). Philadelphia, Lippincott Co

Holmes FA, Hwee-Yong YAP, Esparza L, et al (1987) Mitoxantrone, cyclophosphamide, and fluorouracil in metastatic breast cancer unresponsive to hormonal therapy. *Cancer* 59(12): 1992–1999 (Jun 15)

Hubbard SM, Seipp C (1985) Administration of cancer treatments: Practical guide for physicians and oncology nurses, in DeVita VT, Hellman S, Rosenberg SA (eds): *Cancer: Principles and Practice of Oncology* (ed 2). Philadelphia, Lippincott Co

Hudes GR, Comis RL (1988) Phase I and II studies of trimetrexate administered in combination with flurorouracil to patients with metastatic cancer. *Seminars in Oncology* (15 suppl 2): 41–45

Johnson BL, Gross J (1985) *Handbook of Oncology Nursing*. New York, John Wiley and Sons

Kemeny N, Daly J, Reichman B, et al (1987) Intrahepatic or systemic infusion of fluorodeoxyuridine in patients with liver metastases from colorectal carcinoma. *Annals Internal Medicine* 104: 459–465

Knight WA, Livingstone RB, Fabian C, Costanzi J (1979) Phase I–II trial of methyl-GAG: A SWOG Pilot. *Cancer Treatment Report* 63(11–12): 1933

Knobf MKT, Fischer DS, Welch-McCaffrey D (1984) *Cancer Chemotherapy: Treatment and Care* (ed 2). Boston, GK Hall Medical Publishers

Koeller JM, Earhart RH, Davis TE, et al (1983) Phase I trial of CBDCA (NSC #241–240) by bolus intravenous injection. *AACR Proceedings* 24(642): 162 (abstract)

Kris MG, D'Acquisto RW, Gralla RJ, et al (1989) Phase II trial of trimetrexate in patients with stage III and IV non-small cell lung cancer. *American Journal of Clinical Oncology* 12(1): 24–26

Kufe D, Major P, Agarwal R, et al (1980) Phase I–II trial of deoxycoformycin (DCF) in T-cell malignancies. *AACR Proceedings* 21(C-39): 328

Lambertenghi-Deleliers G, Pogliani E, Maiolo AT, et al (1983) Therapeutic activity of 4-demethoxydaunorubicin (DMDR) in adult leukemia. *TUMORI*, 69, 515–519

Lasley K, Ignoffo RJ (1981) *Manual of Oncology Therapeutics*. St. Louis, CV Mosby Co

Lederle Laboratories (1988) *Novantrone Formulary Brochure*. Wayne, NJ

Ligha SS, Gutterman JV, Hall SW, et al (1978) Phase I clinical investigation of 4'-(9-acidinylamino) methanesulfon-m-aniside (NSC-249992), a new acridine derivative. *Cancer Research* 38(11): 3712–3716

Lu K, Savaraj J, Kavanaugh J, et al (1984) Clinical pharmacology of 4-demethoxydaunorubicin. *ASCO Proceedings* 3(C-147): 88 (abstract)

MacElveen-Hoehn P (1985) Sexual assessment and counselling. *Seminars in Oncology Nursing* 1(1): 69–75

Major PP, Agarwal RP, Kufe DW (1981). Clinical pharmacology of deoxycoformycin. *Blood* 58(1): 91–96

Malspers L, Weinrib AB, Staubus AE, et al (1984) Clinical pharmacokinetics of 2'-deoxycoformycin. *Cancer Treatment Symposium* 2: 7–15

Marsh KC, Liesman J, Patton TF, et al (1981) Plasma levels and urinary excretion of methyl-GAG following IV infusion in man. *Cancer Treatment Reports* 65(3–4): 253

Mead Johnson Oncology Products (1989) *The Introduction of Ifex and Mesna*. Evansville, Ind

Melmon KL, Morelli HF (1978) *Clinical Pharmacology: Basic Principles in Therapeutics* (ed 2). New York, MacMillan Publishing Co

Micetrick KC, Barnes D, Erickson LC (1985) A comparison of the cytotoxicity and DNA damaging effects of carboplatin and cisplatin (II). *AACR Proceedings* 26(1036): 263 (abstract)

National Cancer Institute Investigational Drugs—Pharmaceutical Data 1988. US Department of Health and Human Services. NIH Publication #89-2141

Nichols C, Williams S, Tricot G, et al (1988) Phase I study of high dose etoposide plus carboplatin with autologous bone marrow rescue (ABMT) in refractory germ cell cancer. *ASCO Proceedings* 7(454): 118 (abstract)

Paciarini A, et al (1983) Pharmacokinetic studies of IV and oral 4-demethoxydaunorubicin in man. 13th International Congress of Chemotherapy. Vienna, Austria

Patty Z, Boddie AW, Charnsagerej C, et al (1986) Hepatic arterial infusion with floxuridine and cisplatin: overriding importance of antitumor effect vs. degree of tumor burden as determinants of survival among patients with colorectal cancer. *Journal of Clinical Oncology* 4: 1356–1364

Perry MC, Yarbro JW (1984) *Toxicity of Chemotherapy*. New York, Grune and Stratton

Peters FTM, Beijnen JH, ten Bokkel Huinink WW (1987) Mitoxantrone extravasation injury. *Cancer Treatment Reports* 71(10): 992–993

Physician's Desk Reference (1986) (ed 40). Oradell, NJ, Barnhart ER (publisher), Medical Economics

Pratt WB, Ruddon RW (1979) *The Anticancer Drugs*. New York, Oxford University Press

Rodriques V, Cabanillas F, Bodey GP, Freireich EJ (1982) Studies with ifosfomide in patients with malignant lymphoma. *Seminars in Oncology* IX(4) (suppl 1, December): 87

Silver RT, Lauper RD, Jarowski CI (1987) *A Synopsis of Cancer Chemotherapy* (ed 2). New York, Yorke Medical Books

Skeel RT (ed) (1982) *Manual of Cancer Chemotherapy.* Boston, Little, Brown and Co

Skidmore-Roth L (1989) *Mosby's 1989 Nursing Drug Reference.* St. Louis, CV Mosby Co

Smith IE, Evans BD, Gore ME, et al (1987) Carboplatin (Paraplatin, JMB) and etoposide (VP-16) as first line combination therapy for small cell lung cancer. *Journal of Clinical Oncology* 5(2): 186 (February)

Stewart JA, McCormack JJ, Tong W, et al (1988) Phase I clinical and pharmacokinetic study of trimetrexate using a daily × 5 schedule. *Cancer Research* 48(17): 5029–5035

Tamassia V, Goldaniga R, Moroma A, et al (1983) Pharmacokinetic studies on three new anthracyclines: epirubicin, DMDR, esorubicin, in *Fourth NCI-EORTC Symposium in New Drugs in Cancer Therapy,* December 14–17, 1983, p. 16 (abstract)

Tenebaum L (1989) *Cancer Chemotherapy: A Reference Guide.* Philadelphia, WB Saunders

Von Hoff DD (1987) Whether carboplatin? A Replacement for or an alternative to cisplatin. *Journal of Clinical Oncology* 5(2): 169 (February)

Warrell RP, Burchenal JH (1983) Methyl glyoxolal-Bi(Guanylhydrazone) (Methyl-GAG): Current status and future prospects. *Journal of Clinical Oncology* 1(1): 54

Warrell RP, Lee BJ, Kempin SJ, et al (1981) Effectiveness of methyl-GAG (methyl glyoxal-bis-[guanylhydrazone]) in patients with advanced malignant lymphoma. *Blood* 57(6): 1011

Warrell RP, Lee BJ, Kempin SJ, et al (1981) Clinical evaluation of methyl-GAG (methyl glyoxal-bis-[guanylhydrazone]) alone and in combination with VM-26 (Teniposide), in advanced malignant lymphoma. *AACR and ASCO Proceedings* 22(C-738): 521

Whitacre MY, Finley RS (1989) *Paraplatin Administration Guide.* Evansville, Ind, Bristol Myers Co

Yarbro CH (1989) Carboplatin: A clinical review. *Seminars in Oncology Nursing* 5(2) (suppl 1, May): 63–69

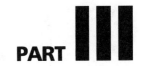

CLINICAL APPLICATION

6

PRINCIPLES OF CHEMOTHERAPY ADMINISTRATION

THE ADMINISTRATION of chemotherapy has not always been as it is today. As recently as the 1950s, the physician administered the medications and the nurse was left to care for any side effects (Lind and Bush 1987). The first chemotherapy drug, a nitrogen mustard (mechlorethamine), was discovered in the 1940s, and in comparison to other areas of medicine, the field of oncology was still in its infancy. As the number of available drugs increased and the technology of chemotherapy administration became more complex, the nurse assumed the primary role in drug delivery. Today there is a specialized field of oncology nursing. Nurses are involved in developing policies, procedures, and national standards for the safe administration of drugs, and in political lobbying as patient advocates.

The formal, national organization of oncology nurses, the Oncology Nursing Society (ONS), has recommended that only adequately prepared professional registered nurses who are proficient in chemotherapy administration assume the responsibility for actual drug delivery (ONS Module II 1988). This recommendation helps to ensure the highest possible quality of care and safety for the cancer patient. The process to become qualified to administer chemotherapy is variable, differing from institution to institution depending on their policies and influenced by their state's nurse practice act. Usually qualified nurses teach their peers the specialized techniques that are necessary to become proficient. Some of the guidelines currently in use were developed in the late 1960s, but are as pertinent to nursing practice today as they were when they were written (Lind and Bush 1987).

To prepare nurses to administer chemotherapy, the educational programs should be comprehensive, including both didactic theory and supervised clinical experience. The *didactic component* must include a review of cancer pathophysiology while focusing on the pharmacology of antineoplastic agents, principles of safe handling and administration, as well as problem assessment and management of potential treatment side effects. *Clinical experience* must provide skills in intravenous therapy, e.g., venipuncture and site selection; administration techniques and guidelines; management of various venous access devices, such as silastic catheters and implantable ports; as well as the more complex drug delivery techniques of intraperitoneal, intracavitary, and intrathecal therapies; arterial lines; and the internal and external infusion pumps. Today's complex drug regimens and clinical trials demand the nurse understand the principles and practice of chemotherapy administration, not just simply memorize the different drugs (Lind and Bush 1987). There is a difference between remembering the side effects listed in a book or protocol and being able to accurately anticipate and prevent the ones the patient is actually at risk of developing. Pain control and antiemetic therapies must also be understood and proficiently managed as they are important to the quality care a patient should receive, as important as the actual chemotherapy protocol (Lind and Bush 1987).

CHEMOTHERAPY CHECKLIST

It is of major concern to oncology nurses that chemotherapeutic agents are given safely. This concern includes safe handling as well as proficient skills in intravenous technique and therapy (Lind and Bush 1987). As with the administration of any medication, it is essential with chemotherapeutic agents to verify that the medication to be given is correct. This is important regardless of the setting in which you administer chemotherapy. One step that can be taken to make this responsibility somewhat easier is a chemotherapy checklist. Table 6.1 is an example of such a checklist.

ISSUES IN CHEMOTHERAPY ADMINISTRATION IN AMBULATORY AND HOME SETTINGS

In light of current economic factors, chemotherapy today is being administered in locations outside the typical inpatient setting. These locations include hospital-based clinics, private physician offices, and the client's home or place of business. The basic principles of chemotherapy administration are the same despite the setting, but there are some slight differences (e.g., patient education regarding self-care measures). Issues of handling and disposing of chemotherapy drugs will be presented in chapter 8.

One factor that is key to the success of chemotherapy administration outside the hospital is *patient selection* (Garvey 1987). The health care team must make a careful assessment of many variables (see table 6.2). The team must be con-

fident that all these considerations can be safely controlled before selecting a patient for outpatient therapy. Otherwise, it might be more appropriate for the patient to receive the therapy in the hospital, or at least receive one course of therapy as an inpatient so the team can assess drug tolerance. The nurse must continually assess the patient, and his or her environment, so the health care team has a basis for clinical judgments relating to continuing the therapy in an ambulatory setting.

Currently a *variety of chemotherapeutic agents* is being successfully administered in ambulatory settings (see table 6.3). As practitioners become more sophisticated in handling treatment side effects and with more innovative equipment to help in administration, this list of drugs will increase. Besides chemotherapy, ambulatory care nurses are now administering blood products, antibiotics, various nutritional support products, and pain medications. The nurse cannot successfully administer any of these therapies alone in an outpatient setting without support. The assistance of the patient, the family, and potentially other community-based support services are required. Once the nurse gives the chemotherapy (for example) and waits for 30 to 60 minutes to complete an assessment for potential complications, it is the patient or the family who must be capable of providing self-care measures to minimize side effects (Garvey 1987). They must be aware of and know how to recognize a reaction, who to report it to, and which reactions must be reported immediately.

The *education of the patient and the family* is within the realm of nursing practice. It is one of our most important responsibilities. Nurses must always provide the clients with carefully planned and thorough self-care education programs. Many times how patients handle a situation is based on the information given to them by the nurse and how well this information is understood by the patient. The nurse must be able to evaluate whether the patient and family are adequately prepared for the chemotherapy

Table 6.1   Chemotherapy Checklist

1. Verify informed consent. May be written or oral depending on institution policy, but it is required before chemotherapy administration.
2. Know the drug pharmacology: mechanism of action, usual dosage, route of administration, acute and long-term side effects, and route of excretion.
3. Review laboratory data keeping in mind acceptable parameters. Report abnormalities to the physician.
4. Check physician order for name of drug(s); dosage; route; rate; and timing of drug(s) administration. (Question anything that seems out of the ordinary.)
5. Recalculate dosage. Check height and weight; calculate body surface area (BSA).
6. Verify physician orders and dosage calculations with another nurse.
7. *Premedication*: Administer any premedications at least 20–30 minutes before chemotherapy starts. In some cases, may want to start the patient on antiemetic therapy the night before or the morning of therapy.
8. *Patient Education*: Teach and review with the patient and family details of the chemotherapy schedule, expected side effects, and self-care preventative management suggestions to minimize untoward side effects. Provide written explanations the patient can refer to later since all this information at once may be overwhelming. Refer questions to physician as necessary.
9. Reconstitute drug(s) according to manufacturer suggestions, OSHA guidelines, and institution procedures. May be the responsibility of the nursing or the pharmacy department depending on the institution's policy.
10. Gather appropriate equipment. D_5W or normal saline (NS) are commonly used to infuse chemotherapy, but not exclusively. Use the correct solution and volume. Protect from direct sunlight if applicable.
11. Administer chemotherapy agents according to written policies and procedures using proficient intravenous therapy skills and techniques.
    a. Administer all medications using the 5 rights: (Tenenbaum 1987)
       (1) Right Patient
       (2) Right Drug
       (3) Right Dose
       (4) Right Route
       (5) Right Time
    b. If no information is available, assume the drug you are giving is a vesicant and administer it with caution.
    c. Avoid drug infiltration. If unsure whether the IV is infiltrated, discontinue it, and restart another IV rather than risk extravasation. WHEN IN DOUBT, PULL IT OUT.
    d. Do not mix drugs together when administering combination therapy. Use syringe or intravenous of NS to flush before first drug, in between drugs, and upon completion of all drugs.
    e. It is not optimal to administer vesicant drugs through an indwelling peripheral IV (one that has been in place 4–6 hours or more). It is important to preserve veins, but it is more important to prevent potential extravasation.
    f. Nonvesicant chemotherapy drugs may be administered through an existing IV, once the site has been fully assessed for patency and lack of infiltration.
    g. If unable to start an IV after two attempts, consult a colleague for assistance.
12. Do not allow anyone to interrupt you during the preparation or administration of chemotherapy.
13. Do not foster a patient's dependency on one nurse.
14. Have emergency drugs and an extravasation kit readily available should an adverse reaction occur.
15. *Always listen to the patient*. The patient's knowledge and preference should be utilized as frequently as possible. As the patient becomes more knowledgeable regarding IV techniques, his or her personal experience with successful IV sites, methods, and sensations can be a great aid to the nurse. There are times when the patient's preference may not be the best choice, but his or her participation should always be encouraged.
16. Dispose of intravenous supplies according to OSHA guidelines, and institution policy and procedure. (See chapter 8.)
17. Document drug administration according to institution policy and procedures. Use time savers in documentation, e.g., instead of writing step-by-step how a vesicant was given, write "(Name of drug) administered according to institution policy and procedure for vesicants."
18. Observe for adverse reactions.
19. Use the opportunity to teach and counsel the patient and the family while administering the chemotherapy.

Sources: ONS Module II 1988; Morra 1981; Miller 1980

Table 6.2 Patient Assessment for Ambulatory and Home Chemotherapy

I. The Patient
  A. Physical history
    1. Disease status
    2. Performance status
    3. Abnormal findings—correctable?
    4. Venous access
  B. Psychosocial history
II. Patient's Environment
  A. Support services
  B. Physical aspects of the setting
III. Therapy
  A. Chemotherapy drugs to be given
  B. Special issues:
    1. Hydration
    2. Emetic potential
    3. Potential toxicities
    4. Anticipated tolerance
    5. Technical issues in administration
  C. Required laboratory tests

Table 6.3 Chemotherapeutic Agents Used in Ambulatory Care Settings

bleomycin	cisplatin
DTIC (dacarbazine)	Cytoxan
Adriamycin (doxorubicin)	(cyclophosphamide)
thiotepa	5-FU (5-fluorouracil)
mithramycin	methotrexate
vinblastine	mitomycin
cytosine arabinoside	vincristine
(cyclophosphamide)	

Source: Garvey 1987, p. 144. Reprinted with permission.

treatment. This can be measured when the patient can: 1) perform return demonstrations, or 2) verbally repeat the information. Written materials such as the NCI booklets: *Chemotherapy and You* and *Caring for the Patient with Cancer at Home—A Guide for Patients and Families* are valuable resources.

Legal and ethical issues in chemotherapy administration are the same in the ambulatory care and home settings as they are in the hospital setting

(Garvey 1987). Only a registered nurse proficient in administering chemotherapy should take on such a responsibility regardless of the setting. The nurse should utilize written standards of care and policies and procedures. Otherwise, should an incident occur (e.g., extravasation or anaphylaxis), the nurse would not have a formal basis for the clinical judgments or actions used. Obviously the nurse must know if the drug being administered has the potential for tissue damage if extravasated or for an anaphylactic reaction. The nurse must have rapid access to the necessary medications (see table 6.4) and know how to handle these problems according to written policy. The patient's physician must be notified of a reaction and backup medical assistance, such as EMTs or paramedics, should be called as necessary (Garvey 1987).

NURSING ASSESSMENT: PRE- AND POSTCHEMOTHERAPY

Before administering chemotherapy to a patient (in any setting), especially a new patient, it is very important to establish a pretreatment profile of the person and their disease status. This assessment should completely review physical and psychosocial functioning. The profile will

Table 6.4 Emergency Home Care Kits

Anaphylaxis Kit	Extravasation Kit
Epinephrine (1:1000 IV)	Cold and hot compresses
Benadryl (50 mg IV)	Solumedrol (80 mg
Benadryl (50 mg PO)	ampule)
Tylenol tablets	Specific antidote, e.g.,
Airway	sodium thiosulfate for
IV fluid solution and	nitrogen mustard
tubing	(mechlorethamine)
	Needles and syringes
	(22-gauge, 3-mL, and
	5-mL)
	Alcohol swabs

Source: Adapted from Garvey 1987, p. 145. Reprinted with permission.

serve as a basis for current issues or abnormalities as well as to serve as a means of evaluating any changes that might be due to the therapy.

For example, during the pretreatment assessment the nurse identifies that the patient, a 25-year-old male with Hodgkin's disease, is getting married after his treatments and has always wanted a large family. The decision to treat him with MOPP (mechlorethamine (nitrogen mustard), Oncovin, prednisone, and procarbazine) or ABVD (Adriamycin, bleomycin, vincristine, and DTIC) has not been made yet by his physician. Knowing that the patient has a good chance of long-term disease-free survival with either treatment, and that MOPP has a higher incidence of causing sterility than ABVD, the nurse brings this information to the physician. The physician can then consider it when choosing the best treatment for this young man (Bonadonna and Santoro 1985). If this information had not been identified prior to treatment, the patient would not be able: 1) to use sperm banking, or 2) to have a chance to receive therapy with a lower risk of sterility. This level of assessment is within the realm of expert practice mentioned in chapter 1. Not all nurses participate in such treatment decisions. However, the assessment of potential reproductive toxicity to the patient is an expectation of a nurse administering chemotherapy.

Table 6.5 is a general outline for a nursing assessment. Another example of prechemotherapy nursing assessment guidelines is that described by Engelking and Steele (1984). These very detailed guidelines identify:

1. Nursing diagnoses organized by body systems

2. Diagnosis-appropriate parameters

3. Abnormal findings and appropriate collaborative actions prior to drug administration

Table 6.6 is an example of a multisystem assessment organized in a nursing diagnosis framework. A general assessment guideline may be appropriate for the experienced oncology nurse as it augments her existing practice. A nurse new to the oncology field may benefit from more detailed guidelines as a tool to develop strong assessment skills.

Regardless of the tool utilized, clinical assessment of the patient and the disease must be an ongoing process, so that interventions and management plans can be changed as soon as appropriate. The assessment is just as important

Table 6.5 Nursing Assessment for Chemotherapy

I. **Prechemotherapy Assessment**
  A. *Physical evaluation*
    1. Pertinent past history
      a) Diagnosis and disease presentation
      b) Concomitant health conditions and allergies
    2. System review
      a) Pertinent laboratory data (hematopoietic function)
      b) Neurologic function
      c) Oral cavity and integumentary status
      d) Cardiovascular function
      e) Respiratory function
      f) Urologic function
      g) Gastrointestinal function
      h) Sexual function
      i) Dermatologic status
    3. Presence of prior cancer therapy toxicities
      a) Surgery
      b) Radiation therapy
      c) Chemotherapy
  B. *Psychosocial evaluation*
    1. Knowledge of cancer and chemotherapy
      a) Dispel myths
      b) Address feelings of anxiety and fear
    2. Prior (personal) experience with chemotherapy
    3. Support system and significant others
    4. Informed consent (see chapter 2)
  C. *Patient and family education*

II. **Postchemotherapy Assessment**
  A. *Review assessment as above for changes*
    1. Tumor response
    2. Status improvements
    3. Abnormal findings
  B. *Management of side effects (see chapter 4)*
  C. *Patient/family education*

Table 6.6 Prechemotherapy Nursing Assessment Guidelines

Potential Problems/ Nursing Diagnoses	Physical Status: Assessment Parameters/Signs & Symptoms	Drug & Dose- Limiting Factors
Hematopoietic System		
1. Impaired tissue perfusion related to chemotherapy-induced anemia	• Hgb g (norms 12–14; 14–16) • Hct% (norms 32–36; 36–40) • Vital signs ($\downarrow$ BP, $\uparrow$ pulse, $\uparrow$ respiration) • Pallor (face, palms, conjunctiva) • Fatigue or weakness • Vertigo	Hgb <8 g Hct <20% and blood transfusions not initiated
2. Impaired immunocompetence and potential for infection related to chemotherapy-induced leukopenia	• WBC (norm 4,500–9,000/mm^3) • Pyrexia/rigor, erythema, swelling, pain any site • Abnormal discharges, draining wounds, skin/mucous membrane lesions • Productive cough, SOB, rectal pain, urinary frequency	WBC $\leq$ 3,000/mm^3 Fever > 101°F • Hold all myelosuppressive agents (Exceptions may include leukemia, lymphoma, and/or situations in which there is neoplastic marrow infiltration.)
3. Potential for injury (bleeding) related to chemotherapy-induced thrombocytopenia	• Platelet count (150,000–400,000/mm^3) • Spontaneous gingival bleeding or epistaxis • Presence of petechiae or easy bruisability • Hematuria, melena, hematemesis, hemoptysis • Hypermenorrhea • Signs & sx intracranial bleed (irritability, sensory loss, unequal pupils, headache, ataxia)	Platelet count $\leq$ 100,000/mm^3 • Hold all myelosuppressive agents (Exceptions may include leukemia, lymphoma, and/or situations in which there is neoplastic marrow infiltration.)
Integumentary System		
Alteration in mucous membrane of mouth, nasopharynx, esophagus, rectum, anus, or ostomy stoma related to chemotherapy-induced tissue changes	Mucositis Scale* 0 = pink, moist, intact mucosa: absence of pain or burning +1 = generalized erythema with or without pain or burning +2 = isolated small ulcerations and/or white patches +3 = confluent ulcerations with white patches on $\geq$ 25% mucosa +4 = hemorrhagic ulcerations	+2 mucositis • Hold antimetabolites (esp. methotrexate, 5-FU) • Hold antitumor antibiotics (esp. doxorubicin, dactinomycin)
Gastrointestinal System		
Discomfort, nutritional deficiency, and/or fluid and electrolyte disturbances related to chemotherapy-induced: A. Anorexia	• Lab values: albumin & total protein • Normal weight/present weight & % of body weight loss • Normal diet pattern/changes in diet pattern • Alterations in taste sensation • Early satiety	

B. Nausea & vomiting	• Lab values: Electrolytes
	• Pattern of n/v (incidence, duration, severity)
	• Antiemetic plan
	   Drug(s), dosage(s), schedule, efficacy
	   Other (dietary adjustments, relaxation techniques, environmental manipulation)
		Intractable n/v × 24 h if IV hydration not initiated

C. Bowel disturbances 1. Diarrhea	• Normal pattern of bowel elimination • Consistency (loose, watery/bloody stools) • Frequency & duration (#/day and # of days) • Antidiarrheal drug(s), dosage(s), efficacy	Diarrheal stools × 3/24 h • Hold antimetabolites (esp. methotrexate, 5-FU)
2. Constipation	• Normal pattern of bowel elimination • Consistency (hard, dry, small stools) • Frequency (hours or days beyond normal pattern) • Stool softener(s), laxative(s), efficacy	No BM × 48 h past normal bowel patterns • Hold vinca alkaloids (vinblastine, vincristine)

D. Hepatotoxicity	• Lab values: LDH, SGOT, alk phos, bilirubin
	• Pain/tenderness over liver, feeling of fullness
	• Increase in nausea/vomiting or anorexia
	• Changes in mental status
	• Jaundice
	• High-risk factors:
	  Hepatic metastasis Concurrent hepatotoxic drugs
	  Viral hepatitis Graft vs. host disease
	  Abdominal XRT Blood transfusions
		Evidence of chemical hepatitis
		• Hold hepatotoxic agents (esp. methotrexate, 6-MP) until differential dx established

Respiratory System
Impaired gas exchange or ineffective breathing pattern related to chemotherapy-induced pulmonary fibrosis
	• Lab values: PFT's CXR
	• Respirations (rate, rhythm, depth)
	• Chest pain
	• Nonproductive cough
	• Progressive dyspnea
	• Wheezing/stridor
	• High-risk factors:
	  Total cumulative dose of bleomycin Age >60 yr
	  Preexisting lung disease Concomitant use of other pulmonary toxic drugs
	  Prior/concomitant XRT Smoking hx
		Acute unexplained onset respiratory symptoms
		• Hold all antineoplastic agents until differential dx established

(continued)

Table 6.6 *(continued)*

Potential Problems/ Nursing Diagnoses	Physical Status: Assessment Parameters/Signs & Symptoms	Drug & Dose- Limiting Factors
Cardiovascular System		

Decreased cardiac output related to chemotherapy-induced:
 A. Cardiac arrhythmias
 B. Cardiomyopathy
	• Lab values: cardiac enzymes, electrolytes, ECG, ECHO, MUGA
	 • Vital signs
	 • Presence of arrhythmia (irregular radial/apical)
	 • Signs/sx CHF (dyspnea, ankle edema, nonproductive cough, rales, cyanosis)
	 • High-risk factors:
	   Total cumulative Prior/concurrent
	   dose anthracyclines mediastinal XRT
	   Preexisting cardiac disease Bolus administration
	                higher drug doses
		Acute sx CHF and/or cardiac arrhythmia
		 • Hold all antineoplastic agents until differential dx established
		 Total dose doxorubicin or daunorubicin > 550 mg/m^2
		 • Hold anthracyclines

Genitourinary System		

1. Alteration in fluid volume (excess) related to chemotherapy-induced:
 A. Glomerular or renal tubule damage
 B. Hyperuricemic nephropathy
	• Lab values: BUN, creatinine clearance, serum creatinine, uric acid, electrolytes, urinalysis
	 • Color, odor, clarity of urine
	 • 24-h fluid intake & output (estimate/actual)
	 • Hematuria; proteinuria
	 • Development of oliguria or anuria
	 • High-risk factors:
	   Preexisting renal disease
	   Concurrent treatment with nephrotoxic drugs (esp. aminoglycoside antibiotics)
		Hematuria
		 • Hold cyclophosphamide
		 Serum creat > 2.0 and/or
		 Creat clear < 70 mL/min
		 • Hold *cis*-platinum, streptozotocin
		 Anuria $\times$ 24 h
		 • Hold all antineoplastic agents

2. Alteration in comfort related to chemotherapy-induced hemorrhagic cystitis		
Nervous System		
1. Impaired sensory/motor function related to chemotherapy-induced 1. Peripheral neuropathy 2. Cranial nerve neuropathy	• Paresthesias (numbness, tingling in feet, fingertips) • Trigeminal nerve toxicity (severe jaw pain) • Diminished or absent deep tendon reflexes (ankle and knee jerks) • Motor weakness/slapping gait/ataxia • Visual and auditory disturbances	Presence of any neurologic signs & symptoms • Hold vinca alkaloids, *cis*-platinum, hexamethyl melamine, procarbazine until differential dx established

2. Impaired bowel and bladder elimination related to chemotherapy-induced autonomic nerve dysfunction	• Urinary retention
	 • Constipation/abdominal cramping & distention
	 • High-risk factors:
	   Changes in diet or mobility
	   Frequent use of narcotic analgesics
	   Obstructive disease process
		Presence of any neurologic signs & symptoms
		 • Hold vinca alkaloids until differential dx established

*Adapted from "Guidelines for Nursing Care of Patients with Altered Protective Mechanisms." Oncology Nursing Society Clinical Practice Committee.
 Source: Engelking 1988. Reprinted with permission from World Health Communications, Inc.

once treatment is finished, to watch for signs of recurrence, as it is during treatment to evaluate toxicities and response. It is essential to remember the patient is a person, not a disease entity, and deserves to be treated in a holistic fashion. One of nursing's roles is to assist clients to resume the activities in life that were important before the illness. Without being unnecessarily fearful of the disease, the patient must also know when to seek medical attention.

REACTIONS: EXTRAVASATION, ANAPHYLAXIS, AND HYPERSENSITIVITY

Extravasation

Extravasation is tissue damage as a result of an infiltrated chemotheraputic agent. Drugs with this potential are called vesicants (see table 6.7). The reactions range from mild to severe depending on the specific drug, the amount of drug infiltrated, and the length of the exposure (Brown 1987). Injuries from extravasation consist of hyperpigmentation, burning, erythema, inflammation, ulceration, necrosis, prolonged pain, tissue sloughing, infection, or loss of mobility (Brown 1987; Montrose 1987).

These injuries are most often obvious immediately after treatment or at least within 7 to 10 days, and may last for several months (Brown 1987) (see figures 6.1 and 6.2).

The treatment of extravasation is controversial. The incidence of this reaction ranges from 0.1% to 6%, so our clinical experience is relatively limited (Montrose 1987). More documentation is needed, but it is unethical to conduct a clinical study that would 1) have a no-treatment control arm or 2) knowingly infiltrate a vesicant agent for patient accrual to such a study (ONS Module V 1988). Prompt recognition of an infiltrate is required so interventions can be started immediately. Antidotes are generally recommended based on the manufacturer's directions or on theoretical rationale only.

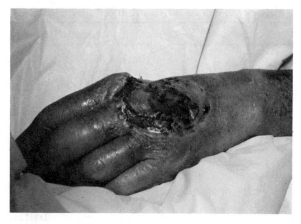

Figure 6.1 Untreated doxorubicin extravasation
Source: Groenwald 1990.

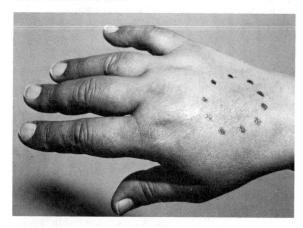

Figure 6.2 Steroid-treated doxorubicin extravasation
Source: Groenwald 1990.

There is only one known antidote—sodium thiosulfate for mechlorethamine (nitrogen mustard). All other medications used in the setting of an extravasation have also been coined "antidote," even though scientifically they are not true antidotes (see table 6.8).

The Oncology Nursing Society has developed guidelines (not standards) for the treatment of an extravasation. These guidelines are generally followed by a number of institutions across the country. ONS membership is continually involved

Table 6.7   Vesicant/Irritant and Nonvesicant Cancer Chemotherapeutic Agents

Vesicant Drugs (Commercial Agents)

Generic Name	Other Name	Generic Name	Other Name
dactinomycin	Actinomycin D	mitomycin C	Mutamycin
daunomycin	Cerubidine	estramustine	Estracyte
doxorubicin	Adriamycin	mechlorethamine	Nitrogen Mustard
		vinblastine	Velban
		vincristine	Oncovin

Vesicant Drugs (Investigational Agents)

Generic Name	Other Name	Generic Name	Other Name
amsacrine	M-AMSA	bisantrene	—————
maytasine	—————	pyrazofurin	Pyrazomycin
vindesine	Eldisine		

Irritant Agents

Generic Name	Other Name	Generic Name	Other Name
carmustine	BCNU	teniposide I+	(VM-26)
dacarbazine	DTIC	mitoguazone I+	Methyl-GAG
etoposide	VP-16-213/VePesid		
streptozocin	Zanosar		

Non-Vesicant Agents

Generic Name	Other Name	Generic Name	Other Name
bleomycin*	Blenoxane	methotrexate	Mexate
cyclophosphamide	Cytoxan	cisplatin**	Platinol
cytarabine	ARA-C	thiotepa	
floxuridine	FUDR	mitoxantrone+	Novantrone
fluorouracil*	5-FU	asparaginase	Elspar
tegafur I+	Ftorafur	thioguanine injection I+	
mithramycin/plicamycin	Mithracin		

Definitions

Vesicant:	A cancer chemotherapeutic agent capable of causing or forming a blister or causing tissue destruction.
Irritant:	A cancer chemotherapeutic agent capable of producing venous pain at the site and along the vein, with or without an inflammatory reaction.
Extravasation:	The leakage of a vesicant or irritant drug into the subcutaneous tissue that is capable of causing pain, necrosis, or sloughing of tissue.

I+ Indicates Investigational Drugs now in clinical trials.
*   Occasionally causes mild phlebitis.
** Single case report each of cellulitis and fibrosis (*Ca. Treat. Rep.* 64:10 1164-1164, 1980).
Source: ONS Cancer Chemotherapy Guidelines Module V. Reprinted with permission.

in refining the ONS guidelines. In a letter to the editor of *Oncology Nursing Forum,* Brown (1987) took issue with using DMSO as an antidote for doxorubicin (Adriamycin) extravasations. They presented the pros and cons of this issue using references sited by the ONS as well as others. They also recommended an additional column in the ONS antidote table: "Negative Studies." This column would be used to list available extravasation research reports, thus more clearly acknowledging the existing controversies.

Table 6.8 Antidotes for Vesicant/Irritant Drugs

Drug Classification	Specific Agent	Local Antidote	Positive Effect animal studies	Positive Effect clinical case reports	Antidote Preparation	Method of Administration	Comments
Alkylating Agent	mechlorethamine (Nitrogen Mustard)	Isotonic Sodium Thiosulfate 1 g/10 mL (Manufacturer's recommendations)	none	yes	Mix 4 mL of 10% Na Thiosulfate with 6 mL sterile water for injection. (⅙ molar solution results)	1. Inject 5–6 mL (0.2–0.24 g) IV through the existing line and SQ into the extravasated site with multiple injections. 2. Repeat dosing SQ over the next several hours. 3. Apply cold compresses. 4. No total dose established.	1. ACTION: chemical neutralization 2. Initiate treatment immediately and liberally.
	mitomycin C (Mutamycin)	Topical DMSO (RIMSO)	yes	none	1–2 mL of 1 mmol DMSO 50%–100%	1. Apply topically one time to the site.	1. Probably not effective for distal or delayed ulcers. 2. Initiate treatment immediately. 3. ACTION: carrier solvent or oxygen radical scavenger.
Plant Alkaloids	vinblastine (Velban) vincristine (Oncovin)	Hyaluronidase (Wydase) 150 u/mL (Manufacturer's recommendations)	yes	none	Add 1 mL USP Sodium Chloride (150 U/mL results)	1. Inject 1–6 mL (150–900 U) SQ into the extravasated site with multiple injections. 2. Repeat dosing SQ over the next several hours. 3. Apply *warm* compresses. 4. No total dose established.	1. ACTION: enhances absorption and dispersion of the extravasated drug. 2. Corticosteroids and topical cooling appear to worsen toxicity. 3. Warm compresses increase systemic absorption of the drug.
	vindesine (Eldisine) teniposide (VM-26) etoposide (VP-16-213 VePesid)	Hyaluronidase (Wydase) 150 U/mL	yes	none			

(continued)

Table 6.8 (continued)

Drug Classification	Specific Agent	Local Antidote	Positive Effect animal studies	Positive Effect clinical case reports	Antidote Preparation	Method of Administration	Comments
Anthracycline Antibiotics	doxorubicin (Adriamycin) daunomycin (Cerubidine)	Topical cooling	yes	yes	Topical cooling may be achieved using 1. ice packs 2. cooling pad with ice water circulating 3. cryogel packs changed frequently	1. Cooling of site to pt tolerance for 24 hrs. 2. Elevate and rest extremity 24–48 hrs then resume normal activity as tolerated. 3. If pain, erythema, or swelling persist > 48 hrs, refer to plastic surgeon.	1. Application of cold compresses inhibits cytotoxicity of drug. 2. Some studies suggest a role for topical dimethyl sulfoxide (DMSO) while others show no benefit or delayed healing. 3. Local singular injections of low-dose (<50 mg) soluble hydrocortisone may be beneficial.
	bisantrene	Sodium Bicarbonate 1 mEq/1 mL (premixed)	yes	yes	Mix equal parts of 1 mEq/mL Sodium Bicarbonate with sterile normal saline (1:1 solution). Resulting solution is 0.5 mEq/mL	1. Inject 2–6 mL (1.0–3.0 mEq) IV through the existing line and SQ into the extravasated site with multiple injections. 2. Apply cold compresses. 3. Total dose not to exceed 10 mL of 0.5 mEq/mL solution (5.0 mEq).	1. ACTION: chemical activation. 2. Dilute bicarbonate chemically degrades the drug.

Sources: Adapted from ONS Module V 1988; ONS Clinical Practice Committee 1989. Reprinted with permission.

This difference in opinion highlights how important it is for an institution to have an extravasation policy and procedure, and to stay current with the literature so the procedure continues to be appropriate. If there is not a policy or standing order at the institution, the nurse should take an active role in developing one so there is a basis for his or her actions in case of an extravasation. It is comforting to know though, that current clinical experience indicates that 89% of all extravasations never progress beyond a mild reaction, even without a pharmacologic treatment (Birdsall and Naleboff 1988). If severe necrosis occurs, the only successful treatment is surgical debridement with skin grafting or if extremely extensive necrosis occurs amputation may be required (Harwood et al. 1989).

Prevention of extravasation is the best treatment a nurse can offer the patient (see table 6.9). As mentioned, only qualified registered nurses should administer chemotherapy. The nurse must always be aware if the drug being administered is a vesicant drug. Vesicant drugs need to be delivered with caution, and with the utmost proficiency in intravenous therapy technique. Each institution has the responsibility of developing written procedures for administering vesicant agents, both through a peripheral IV and

Table 6.9 Prevention of Extravasation

Use experienced personnel

Use patient education

Use single venipuncture—new site

Avoid areas of compromised circulation (phlebitis, lymphedema, mastectomy side, lower extremities, hematomas)

Avoid areas with underlying tendons and nerves

Ensure adequate drug dilution—sideport injection through freely flowing IV

Maintain careful observation—visualize entire limb continuously throughout procedure

Consider the use of venous access devices in cases of difficult peripheral access

Source: Adapted from Montrose 1987. Reprinted with permission.

through a venous access device, for the safety of the patient, the nurse, and the institution itself.

Table 6.10 outlines the procedure recommended by the ONS for the management of an extravasation.

Hypersensitivity and Anaphylactic Reactions

Allergic or hypersensitivity reactions to chemotherapy drugs vary from mild to life-threatening. The reactions result when the immune system is overstimulated by a foreign substance resulting in the formation of antibodies. The reaction occurs, and may worsen, with each exposure to the foreign substance (Brown 1987). Hypersensitivity reactions may be classified into four types: Types I-IV (see table 6.13) (Weiss 1984). Type I reactions, *anaphylaxis* and anaphylactoid, are the ones most frequently seen in the oncology setting (Brown 1987). Signs and symptoms of this reaction may include agitation, dizziness, nausea, urticaria, chest tightness, rhinitis, and cramping abdominal pains. Respiratory distress, hypotension, and edema of the eyes or face may also be noted (Brown 1987; Garvey 1987). Hypersensitivity reactions have been reported with IV L-asparaginase, cisplatin, cyclophosphamide (Cytoxan), mechorethamine (nitrogen mustard), methotrexate, and melphalan (Brown 1987).

A localized hypersensitivity reaction, called "flare," has been described with doxorubicin (Adriamycin) and daunorubicin (Goodman 1986). In a flare reaction urticaria usually develops at the injection site and potentially along the vein. This reaction usually remains localized, not spreading systemically. Flare may occur only with the first treatment of doxorubicin (Adriamycin) or daunorubicin and not any subsequent doses or it may only appear with subsequent doses, not the first one (Brown 1987).

Bleomycin has been associated with hyperpyrexia. These high fevers usually last for 24 hours from the time of bleomycin administration

Table 6.10 Management of Extravasation

1. Assess site for signs and symptoms of extravasation (see table 6.11).
2. Manage extravasation of drugs with known intravenous antidotes (see table 5.9) or with subcutaneous antidote
   a) Stop the chemotherapy administration.
   b) Leave the needle in place.
   c) Aspirate any residual drug and blood in the intravenous tubing, needle, and infiltration site.
   d) Instill the intravenous antidote (see table 6.8).
   NB: If unable to aspirate the residual drug from the intravenous tubing, **DO NOT** instill the antidote through the needle. Proceed directly to the next step.
   e) Remove the needle.
   f) Inject the subcutaneous antidote in a clockwise fashion into the infiltrated area, using a 25-gauge needle. Change the needle with each new injection as needed.
   g) Avoid applying pressure to the suspected infiltration site.
   h) Apply topical ointment as needed, if ordered.
   i) Cover lightly with an occlusive sterile dressing.
   j) Apply warm or cold compresses as indicated (see table 5.9).
   k) Elevate the arm.
   l) Observe the site regularly for reaction.
   m) Document the following information in the patient's medical record:
      1) Date
      2) Time
      3) Needle size and type
      4) Insertion site
      5) Drug sequence
      6) Drug administration technique
      7) Approximate amount of drug extravasated
      8) Nursing management of extravasation
      9) Patient complaints and statement
      10) Appearance of the site
      11) Physician notification
      12) Follow-up measures
   n) Document the incident on a report form according to institution policy and procedures (see figure 6.3).

Source: ONS Module V 1988

and respond well to conservative therapies (Brown 1987). Also with bleomycin, patients with lymphoma may experience, though rarely (1%–8%), an anaphylactoid reaction (Dorr and Fritz 1980).

The nurse must always be aware of a drug's potential to cause hypersensitivity reactions. Drugs with a documented reaction must be delivered with caution. Emergency medications must be readily available in case an anaphylactic reaction should occur (see table 6.4). Nursing assessment prior to administration is important to elicit any prior allergies or chemotherapy reactions. Table 6.14 outlines the ONS procedure recommended for the management of hypersensitivity and anaphylactic reactions. (Also see table 6.15.)

Table 6.11 Nursing Assessment of Extravasation versus Other Reactions

Assessment Parameter	Extravasation	Irritation of the Vein	Flare Reaction
Pain	Pain, burning, or stinging are common and can occur while the drug is being given and around the needle site.	Aching and tightness along the vein.	Itching
Redness	Redness may occur around the needle site.	The full length of the vein may be reddened or darkened.	Either red blotches or red streaks can occur as the drug is being given. The blotches and streaks appear along the vein.
Swelling	Swelling may occur around the needle site, either immediately or hours later.	Swelling is not likely.	Swelling is not likely.
Blood Return	Blood return may still be present.	Blood return is usually, but not always present.	Blood return is usually, but not always present.

Source: ONS Cancer Chemotherapy Guidelines Module V 1988. Reprinted with permission.

STANFORD UNIVERSITY HOSPITAL and CLINICS
Stanford University Medical Center
Stanford, California 94305

723-7621

CHEMOTHERAPY DRUG EXTRAVASATION RECORD

(addressograph stamp)

Date: _____ Time: _____   Infiltration Site: _____

Drug Regimen: _____

Order Drugs Given: _____

_____

Drug/Amount Extravasated: _____

Size of Needle: _____

NARRATIVE OF EVENT: (including condition of veins, appearance of infiltration
    site, patient comments)

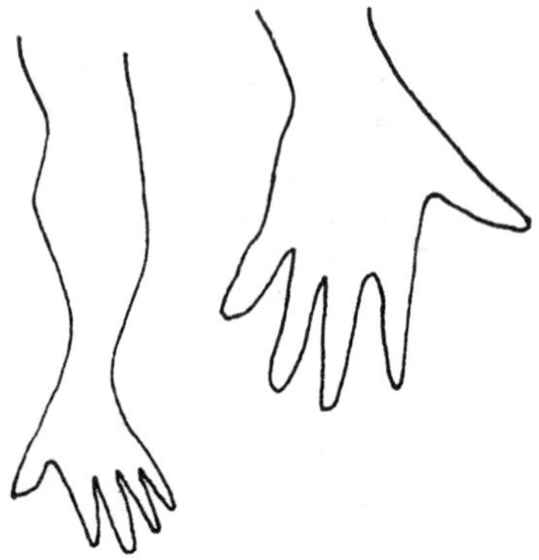

NURSING INTERVENTIONS

a)   MD Notified _____ Time: _____

b)   Antidote and Technique Used:

c)   Instruction to Patient:

d)   Follow-up Plan:
     (Include referral — if made)

_____
Signature

15-30 (Rev. 9/88)   **WHITE - Medical Records   CANARY - Oncology Chart   PINK - Extravasation Rand**

Figure 6.3   Institutional Extravasation Record

Source: Stanford University Hospital and Clinics. Reprinted with permission.

390

Table 6.12 Standardized Nursing Care Plan for Patient Experiencing Extravasation (Based on ONS Cancer Chemotherapy Guidelines)

Nursing Diagnosis	Defining Characteristics	Expected Outcomes	Nursing Interventions
A. Potential alteration in skin integrity related to extravasation	A. Vesicant drugs may cause erythema, burning, tissue necrosis, tissue sloughing	A. Extravasation, if it occurs, is detected early with early intervention	A. Careful technique is used during venipuncture (see chap. 7) 1. Select venipuncture site away from underlying tendons and blood vessels. 2. Secure IV so that catheter/needle site is visible at all times. 3. Administer vesicant through freely flowing IV, constantly monitoring IV site and pt response. Nurse should be thoroughly familiar with *institutional policy and procedure* for administration of a vesicant agent. 4. If vesicant drug is administered as a continuous infusion, drug must be given through a patent central line.

B. Potential pain at site of extravasation	B. Vesicant drugs include
	1. Commercial agents
	  a. dactinomycin
	  b. daunomycin
	  c. doxorubicin
	  d. mitomycin C
	  e. estramustine
	  f. mechlorethamine
	  g. vinblastine
	  h. vincristine
	2. Investigational agents
	  a. amsacrine
	  b. Maytansine
	  c. vindesine
	  d. Bisantrene
	  e. Pyrazofurin
		B. Skin and underlying tissue damage is minimized	B. If extravasation is *suspected:*
			1. Stop drug administration.
			2. Aspirate any residual drug and blood from IV tubing, IV catheter/needle, and IV site if possible.
			3. Instill antidote if one exists through needle if able to remove remaining drug in previous step. If standing orders are not available, notify physician and obtain order.
			4. Remove needle.
			5. Inject antidote into area of apparent infiltration if antidote is recommended, using 25-gauge needle into subcutaneous tissue.
			6. Apply topical cream if recommended.
			7. Cover lightly with occlusive sterile dressing.
			8. Apply warm or cold applications as recommended.
			9. Elevate arm.
			10. Assess site regularly for pain, progression of erythema, induration, and for evidence of necrosis:
			  a. If outpatient, arrange to assess site or teach pt to and notify provider if condition worsens. Arrange next clinic visit for assessment of site depending on drug, amount infiltrated, extent of potential injury, and pt variables.

(continued)

Table 6.12 (continued)

Nursing Diagnosis	Defining Characteristics	Expected Outcomes	Nursing Interventions
			B. 10. *b.* Discuss with MD plastic-surgical consult if erythema, induration, pain, tissue breakdown occurs.
			11. When in doubt about whether drug is infiltrating, treat as an infiltration.
			12. Document precise, concise information in patient's medical record:
			a. Date, time
			b. Insertion site, needle size and type
			c. Drug administration technique, drug sequence, and approximate amount of drug extravasated
			d. Appearance of site, pt's subjective response
			e. Nursing interventions performed to manage extravasation, and notification of physician
			f. Photo documentation if possible
			g. Follow-up plan
			h. Nurse's signature
			i. Institutional policy and procedure for documentation should be adhered to.
C. Potential loss of function of extremity related to extravasation			
D. Potential infection related to skin breakdown			

Table 6.13 Hypersensitivity Reactions

TYPE I:	Either an antigen–antibody reaction (anaphylaxis) or a direct antigen (anaphylactoid) reaction
TYPE II:	An antigen–antibody reaction that occurs on the cell surface
TYPE III:	An intravascular antigen–antibody reaction
TYPE IV:	Reaction is a delayed response in the form of contact dermatitis

Source: Goodman 1986, p. 31. Reprinted with permission.

Table 6.14 Management of Hypersensitivity and Anaphylactic Reactions

1. Review the patient's allergy history.
2. Consider prophylactic medications with hydrocortisone or an antihistamine in atopic/allergic individuals (this requires a physician's order).
3. *Patient and family education:* Assess the patient's readiness to learn. Inform patient of the potential of an allergic reaction and to report any unusual symptoms such as:
   a) Uneasiness or agitation
   b) Abdominal cramping
   c) Itching
   d) Chest tightness
   e) Lightheadedness or dizziness
   f) Chills
4. Ensure emergency equipment and medications are readily available.
5. Obtain baseline vital signs and note patient's mental status.
6. As appropriate, perform a scratch test, intradermal skin test, or test dose before administering the full dosage (this requires a physician's order). If there is no reaction, the remaining dose can be administered. If an allergic response is suspected, discontinue the test dose (unless it has been completed), maintain the intravenous line, and notify the physician.
7. For a *localized allergic* response:
   a) Evaluate symptoms; observe for urticaria, wheals, localized erythema.
   b) Administer diphenhydramine or hydrocortisone as per physician's order.
   c) Monitor vital signs every 15 minutes for 1 hour.
   d) Continue subsequent dosing or desensitization program according to a physician's order.
   e) If a "flare" reaction appears along the vein with doxorubicin (Adriamycin) or daunorubicin (see table 6.12), flush the line with saline.
      (1) Ensure that extravasation has not occurred.
      (2) Administer hydrocortisone 25–50 mg intravenously with a physician's order followed by a Normal Saline flush. This may be adequate to resolve the "flare" reaction.
      (3) Once the "flare" reaction has resolved, continue *slow* infusion of the drug.
      (4) Monitor for repeated "flare" episodes. It is preferable to change the intravenous site if possible.
8. For a *generalized allergic* response, *anaphylaxis* may be suspected if the following signs or symptoms occur (usually within the first 15 minutes of the start of the infusion or injection):
   a) Subjective signs and symptoms
      (1) Generalized itching
      (2) Chest tightness
      (3) Difficulty speaking
      (4) Agitation
      (5) Uneasiness
      (6) Dizziness
      (7) Nausea
      (8) Crampy abdominal pain
      (9) Anxiety
      (10) Sense of impending doom
      (11) Desire to urinate or defecate
      (12) Chills
   b) Objective signs
      (1) Flushed apperance (edema of face, hands, or feet)
      (2) Localized or generalized urticaria
      (3) Respiratory distress with or without wheezing
      (4) Hypotension
      (5) Cyanosis
9. For a *generalized allergic* response:
   a) Stop the infusion immediately and notify the physician.
   b) Maintain the intravenous line with appropriate solution to expand the vascular space, e.g., normal saline.
   c) If not contraindicated, ensure maximum rate of infusion if the patient is hypotensive.
   d) Position the patient to promote perfusion of the vital organs, the supine position is preferred.
   e) Monitor vital signs every 2 minutes until stable, then every 5 minutes for 30 minutes, then every 15 minutes as ordered.
   f) Reassure the patient and the family.
   g) Maintain the airway and anticipate the need for cardiopulmonary resuscitation.
   h) All medications must be administered with a physician's order.
10. Document the incident in the medical record according to institution policy and procedures.
11. Physician-guided desensitization may be necessary for subsequent dosing.

Source: ONS Module V 1988. Reprinted with permission.

Table 6.15 Standardized Nursing Care Plan for Patient Experiencing Hypersensitivity or Anaphylaxis

Nursing Diagnosis	Defining Characteristics	Expected Outcomes	Nursing Interventions
I. *Potential for injury related to hypersensitivity and anaphylaxis*	I. A. Allergic or hypersensitivity reactions to chemotherapy vary from simple allergic reactions to life threatening ones	I. A. Allergic reactions (hypersensitivity and anaphylaxis), if they occur, will be detected early	I. A. Review standing orders for management of allergic reactions (hypersensitivity and anaphylaxis) per institutional policy and procedure.
	B. The reactions are the result of a foreign substance being introduced to the body with resultant antibody formation	B. Airway will remain patent	B. Identify location of anaphylaxis kit. The kit should contain: 1. epinephrine 1:1000 2. hydrocortisone sodium succinate (SoluCortef) 3. diphenhydramine HCl (Benadryl) 4. aminophylline 5. similar emergency drugs
	C. The reactions may worsen with subsequent exposure to the foreign substance (chemotherapeutic agent)	C. B/P will remain within 20 mm Hg of baseline	C. Prior to drug administration obtain baseline vital signs and record mental status
		D. Future allergic responses will be prevented	D. Observe for following s/s, usually occurring within the first 15 mins of infusion *Subjective* nausea generalized itching crampy abdominal pain chest tightness anxiety agitation sense of impending doom wheeziness desire to urinate/defecate dizziness chills

I. D. *Objective*

flushed appearance (angioedema of the face, neck, eyelids, hands, feet)

localized or generalized urticaria

respiratory distress ± wheezing

hypotension

cyanosis

E. ONS recommendations for generalized allergic response:

1. Stop infusion and notify MD
2. Obtain orders for infusion of NS to maintain vascular volume and titrate infusion rate to maintain adequate B/P (i.e., within 20 mm Hg of baseline systolic B/P)
3. Place pt in supine position to promote perfusion of visceral organs
4. Monitor vital signs q 2 min until stable, then every 5 min for 30 mins, then every 15 min
5. Provide emotional reassurance to pt and family
6. Maintain patent airway and have equipment ready for CPR if needed
7. Medications per MD order and institutional policy and procedure

F. Document incident

G. Discuss with MD desensitization versus drug discontinuance for further dose

BIBLIOGRAPHY

Birdsall C, Naleboff AF (1988) How do you manage chemotherapy extravasation? *American Journal of Nursing* Feb: 228–230

Bonadonna G, Santoro, A (1985) Clinical evolution and treatment of Hodgkin's disease, in Wiernik PH, et al (eds.): *Neoplastic Diseases of the Blood*, Vol 2. New York, Churchill Livingstone

Brown J (1987) Chemotherapy, in Groenwald SL (ed.): *Cancer Nursing Principles and Practice*. Boston, Jones and Bartlett

Burkhalter P, Donley D (1978) *Dynamics of Oncology Nursing*. New York, McGraw-Hill

Dana W (1985) *Outpatient and Home Chemotherapy: Offering the Cancer Patient a More Normal Life*. Houston, MD Anderson Hospital and Tumor Institute

Dorr RT, Fritz W (1980) *Cancer Chemotherapy Handbook*. New York, Elsevier

Engelking C (1988) Prechemotherapy nursing assessment in outpatient settings. *Outpatient Chemotherapy* 3(1): 9–11

Engelking CH, Steele NE (1984) A model for pretreatment nursing assessment of patients receiving cancer chemotherapy. *Cancer Nursing* 7: 203–212

Garvey EC (1987) Current and future nursing issues in the home administration of chemotherapy. *Seminars in Oncology Nursing* 3(2): 142–147

Goodman MS (1986) *Cancer: Chemotherapy and Care*. Evansville, Bristol Laboratories

Harwood K, et al (1989) Management of doxorubicin extravasation. *Oncology Nursing Forum* 16(1): 10–11

Hilkemeyer R (1982) A Historical perspective in cancer nursing. *Oncology Nursing Forum* 9(2): 47–56

Hubbard SM (1987) Reflections on the oncology nurse's role in cancer therapy: future challenges. *Seminars in Oncology Nursing* 3(2): 154–158

Krakoff IN (1987) Cancer chemotherapy agents. *CA: A Cancer Journal for Clinicians* 37(2): 93–105

Lind J, Bush NJ (1987) Nursing's role in chemotherapy administration. *Seminars in Oncology Nursing* 3(2): 83–86

Meeske K, Ruccione K (1987) Cancer chemotherapy in children: nursing issues and approaches. *Seminars in Oncology* 3(2): 118–127

Miller SA (1980) Nursing actions in cancer chemotherapy administration. *Oncology Nursing Forum* 7(4): 8–16

Montrose PA (1987) Extravasation management. *Seminars in Oncology Nursing* 3(2): 128–132

Moore JM (1982) The influence of the time of administration on cisplatinum-induced nausea and vomiting. *Oncology Nursing Forum* 9(3): 26–32

Morra ME (ed) (1981) *Cancer Chemotherapy Treatment and Care*. Boston, GK Hall Medical

Oncology Nursing Society (1988) *Cancer Chemotherapy Guidelines: Module II*. Pittsburg, ONS

Oncology Nursing Society (1988) *Cancer Chemotherapy Guidelines: Module V. Recommendations for the Management of Extravasation and Anaphylaxis*. Pittsburg, ONS

ONS Clinical Practice Committee (1989) Revision of Module V. *ONF* 6(2): 275

Perri J (1981) Nursing care of the cancer patient: chemotherapy, in Bouchard-Kurtz R, Speese-Owens N (eds.): *Nursing Care of the Cancer Patient* (ed 4). St. Louis, CV Mosby Co

Stuart M (1981) *Cancer: Chemotherapy and Care, Part I and II*. Chicago, Bristol Laboratories

Tenenbaum L (1987) Nursing administration of chemotherapy, in Ziegfeld CR (ed.): *Core Curriculum for Oncology Nursing*. Philadelphia, WB Saunders

Weiss RB (1984) Hypersensitivity reactions to cancer chemotherapy, in Perry MC, Yarbo JW (eds.): *Toxicity of Chemotherapy*. New York, Grune and Stratton

7

DRUG DELIVERY SYSTEMS

As was discussed in the previous chapter, physicians originally administered all chemotherapy drugs. Nurses gradually assumed this role. At first administration was very basic, as there were only a few drugs in use. Now nurses administer over forty drugs and utilize technologically advanced drug delivery systems. This chapter will present information related specifically to drug administration, including a review of drug delivery systems. Throughout this section various products will be featured. By no means do those highlighted constitute a full list of products. Instead, they only represent a sampling of what is currently available in today's market and do not constitute an endorsement of any product.

ROUTES OF ADMINISTRATION

The goal of chemotherapy administration is to optimize drug availability. In an attempt to deliver drugs in high concentrations to areas of greatest clinical need and to improve the antitumor effects, many diverse routes of drug administration have been developed (Haskell 1980). The current routes of administration include:

intrathecal (IT)
intra-arterial (IA)
intracavitary (IC)

subcutaneous (SQ)
intramuscular (IM)
topical (TOP)
oral (PO)
intravenous (IV)

The following three routes of administration allow for high drug concentrations in the disease area while minimizing the systemic concentrations, and thus the side effects:

intrathecal
intra-arterial
intracavitary

Administering chemotherapy *intrathecally* allows the drugs to reach the central nervous system to prevent or treat local disease. The majority of chemotherapy agents do not cross the blood-brain barrier, so they must be delivered directly into the cerebrospinal fluid. This is accomplished by either: 1) a lumbar puncture or 2) utilizing an indwelling subcutaneous cerebrospinal fluid reservoir, such as the Ommaya reservoir (Heyer–Schulte del Caribe, Anasco PR). The benefits and risks to the patient must be determined before either method of administration is chosen. To put it concisely, the benefits and risks a patient must consider include: 1) having a lumbar puncture performed for each treatment (weighing the pain and potential complications that procedure involves) or 2) the potential complications of surgically inserting an Ommaya reservoir, but utilizing a consistent port for each treatment. The Ommaya reservoir is a mushroom-shaped, reusable, self-sealing, silicone port which is connected to a catheter placed in the ventricle (figure 7.1). The reservoir is accessed by inserting a hypodermic needle, usually a small-gauged butterfly needle with an attached three-way stopcock and syringe, directly into the dome. During the procedure an amount of cerebrospinal fluid, equal to the amount of

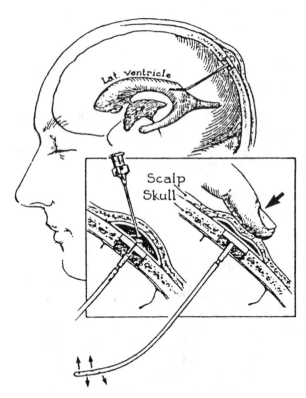

Figure 7.1 Cerebrospinal fluid reservoir and mode of use

Source: Ratcheson, R.A., and Ommaya, A.K. Experience with the subcutaneous cerebrospinal fluid reservoir. *New England Journal of Medicine,* 1968, 279, 1025–1031. Copyright © 1968 by the *New England Journal of Medicine.* Reprinted by permission.

medication to be injected, is removed. The medication is injected into the reservoir and, once the needle is removed, the domed reservoir is manually compressed and released to mix the medication with the cerebrospinal fluid (Brown 1987). This procedure is usually performed by a physican using strict aseptic technique.

Intra-arterial infusions treat an isolated organ or inoperable tumor. The chemotherapy agents are administered through a catheter inserted into an artery usually in the liver, head, neck, or brain. The celiac artery is used to treat the liver, the external carotid artery for the head and neck area, and the internal carotid artery for brain tumors (Johnston and Pratt 1981). The catheters are inserted into the artery surgically with general anesthesia or using angiographic catheterization and a local anesthetic. The catheters are then connected to either an implanted or portable pump. There are two implantable pumps currently being used: the Infusaid pump (Shiley Infusaid Inc, Norwood, MA), and the Medtronic pump (Medtronic, Minneapolis). The Auto-syringe pump (Baxter Health Care Corp, Auto-syringe Division, Hooksett, NH), (see figure 7.2) is an example of a portable system used for intra-arterial infusions. (These pumps will be described in more detail later in this section).

Intracavitary administration is a broad term used to describe the administration of chemotherapy directly into a body cavity. This is commonly done to treat malignant effusions or microscopic localized disease in the bladder, peritoneum, or pleura. The chemotherapy is infused via a catheter, placed directly into one of these areas. The drugs remain in the area for a specific amount of time, then may or may not be drained out via the same catheter. Either an *external catheter,* such as the Tenckhoff catheter (Cobe Laboratory, Lakewood, CO) (see figure 7.3), or a *subcutaneous intravenous port,* such as the Port-A-Cath (Pharmacia Nu Tech, Piscataway, NJ) (see figure 7.4) is used in intraperitoneal chemotherapy. Foley catheters are used for bladder instillations, while a chest tube is used for treating the pleura.

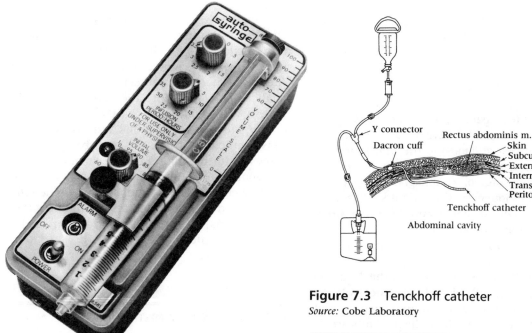

Figure 7.2 Portable infusion pump
Source: From Auto-Syringe, Inc. Reprinted by permission.

Figure 7.3 Tenckhoff catheter
Source: Cobe Laboratory

Three other modes of drug administration are used less frequently:

subcutaneous
intramuscular
topical

Many of the antineoplastic agents are irritating or damaging to body tissue, so it is inadvisable to give a subcutaneous or intramuscular injection of these agents. Some drugs that can be given by the subcutaneous route are cytosine arabinoside (ARA-C) and the interferons, while bleomycin and methotrexate can be given intramuscularly. L-asparaginase is one drug that may be given either by the subcutaneous or intramuscular route. Topical administration has limited usefulness with only mechlorethamine and 5-fluorouracil cream having this method as one

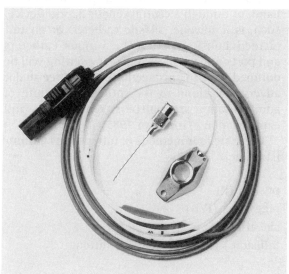

Figure 7.4 Port-A-Cath
Source: Pharmacia Deltec.

of their routes of administration, (Dorr and Fritz 1980). Occasionally, a specific protocol or drug may be administered using one of these methods.

The last two routes of chemotherapy administration are the most common:

oral
intravenous

The *oral* route is usually preferred but absorption can be unpredictable. Several factors must be considered before choosing the oral route: patency and functioning of the GI tract, presence of nausea, vomiting, or dysphagia, the patient's state of consciousness, the patient's willingness to comply to the schedule, and the availablity of the medication in oral form.

The *intravenous* (IV) route of administration is the most common method used to deliver chemotherapy. It allows absorption of the drug thus providing predictable blood levels (Brown 1987). Intravenous drugs may be administered through a peripheral access, a vein in the patient's arm or hand, or through a central venous access device, such as a silicone, silastic catheter, or an implanted infusion port. (The various catheters and ports utilized in the oncology setting will be outlined later in this section). The three major adverse reactions to the intravenous route of administration are: phlebitis, venous flare, and extravasation (Troutman 1985).

There are four methods of intravenous administration:

push (IVP)
piggyback (IVB)
sidearm
infusion, continuous or intermittent

Intravenous *push* refers to directly administering the medication into the intravenous cannula, through either an angiocath or a butterfly needle. A *piggyback* method denotes there is a main line of intravenous fluid connected into the intravenous cannula. The solution to be piggybacked is connected, usually in the port closest to the patient, into the main intravenous line. The *side-arm* method of administration is the route of choice for chemotherapy with vesicant properties. Again, a main line of intravenous fluid, freely flowing, is connected into the intravenous cannula. The nurse directly administers the medication, slowly, into the port closest to the patient while continually assessing the peripheral IV site for complications and extravasation. This method, as could the piggyback method, allows for further dilution of the chemotherapeutic agent with the main fluid. The two solutions *must* be compatible (see appendix 4). The *infusion* method may last from several minutes (bolus infusions) to several days, 24 hours a day (continuous infusions).

INTRAVENOUS ADMINISTRATION

With the intravenous route of chemotherapy being the most common route, the nurse must be knowledgeable and skilled in IV therapy (Crudi and Larken 1984). IV therapy proficiency must include such basics as: knowledge of the usual venous patterns (see figures 7.5 and 7.6), criteria for vein selection, and actual venipuncture skills.

Vein Selection

Selecting the best available vein is essential for patient comfort, ease of drug delivery, and prevention of extravasation (see table 7.1):

1. Always use veins in a distal location, moving proximal with each venipuncture.
2. Look for veins that are smooth and pliable, not inflamed, sclerosed, phlebitic, or bruised. Avoid areas with decreased circulation, impaired lymphatic drainage, and the veins in the legs and feet.

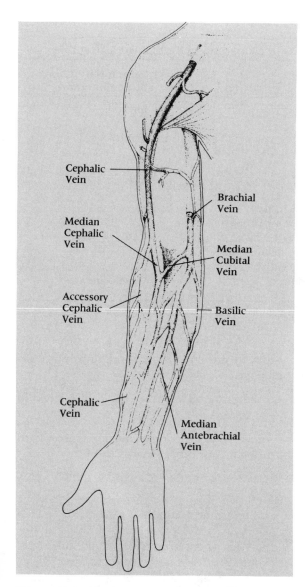

Figure 7.5 Venipuncture sites on the arm
Reprinted with permission, Bristol Laboratories.

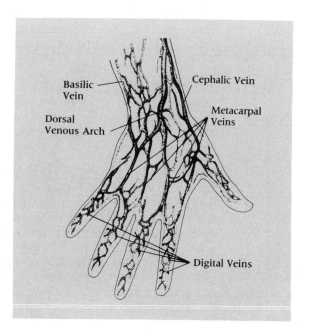

Figure 7.6 Venipuncture sites on the dorsum of the hand
Reprinted with permission, Bristol Laboratories.

Intravenous Therapy Techniques

The choice of an angiocath or a butterfly needle must be based on the individual patient, the goal of the therapy, the length of time the needle is required to be in place, the risk of vein perforation with the steel cannula of a butterfly needle, and the type of therapy to be given (Knobf 1982). The size of the needle to be used is a result of the same factors as choosing the type of needle (see figure 7.7). Usually a 21-gauge needle is acceptable for most intravenous therapies. Large-bore needles, 18 or 19 gauge, are usually required for blood transfusions and viscous fluids. Small-bore needles, 23 and 25 gauge, are used in patients with small fragile veins and for IV fluids of short duration (Knobf 1982). The selection is not this simple though. Controversy exists within the oncology nursing community as to whether larger gauge needles are, or are not, better than smaller gauge needles for chemotherapy admin-

3. The size and anatomical location of the appropriate vein is a function of the chemotherapy agent to be used and the length of the infusion.

Table 7.1 Selecting a Vein

Assess veins in both arms and hands. Do not use veins in compromised limbs/lower extremities.

	Criteria for Vein Selection	Appropriate Choice of Venipuncture Site
Most Desirable	IDEAL VEIN/BEST LOCATION large, soft resilient veins in forearm, hand	forearm
	IDEAL VEIN/UNDESIRABLE LOCATION large, soft, resilient veins in hand/antecubital fossa; small, thin veins in forearm	hand
	SATISFACTORY VEIN/BEST LOCATION small, thin veins in forearm/hand	forearm
	SATISFACTORY VEIN/UNDESIRABLE LOCATION small thin veins in hand; veins in forearm not palpable or visible	hand
	UNSATISFACTORY VEIN/UNDESIRABLE LOCATION small, fragile veins, which easily rupture, in hand/forearm	Consider central venous line*
Least	UNSATISFACTORY VEIN/UNDESIRABLE LOCATION veins in forearm/hand not palpable or visible	Consider central venous line*

*In some situations, central venous lines are inserted before the patient is started on a chemotherapy protocol.
Source: Hughes 1986, 37.

istration. Briefly, many believe large gauge needles provide a more rapid access to the general circulation, thus decreasing the potential of vein irritation. Small gauge needles are believed to be less likely to cause vein perforation and scar tissue, while providing an increase in blood circulation and thus better drug dilution during administration. Controversial issues of chemotherapy administration will be discussed in more detail later in this chapter.

Once the vein has been selected, and venipuncture has been performed, it is important to perserve the vein's integrity. Because chemotherapy treatments may go on for months, if not years, it is important to take care of the existing veins in order to prolong their quality for use later. There are a few steps that can be taken to preserve venous integrity:

- Prevent infections with the use of institutional skin preparation and dressing procedures.
- Flush the IV line with normal saline before each medication, after each medication in a combination, and after the last medication, in

order to prevent drug mixing and thus vein damage.

- Securely tape all junctures and tubing to avoid local trauma.
- Protect IV lines and needle placement with arm boards or other devices.
- Preserve the number of available quality veins by:
  —Using veins sparingly
  —Doing all available laboratory work by fingerstick or drawing bloods at the time IV is started (i.e., a single venipuncture)
  —Using veins sequentially, starting distally (near the hand) and proceeding proximally (toward the elbow) (Lokich 1978) with each venipuncture

Once it is appropriate to administer the chemotherapy drugs, the procedure in table 7.2 is recommended by the Oncology Nursing Society Cancer Chemotherapy Guidelines, for establishing a new intravenous line.

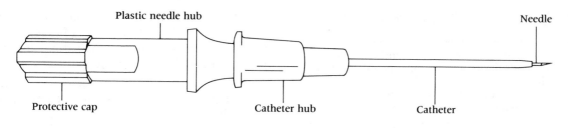

Over-the-needle catheter
(ONC) (Angiocath)

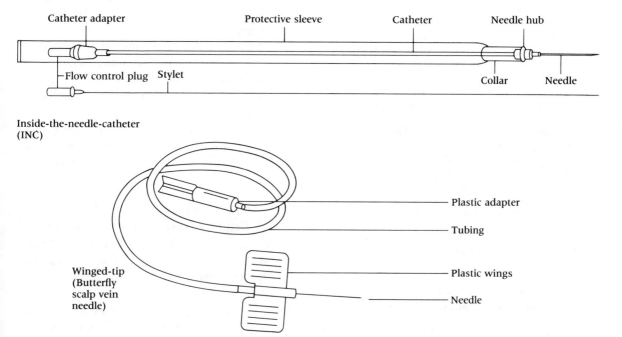

Figure 7.7   A comparison of the major types of IV cannulae used in administering IV chemotherapy.

Table 7.2 Establishing a New Intravenous Line

I. Examine the patient's veins and elicit the patient's desire in selecting a peripheral access site.
  A. Proceed distally (from the hand) to proximally (toward the forearm).
  B. Avoid limbs with compromised circulation, impaired lymphatic drainage (e.g., the side of a prior mastectomy with lymph node dissection), phlebitis, invading neoplasms, hematomas, inflamed or sclerosing areas, the lower extremities and feet (due to an increased risk of phlebitis), and sites distal to a recent venipuncture.
  C. When administering vesicant drugs, avoid using existing peripheral lines and sites of joint flexion for establishing new lines (e.g., antecubital fossa, wrist.)
  D. Alternate arms whenever possible.
  E. Use heat or ask the patient to pump a fist to distend veins.

II. Select appropriate equipment depending upon the venous access route and the method of administration to be used.

III. Exercise safety during venipuncture, drug handling, and administration according to the established policies and procedures of the institution (i.e., wash hands, wear protective clothing, gloves).

IV. Perform venipuncture according to institutional policies and procedures. Figure 7.8 is a pictoral demonstration of venipuncture and administration of chemotherapy by the direct IV push and side-arm methods (Goodman 1986).

Source: Oncology Nursing Society 1988

Dealing with the "Veinless" Patient

One of the most common dilemmas facing oncology nurses is trying to administer chemotherapy to the "veinless" patient (described by Lokich 1978). With the variety of central venous access devices, both catheters and subcutaneous ports, this issue doesn't have to be a problem. There is still that patient that refuses to have another surgical procedure until it is absolutely necessary, even if the benefits dramatically outweigh the risks. The following list of suggestions may prove benefical, to both the patient and the nurse, in ease of venipuncture.

1. The patient should assume a comfortable position.

2. The patient may be anxious about the procedure, so provide explanations of the actions to be taken, emotional support, and relaxation techniques to decrease his or her anxiety.

3. Have the patient exercise his or her hands with a sponge rubber ball daily in between treatments, to develop the veins.

4. Assess both arms before selecting the best vein.

5. Visualize the standard venous patterns (see figures 7.5 and 7.6). Assess the veins by palpation.

6. In an attempt to dilate the veins, apply moist heat to the arms for 5–10 minutes (Johnston-Early, Cohen, and White 1981).

7. Once the soaks are removed, work efficiently while the veins are dilated.

8. Local vein manipulation may also aid dilation:
   a) Appropriate use of a tourniquet or blood pressure cuff to encourage pooling of venous blood
   b) "Milking" the veins from proximal to distal (elbow to hand)
   c) Gently striking the surface of the vein

9. Catheter selection is very important in this setting. The veins may well be small and an appropriately sized needle will decrease trauma.

10. Perform the actual techniques and preparation for venipuncture according to the institution's policies and procedures.

11. After two unsuccessful attempts at the venipuncture, it is sensible to request the assistance of a colleague (Knobf 1982).

12. Patient and family education regarding the benefits and risks of the various central venous access devices could be helpful.

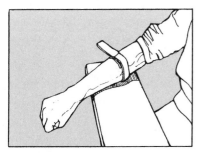

A. Apply tourniquet to mid-forearm, palpate radial pulse and loosen tourniquet if pulse cannot be felt. Have patient open and close fist for venous distention.

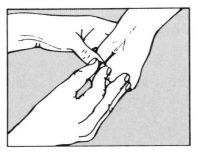

B. Cleanse injection area and hold patient's hand, using thumb to keep skin taut and anchor vein. Place needle in line with vein, bevel up, about one-half inch below proposed entry site.

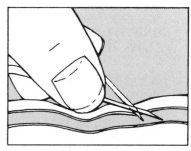

C. Insert needle through skin and tissue at 45° angle, relocate vein, decrease needle angle slightly and slowly enter vein with a downward then upward motion.

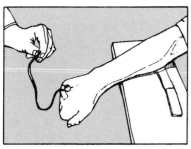

D. Remove touniquet and tape scalp vein tubing.

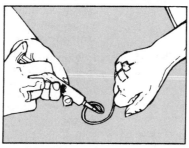

*E. Attach syringe of saline, aspirate to remove air and irrigate.

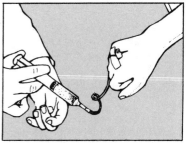

*F. Remove saline syringe, attach chemotherapy syringe and inject slowly, checking for blood return and swelling.

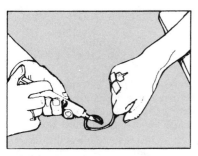

G. Flush catheter with saline solution.

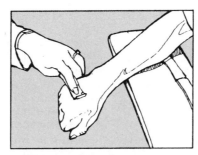

H. Remove needle, apply pressure to prevent bleeding and apply Band-Aid.

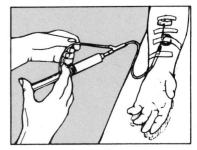

I. If administering agent via sidearm of continuously running IV, establish intravenous access and freely dripping fluid. Cleanse sidearm, insert needle of chemotherapy syringe and administer drug, maintaining even pressure.

Figure 7.8 Venipuncture and administration of chemotherapeutic drugs
*E and F demonstrate the two-syringe technique.
Reprinted with permission, Bristol Laboratories.

CONTROVERSIAL ISSUES IN CHEMOTHERAPY ADMINISTRATION

The Oncology Nursing Society has established guidelines for chemotherapy administration, but recognizes there are some issues that are not easily resolved, e.g., the issue of the antecubital fossa being a reasonable vein to use in chemotherapy administration (see table 7.3). The authors of this book are also aware of these controversies. Like the ONS, our goal in this

Table 7.3 Controversial Issues in Chemotherapy Administration

Issue	Solution	Rationale
Administration site	Use antecubital fossa	Larger veins permit more rapid infusion and administration of drugs Larger veins permit more rapid circulation of potentially irritating drugs
	Avoid antecubital fossa	Mobility of arm restricted Risk of extravasation increased due to patient mobility Early infiltration and extravasation difficult to assess due to subcutaneous tissue Repair of infiltration would be difficult and debilitating for the patient
Needle size	Larger gauge (#19–21 scalp vein needles)	Potentially irritating drugs reach circulation sooner, with less irritation to peripheral veins Decreases administration time
	Small gauge (#23–25)	Smaller gauge needles less likely to puncture wall of vein; less scar tissue at insertion site; and less pain on insertion Increased blood flow around needle increases dilution of the drug Reduced incidence of mechanical phlebitis Slower infusion rate—may reduce side effects, i.e., nausea and vomiting
Sequencing of medications	Administer vesicant first	Vascular integrity decreases over time, i.e., more stable and less irritated at the beginning of treatment Initial assessment of vein patency is most accurate Irritating agents may cause venous spasm and pain
	Administer vesicant last	Vesicants are irritating, may increase vein fragility, and cause spasm at onset of drug administration. The nurse must assess whether the spasm and complaint of pain is an infiltrate or not.
Particular intravenous method of administration	Use sidearm method	Freely running intravenous lines allow for dilution of drugs Can readily stop drug administration while maintaining venous access
	Use direct IV push method	Integrity of the vein can be more easily assessed Extravasation can be noted earlier

Adapted from ONS Module II 1987, 11–12 and 1984, 13.

section is to acknowledge the issues and present the information, thus allowing the readers and their institutions to decide the best method of handling these concerns. Unfortunately, review of the literature does not provide helpful answers.

DOSE CALCULATIONS AND MODIFICATIONS

Dosages of chemotherapeutic agents vary widely. *The standard dosage will vary from the current clinical trial dosage. It is very important to know the usual dosage of each chemotherapy agent and to question any dose that seems incorrect.* The

physician must assess the following areas before prescribing the patient's chemotherapy dosage:

1. Age
2. Nutritional status
3. Any prior chemotherapy or radiation therapy
4. Current blood counts, both hematologic and chemistry profiles
5. Bone marrow reserve
6. Renal and hepatic function
7. Performance status (see table 7.4)
8. Expected drug tolerance

Individual dosages take into consideration the above factors and are based on the patient's body surface area (m^2) which is calculated from his or

Table 7.4 Karnofsky Performance Status Scale

Condition	Percentage	Comments
Able to carry on normal activity and to work. No special care is needed.	100	Normal; no complaints; no evidence of disease
	90	Able to carry on normal activity; minor signs or symptoms of disease
	80	Normal activity with effort; some signs or symptoms of disease
Unable to work. Able to live at home, care for most personal needs. A varying degree of assistance is needed.	70	Cares for self; unable to carry on normal activity or to do active work
	60	Requires occasional assistance but is able to care for most needs
	50	Requires considerable assistance and frequent medical care
Unable to care for self. Requires equivalent of institutional or hospital care. Disease may be progressing rapidly.	40	Disabled; requires special care and assistance
	30	Severely disabled; hosptalization is indicated, although death is not imminent
	20	Hospitalization is necessary; very sick; active supportive treatment necessary
	10	Moribund; fatal processes progressing rapidly
	0	Dead

Source: Karnofsky DA, Burchenol JH 1949; Groenwald 1990.

her height and weight (see figure 7.9). The body surface area is the point of intersection on the middle scale when a straight line joins the height and weight scale. For example, patient A's weight is 109 kg and height is 161 cm. The patient's BSA (m^2) is 2.1.

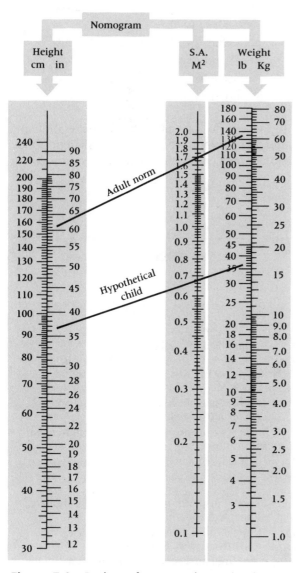

Figure 7.9   Body surface area determination

Source: R.E. Behrman and V.C. Vaughn, eds., *Nelson Textbook of Pediatrics,* 12th ed. (Philadelphia: W.B. Saunders, 1983).

Dose modifications may be made in a situation of renal or hepatic impairment or persistent bone marrow depression. Many issues must be weighed by the physician when considering a dose modification. These include:

- Goal of therapy: cure, control, or palliation. In the setting of cure, drugs must be tolerated in order to maximize possibilities of cure.

- Issues related to routes of metabolism, excretion, and any potential interference by drug interactions.

- Desired antitumor effects: still achievable with a dose modification versus delaying therapy for a short period of time but maintaining maximal doses. (Though a rest period is required for normal body cells to recover from the effects of chemotherapy, it must be noted that the cancer cells still living are also able to replicate during this period.)

- Overall, the benefits and risks to the patient must be considered.

Unfortunately this is not always an easy responsiblity for the physician. Only a few chemotherapeutic agents have established guidelines for dose modifications: those are doxorubicin (Adriamycin), daunorubicin, cisplatin, and methotrexate (Lasley and Ignoffo 1981). There is a fine line between prescribing too little medication and prescribing too much with intolerable side effects.

DRUG INTERACTIONS

There are numerous medications being utilized today within the oncology setting. Various agents are being used to: treat the cancer; control pain, nausea and vomiting, and infections; and correct electrolyte imbalances. Because the median age for developing most cancers is in the sixth decade (Peters 1987), many patients are also taking other medications for concomitant medical problems, as well as self-prescribing over-the-counter medications for numerous reasons. With so many different drugs potentially being used in the same person, it would be reasonable to expect a drug interaction. This interaction could be of benefit, it could worsen the toxicities, or decrease the drugs' effectiveness. Some interactions are quite noticeable, i.e., drug precipitations in IV tubing, but reactions inside the body may not be "seen" at all. An interaction may be noted because of the resultant change but the reaction itself is not obvious. According to Dorr and Fritz (1980) "pharmacologic interactions occur that are manifested by increasing or decreasing efficacy or toxicity by additive and synergistic effects or antagonism." It is important for the nurse and physician to know the potential drug interactions with each medication they are providing. As a rule of thumb, chemotherapy agents should *not* be mixed with any intravenous additive (e.g., heparin, potassium, etc.). Only plain solutions (e.g., 5% Dextrose in Water, Sodium Chloride) should be used as main line infusions for the sidearm and piggyback methods of administration. When a combination of drugs are being administered, normal saline should be used to flush the intravenous line before the medications, in between each medication, and after the last medication is given. When there is a doubt as to whether the medications are compatible, it is safest to assume they are not compatible unless there is information to show otherwise. Reference books and a pharmacist experienced with chemotherapy agents are the best source of information.

DRUG DELIVERY SYSTEMS

One of the fastest growing areas in the oncology setting today is the area of drug delivery systems—catheters, implantable ports, and infusion pumps. By the time this book is published, numerous new products will be available that were only a thought at the time the authors were formulating this section. The tables throughout this section will be useful as basic comparison guides only. They will not provide the practitioner or an institution with the ultimate data needed to decide what products to use in their setting.

Previously, a venous access device was only indicated when the patient had unsatisfactory veins for further cancer therapy. Now there are several indications for early placement of a venous access device (Simon 1987). Patients needing prolonged or extensive intravenous therapies: blood products, antibiotics, and chemotherapy, such as patients with leukemia, usually benefit from venous access devices. Patients receiving continuous infusions of chemotherapy, nutritional supplements, or antibiotics either at home or in the hospital are also ideal candidates for such devices. And of course, devices are still recommended in patients with unsatisfactory venous access.

Two central venous access devices will be discussed in this section: silastic right atrial catheters and implantable venous access ports (VAP).

Silastic Catheters

The Broviac silastic catheter (Davol Inc., Cranston, R.I.) was first reported in 1973. It was a small-bore, 18-gauge catheter that was originally described as being safe for infusing Total Parenteral Nutrition (TPN) on a long-term basis (Simon 1987). In 1979, the larger bored, 16-gauge Hickman catheter (Davol Inc., Cranston, R.I.) was reported to be safe for intravenous infusions including blood transfusions and blood samples (Simon 1987). The Hickman–Broviac catheters became the front runners for not only a type of central venous access device but also for a surgical technique of inserting such catheters. The Hickman-Broviac technique for catheter insertion was designed to reduce an undesirable complication in the long-term use of these catheters: infection (Raaf 1985). Under local anesthesia, two incisions are made. The first for the entry of the catheter tip into the vein and, once the end of the catheter is tunneled into position, a second incision is made for the exit of the catheter from the skin (see figure 7.10). The catheter is inserted into the cephalic, internal, or external jugular veins with the tip resting in either the right atrium or the superior vena cava (Lawson and Finley 1988). Before the catheter is used, its placement must be checked by chest X ray or

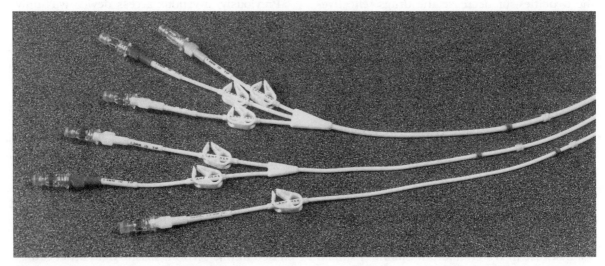

a)

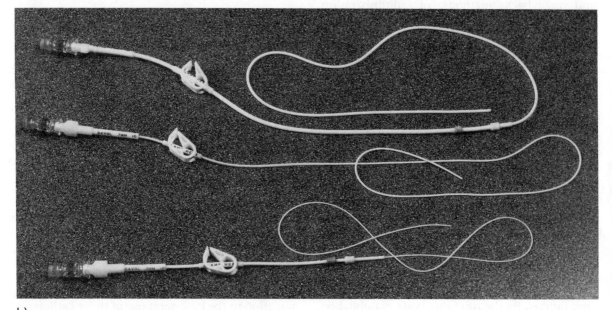

b)

Figure 7.10   a) The Hickman® catheter; b) The Broviac® catheter

fluoroscopy. Some institutions require the placement to be checked before every cycle of chemotherapy.

The only way to access the central venous system was to use an "inside-the-needle" subclavian intravenous catheter (see figure 7.7). There are two main advantages the silastic catheters have over these conventional subclavian lines: 1) the silastic material itself is more flexible and less irritating than the subclavian sheath, and 2) the insertion procedure of "tunneling" helps to decrease the incidence of infection (Simon 1987). Currently there are many silastic catheter companies that utilize the Hickman-Broviac style of insertion, but the characteristics of the individual catheters are somewhat different (see table 7.5). The number and size of the lumens vary from one product to another. The single-lumen catheters are still available, but now there are also double- and triple-lumen catheters with a larger lumen for blood products, a second lumen for intravenous infusions, and perhaps a third lumen for TPN (Simon 1987). A somewhat unique catheter, the Groshong catheter (Catheter Technology Corp., Salt Lake City, Utah), utilizes a two-way valve within the lumen to eliminate the need of daily heparin flushes, to minimize blood backflow problems, and to reduce the risk of air embolism (Catheter Technology 1988) (see figure 7.11).

Care of silastic catheters varies from institution to institution and from product to product. Usually the following care is required to maintain the catheters in good working order:

- Daily heparin flushes through the injection cap
- Changing the injection cap weekly or as indicated by the type and the number of punctures the cap has sustained
- Periodic dressing changes include cleansing the exit site
- Precautions are usually required before showering or bathing

- Consult the physician before swimming, especially in an open lake, pond, or ocean due to risk of infection

---

Implantable Venous Access Ports (VAPs)

Venous access ports (VAPs) consist of two main features: the port housing made of either plastic, stainless steel, or titanium with the resealable silicone septum, and the silastic catheter which is either preattached to the housing or comes as a separate piece needing attachment during the insertion procedure. The insertion procedure is similar to that of the silastic atrial catheters. Under local anesthesia, a pocket is made to house the port. A "tunnel" is made under the skin toward the collarbone for the catheter. The catheter is inserted into the subclavian or internal jugular vein (Lawson and Finley 1988). Both the port and the catheter are sutured into place, including closing the pocket containing the port. Once this is completed, the VAP is completely under the skin. Generally the port looks like a small bump, mostly unnoticeable except to palpation (Wainstock 1987). A dressing may be used initially until the site is completely healed. Placement of the VAP must be verified by chest X ray or fluoroscopy before it is used. As with the silastic catheters, some institutions require placement to be checked before every cycle of chemotherapy.

The port is accessed only by a needle puncture through the skin into the silicone septum. Initially the site may be bruised, swollen, and sore so care should be taken with access. Some institutions apply a local anesthestic such as topical lidocaine to the skin over the septum to decrease the pain of the needle puncturing the skin. A special needle, such as the Huber needle (Vita Needle, Needham, MA), with an offset bevel to prevent coring of the silicone is required for all insertions. These needles are either straight or with a 90° angle and come in a variety of gauges. The 90° angled needles are used mostly for long infusions to allow the needle

Table 7.5 Characteristics of Selected Silicone Silastic Atrial Catheters*

Right Atrial Catheters (Manufacturers)	Features/Internal Diameter	Uses	Maintenance Outpatient Routine Care
Hickman (Davol)	Single/double/triple lumens: 1.6 mm, 1.3 mm Pediatric: 0.7 mm	Blood drawing/administration Total parenteral nutrition Fluids, antibiotics Chemotherapy Double lumen when vascular access is needed frequently for multiple infusates Leukemic Bone marrow recipient Outpatient infusion of chemotherapy and total parenteral nutrition	Irrigation QOD with 3 mL of heparin/saline solution (10–100 units of heparin/mL) Brisk irrigations may help prevent outflow obstruction Routine clamping is not recommended Clamp over protective covering when clamping catheter Dressing changes every other day up until 2-3 weeks after insertion, then dressing is not necessary; apply Band-Aid to exit site Prevent undue tension on the catheter Catheter is taped to the person at all times Change cap(s) every 7 days Showering/bathing is permitted
Broviac (Davol)	Single lumen: 1.0 mm Pediatric: 0.7 mm, 0.5 mm	Broviac is used more for total parenteral nutrition than for blood drawing	Same as above
Chemocath Silastic (HDC)	1.0 mm, 1.6 mm Pediatric: 0.8 mm Single/double lumen		Same as above
Hemed Silicone (Gish)	0.6 mm, 1.0 mm, 1.6 mm Single/doule lumen		Same as above
Quinton Silastic	1.5 mm, 1.0 mm, 0.75 mm		Same as above
Raaf catheter (Quinton)	1.1 or 1.5 each Single/double/triple lumen		Same as above
Groshong (catheter) technology	1.33, 1.1 mm Single/double/triple lumen		• Never clamp the catheter • Requires no heparinization • Pressure-sensitive valve remains closed when not in use • Irrigate briskly with 5 mL of normal saline solution once every 7 days or after use • Irrigate with 20 mL saline solution following blood aspiration or transfusion of blood component • Do not use needle through injection cap

*Catheters are radiopaque or contain a radiopaque strip to visualize on x-ray. All have repair kit and patient-teaching material available.
Source: Adapted from Goodman MS, Wickham R: Venous access devices. *Oncol Nurs Forum* 11(6):25–30, 1984.

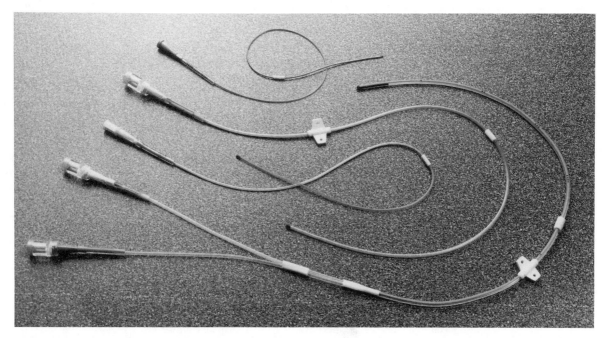

Figure 7.11 The Groshong™ catheter

to be secured and a dressing applied to the access site. One problem with VAP is that the septum can only be punctured 1000–2000 times with a 19-gauge noncoring needle before the port (although not the catheter) has to be changed. The actual procedure for accessing a VAP must be developed in the individual institution and will not be discussed here.

Venous access ports originally came as a single port system (see table 7.6). Due to competition from the double- and triple-lumen silastic catheters, now VAPs are also available as double ports. The double VAPs have one main housing unit with two separate silicone septums and one catheter with two lumens. Most of the double venous access ports have the septums on the surface of the housing. A somewhat unique port, the S.E.A.-Port (Harbor Medical Devices Inc., Boston, MA) is currently under investigation. The S.E.A.-Port differs from the other double venous access ports in that it has a septum on each side of the port housing (see figure 7.12), and its catheter contains two equally large lumens (Harbor Medical

Devices 1988). The S.E.A.-Port also utilizes its own special needles for access, not the Huber needles. The PAS Port system (Pharmacia Nu Tech, Piscataway, NJ) (see figure 7.13) is another development in vascular access ports. It allows ports to be placed peripherally.

The VAPs are considered to have an advantage over silastic catheters in patients who are unable to care for a silastic catheter, who are allergic to tape, or who do not want a noticeable alteration in body image, yet still need long-term venous access (Lawson and Finley 1988). In addition to being used for venous access, the implantable ports can be inserted in an artery, the peritoneum, or the pericardial or pleural cavity for intra-arterial and intracavitary administration of chemotherapy (Hagle 1987).

Care of a VAP is minimal. The ports need to be flushed with heparin after each use or every 3–4 weeks when not in use. Once all incisions are healed, there should be no restrictions on activities including showering, bathing, and swimming. The initial cost of a VAP is greater than the

Table 7.6 Characteristics of Selected Implanted Infusion Ports

Implanted	Reservoir Body	Septum	Catheter	Maintenance
Mediport Mediport II (Davol, Inc.)	Stainless steel Height: 14.2 mm Contoured body Base diameter: 36.6 mm Weight 15 g	Silicone Diameter 11 mm Depth 7.7 mm 1000 punctures 2000 punctures with 22-gauge needles	ID 1.6 mm (arterial) OD 3.0 mm ID 1.0 mm (venous) OD 2.23 mm Radio-opaque Permanently attached	Puncture with Huber point needle only Irrigate every 4 weeks with heparin/saline solution 3–5 cc 100u heparin/mL 20cc normal saline
Mediport DL	Height 14 mm Base diameter: 35.5(w) × 66 mm(l)	Diameter 11 mm As above	OD 4.0 mm ID 2 × 1.5 mm As above	flush following blood drawing For arterial ports irrigate once a week with 3–5 cc 100u heparin/mL Flush catheter after each use No restrictions on the patient because the port is entirely implanted
Infuse-A-Port (Shiley Infusaid Corp.)	Polyethersulfane plastic Contoured body No metal Weight 12.1 g	Rubber septum 2000 punctures (22-gauge needles)	Radio-opaque Preattached or detached system Snap lock fitting ID 0.6 mm (arterial) OD 2.3 mm ID 1.6 mm (venous) OD 2.5 mm	Same as above Use Infusaid needles only
Macroport	Height 12.1 mm Base diameter 38 mm	Diameter 13 mm		
Microport	Height 14 mm Base diameter 30 mm	Diameter 8 mm		
Button port	Height 11 m Base diameter 24 mm	Diameter 9 mm		
Dual Macroport	Height 13 mm Base diameter 33 × 52 mm	Diameter 13 mm		
Port-a-Cath (Pharmacia Nu Tech Inc.)	Stainless steel or titanium body Weight 16–26 g (titanium-stainless steel) Height 13 mm Base diameter 25 mm	Silicone Diameter 11 mm Depth 11.5 mm 2000 punctures (22-gauge needles) 1000 punctures (19-gauge needles)	Silicone or polyurethane Detachable catheter with metal sleeve ID 0.8 mm (arterial) OD 2.3 mm ID 1.3 mm (venous) OD 2.8 mm	Same as above Use Huber needles
Port-A-Cath DL	Base diameter 46 mm		ID 1.4 mm × 2 OD 3.9 mm	
Port-A-Cath Low Profile	Height 10 mm		ID 0.8 mm OD 2.3 mm	

Table 7.6   *(continued)*

Implanted	Reservoir Body	Septum	Catheter	Maintenance
S.E.A.-Port (Harbor Medical Devices, Inc.)	Titanium body Weight 17 g Height 12 mm Base diameter 33 mm	Two rectangular-shaped septa on each side of port Depth 5.1 mm Length 19.1 mm Height 7.1 mm 2000 puctures (19-gauge needle) Silicone	Polyurethane catheter ID 1.42 mm (venous) OD 3.0 mm Modular system with S.E.A.-Lock fitting Radio-opaque	Same as above Use S.E.A.-Port infusion needles with 90° angle only
Groshong Port (Catheter Technology Corp)	Titanium body Weight 9.2 g Height 14.4 mm Base diameter 28.6 mm Rounded contours	Silicone Depth 9.0 mm Diameter 13 mm Minimum 2800 punctures (22-gauge needle) 1500 punctures (19-gauge needle)	Silicone Radio-opaque Modular system with "locking sleeve" mechanism ID 1.52 mm (venous) OD 2.54 mm Groshong two-way valve	Same as above except: 1. In between usage, flush with 10 cc normal saline every 4 weeks 2. Use Huber-like needles 3. 20 cc normal saline flush after medications, TPN, and blood drawing
Q-Port (Davol, Inc.)	Stainless steel Height 12.2 mm Weight 28.8 g Base diameter 31.8 mm Contoured shape	Silicone Diameter 12.7 mm Depth 6.4 mm 2000 punctures (22-gauge needle) 1000 punctures (20/19-gauge needle)	Silicone Radio-opaque ID 3.2 mm (venous) OD 1.5 mm Preattached or detached system (with "bayonet locking ring") Q-Port needle guard to protect catheter	Same as first port listed
Hickman Port (Davol, Inc.)	Titanium or stainless steel Height 14 mm Weight 16–24 g (titanium-stainless steel) Base diameter 31.7 mm	Silicone Diameter 12.7 mm Depth 6.4 mm 2000 punctures (22-gauge needle)	Silicone Radio-opaque Preattached or detached system ID 0.5 mm (arterial) OD 2.0 mm ID 1.6 mm (venous) OD 3.2 mm	Same as first port listed

Note: All ports require usage of noncoring needles to preserve the life of the septum. See individual ports for specific noncoring needle recommendations.
Source: Adapted from Groenwald 1987, 359

silastic catheters, but the care and maintenance costs, including the special needles, are usually minimal (Hagle 1987).

Silastic Catheters Versus Implanted Ports: Choosing the Best System

With each patient considering a venous access device, the benefits and the risks of each system must be fully reviewed. The number of potential systems will be limited by institution and physician preferences. Not all systems are used in every institution. Patients may have heard of a particular system already and developed an opinion on what is best for them. The patient's disease status should be considered in choosing the best type and location for a device (e.g., for a patient with bilateral breast cancer receiving

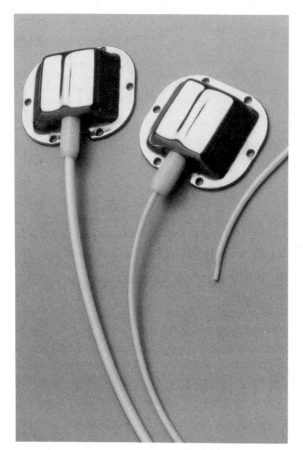

Figure 7.12 The S.E.A.-Port double venous access port

Ambulatory Continuous Infusion Systems

In keeping with the advances in oncology therapy, specialized equipment is required to administer chemotherapy as a continuous infusion, in the home or ambulatory care setting. The continuous infusion method of administration addresses issues of ineffective drug dosing and scheduling, and recent reports suggest this method may substantially affect the therapy results (Mioduszewski and Zarbo 1987). Chemotherapy administered in the home, or at least in an ambulatory setting, increases the patient's comfort with the treatment and decreases the overall cost of the therapy (Garvey 1987). The two types of systems to be discussed in this section are external and implantable pumps.

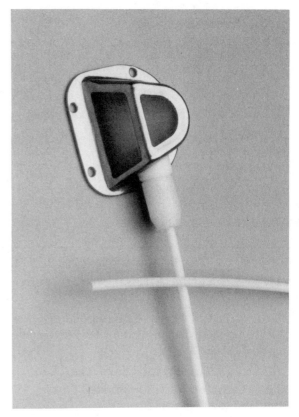

Figure 7.13 The PAS-Port system

adjuvant chemotherapy and radiation therapy the best location of a venous access device may not be on the chest wall; in a leukemic patient, a silastic catheter may be the best choice in light of the extensive chemotherapy, antibiotic coverage, blood support, and risk of infection involved). Other considerations include the type of chemotherapy, the length of the treatments, educational support for the patient and family, the family's ability to provide care for the system at home, and the cost of the system. (See table 7.7 for some general information to help in the comparison of silastic catheters versus implanted ports.)

Table 7.7   General Comparisosn of Venous Access Devices

External Silastic Catheter	Implantable Ports
• May remain inplace as long as trouble-free	• Silicone septum good for 1000–2000 punctures (varies per product and size needle used)
• Technically open system, though catheter closed by injection cap	• Completely closed system
• Barrier against infection: Dacron cuff	• Barrier against infection: skin
• Surgically inserted and removed	• Surgically inserted and removed
• Uses: All intravenous infusions, including transfusions and drawing	• Uses: All intravenous infusions, including blood transfusions and drawing
• Features: Single, double, and triple lumens available	• Features: Single and double lumens available
• Maintenance: Requires daily heparin flushes, regular dressing, and injection cap changes using aseptic techniques. Care is done by the patient or the family. Maintenance costs include heparin, syringes, needles, alcohol, dressing supplies, injection caps, etc.	• Maintenance: Requires heparin flush every 3–4 weeks. Usually done by the nurse. Maintenance cost is minimal
• Appearance: Alteration in body image and physical freedom. Changes are considerable with 4–5 inches of external catheter always present	• Appearance: Usually minimal alteration because the port is totally under the skin. Alteration in body image and physical freedom is limited
• Care must be taken with showering, bathing, and swimming	• No disruption in showering or bathing
• Access: Needle inserted into injection cap at the end of the external catheter. Some clothing displacement during infusions	• Access: Special needle must puncture the skin to access the port. Minimal to significant clothing displacement during infusions depending on site of the port.
• Placement: Can choose exit site for catheter	• Placement: Should be placed over bony prominances to assist in stability during access. Potential areas of placement are limited, especially in overweight patients

• Complications:
  1. Catheter-related infections
  2. Occlusion thrombosis
  3. Infuses, but cannot draw blood (withdrawal occlusion)
  4. Catheter damage, leakage, or dislodgement
  5. Extravasation
  6. Spontaneous blood backflow
	• Complications:
	  1. Port-related infections
	  2. Occlusion thrombosis
	  3. Infuses, but cannot draw blood (withdrawal occlusion)
	  4. Catheter migration
	  5. Extravasation
	  6. Port leakage
	  7. Catheter-needle dislodgement

External Pumps

The external pumps that initially come to mind are the large bulky pumps used in the hospital. With many continuous infusion therapies being delivered in the home or the ambulatory setting, smaller, more practical, external pumps were needed. There are many varieties of these pumps but they fall into three basic designs: 1) the battery-powered syringe-driven pump which moves fluid by the plunger being forced into the syringe barrel, e.g., Autosyringe

(Baxter Health Care Corp., Autosyringe Division, Hooksett, NH); 2) the battery-powered peristaltic pump that moves fluid forward by progressively squeezing the intravenous tubing around a wheel or other pressure point, e.g., CADD pump (Deltec-Pharmacia, Piscataway, NJ) and Pancretec pump (Pancretec Inc., San Diego, CA); and 3) the balloon-powered pump which moves fluid at a constant rate as the balloon deflates, e.g., PCA Infusor (Baxter Health Care Corp., Deerfield, IL) (Mioduszewski and Zarbo 1987). (See table 7.8 for more information on these pumps and others.)

These compact, usually, electronic pumps allow patients to receive intermittent as well as continuous intravenous infusions. They provide the patient with a potentially lower treatment cost as well as control over his or her lifestyle by minimally altering his or her activities during treatment (Brown 1987). All the pumps offer patients unrestricted mobility as they are small, lightweight, and attach to a belt or shoulder holster. A potential disadvantage is that patients must have support in managing these pumps. Family members may be taught the basic functioning of the pump, but on-call medical, nursing, or pharmacy assistance is recommended. Intravenous support services, in the form of either the Visiting Nurse Association, or private community-based companies, are also required for treatment precision and safety and to maintain the central venous access devices, which are frequently used for patient comfort and convenience.

Because there are so many pumps available, a few points must be considered when choosing a system (Lawson and Finley 1988):

- The therapy to be administered
- Length of the proposed therapy
- Drug stability under the proposed conditions
- Issues of infusion capacity, rate, and loading
- Available support services: family or community companies

- Built-in safety features or alarms on the pump
- Issues in cost or reimbursement
- Power source, e.g., battery operated
- The patient's desire for mobility and independence, including issues that may develop due to the size or weight of the pump
- Treatment recommendation for a central venous access device
- Patient and family education in the care of the pump or the central venous access device.

Implantable Pumps

Implantable pumps were first used to deliver continuous infusions of chemotherapy in 1966 (Hagle 1987). The pumps are usually made of titanium with one or two silicone septums and a silastic catheter. The primary septum on the top allows the intravenous solution to be injected into the refillable reservoir, for continuous infusions. A second septum, on the side of the housing, is used for bolus injections. It bypasses the main reservoir thus injected solutions pass directly into the silastic catheter (Hagle 1987).

There are two pumps commonly used in the oncology setting: the Infusaid pumps (Shiley Infusaid Inc., Norwood, MA) and the Medtronic pump (Medtronic Inc., Minneapolis). The Infusaid pumps have a nonreplaceable internal power source, which is recharged every 2–3 weeks when the internal reservoir is refilled with either a chemotherapy drug or heparinized saline. As the internal reservoir is filled it expands to compress the fluorocarbon vapor into a liquid in the outer chamber (see figure 7–14). The drug is forced from the reservoir through the silastic catheter into the artery or vein (Lawson and Finley 1988). The ultimate flow rate is affected by: the drug concentration, the preset length and diameter of the silastic catheter, the pressure at the catheter exit site, and the patient's body temperature (Hagle 1987). Dose modifications may be necessary for extreme changes in the patient's body temperature,

Table 7.8   Ambulatory External Pumps

Name/Model (MFR)	Pumping Mechanism	Drug Reservoir/ Accessories+	Battery	Range of Infusion Rates (mL/hr)	Alarms/ Safety Features*	KVO Rates (mL/hr)	Program Modes	Weight	Dimension
CADD-1 CADD-PLUS (Pharmacia/ Deltec)	Peristaltic	Custom 50- & 100-mL cassettes Remote reservoir adapter	9-V Disposable	0-12.5 0-75	LB; EF; LR; ST; PLO; HP	0-0.9 0-10	Continuous, prime demand Continuous, intermittent prime demand, delay start	15 oz.	1.1" × 6.3" × 3.5" 7.7" × 6.3" × 3.5"
Life Care 1500 (Abbott/Parker)	Volumetric	Custom 60-mL bag; Pumping cassette	2 × 1.5-V lithium	0.1-2.1	LB; AT	none	Continuous, prime	2.5 oz.	2.0" × 3.0" × 0.75"
Autosyringe (Baxter Health Care Corp)	Screw	Most syringes (6-35 mL)	Rechargeable NiCad or AC Line	0.2-88	LR; LF; HF; HP	none	Continuous	19.3 oz.	2.5" × 7.0" × 3.0"
Autosyringe AS30C Infusion Pump (Baxter Health Care Corp)	Peristaltic	Up to 80 mL	9-V Disposable	0.5-9.9	LB; EF	none	Continuous, prime	9.7 oz.	4.0" × 4.4" × 1.5"
Intermedics Model MS-26 (Graseby)	Screw	28-mL in 35-mL syringe	9-V Disposable	0-4.1	LB; LR	none	Prime (bolus), continuous	7.0 oz.	165 × 23 × 53 mm
Corned Liberators (C.R. Bard, Inc)	Peristaltic	Custom 60-mL PVC bag	Rechargeable NiCad	0.17-2.1	none	none	Continuous	17 oz.	3.25" × 5.0" × 1.5"
Corned II (C.R. Bard, Inc)	Peristaltic	Custom 60-mL PVC bag	Rechargeable 5-V NiCad	0.17-2.1	LB; EF; LF; HF	none	Continuous	17 oz.	4.8" × 4.2" × 1.5"
Provider Plus (4000 & 2000) Provider 5000 (Pancretec)	Peristaltic	Separate reservoirs	Rechargeable NiCad Disposable lithium	0.2-200/ 0.2-83 0.1-250	AL; HP; LB; EF; LR; ST; PLO	0-0.2 0-0.1	Continuous, prime, bolus	23 oz. 14 oz.	3.4" × 1.5" × 6.0" 5.2" × 1.3" × 3.4"
PCA Infusor System (Baxter Health Care Corp)	Balloon	60-mL	none	2 or 5	PLO	none	Continuous	30 g	1.5" × 6.0"

Source: Lawson and Finley 1988, 7; Mioduszewski and Zarbo 1987, 106. Reprinted with permission.

+Dependent on model selected

*Abbreviations: AL = air in line; AT = in-line airtrap; EF = electronic fault; HF = high flow; HP = high pressure/occlusion; LB = low battery; LF = low flow; LR = low reservoir; PLO = patient lock-out feature; ST = pump in stop mode

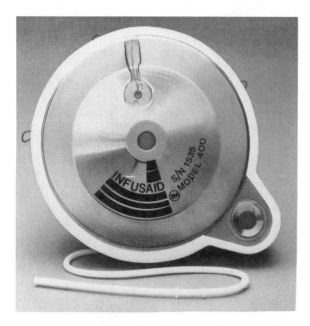

Figure 7.14 The Infusaid pump
Reprinted with permission

Medtronic Synchromed™ Infusion Pump

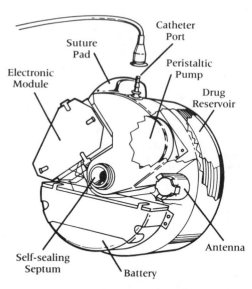

Figure 7.15 The Medtronic pump
Reprinted with permission

(i.e., fever) or for travel to higher altitudes. The only activities patients should refrain from are contact sports, scuba diving, sunbathing, and long, hot baths or saunas (Dangel 1985).

The Medtronic's pump mechanism is slightly different due to its internal lithium battery and computerized electronic microprocessor (see figure 7.15). The battery has an expected life of two years. Unfortunately, to replace it, the entire pump must be removed. The microprocessor regulates the pump. The energy source and flow rates are activated when a hand-held electronic wand transfers signals from the Medtronic desktop computer to the internal microprocessor (Hagle 1987). (For more details on these systems see table 7.9). Shiley Infusaid, Inc. is developing a new pump which combines its fluorocarbon system with a computerized electronic microprocessor. At this time details on this pump are not available as it is in the early stages of investigation.

The treatment most often associated with implantable pumps is intra-arterial infusions of FUDR (floxuridine) to treat primary or metastatic hepatic carcinomas. In addition to the three chemotherapeutic agents (FUDR, 5-fluorouracil, and methotrexate), heparin and morphine have also been administered using the implantable pumps (Hagle 1987). Other uses of these systems include chemotherapy infusions for head and neck cancers, and for CNS disease (Dangel 1985). They have also been used as a central venous access device, utilizing the superior vena cava, for solid and liquid tumors (Brown 1987).

The insertion procedure for these pumps is similar to that for the implanted ports. Through a surgical incision, usually in the abdomen or infraclavicular fossa, a pocket of subcutaneous tissue is made to house the pump (Hagle 1987). The silastic catheter is inserted into the hepatic artery, the subclavian vein, or the superior vena cava. Care must be taken in situating the catheter, so that when accessing the pump the catheter is not accidentally punctured (Hagle 1987).

Table 7.9 Implantable Ports

Name/Model (MFG)	Pumping Mechanism	Drug Reservoir	Battery	Range of Infusion Rates	Alarms/ Safety Features	Program Mode	Weight	Dimensions
Infusaid 100	Self-contained	50 mL hydraulic	none	preset 1.0 and 6.0 mL/d	none	Continuous	187 g	87 × 28 mm
200		35 mL hydraulic		preset 1.0 and 6.0 mL/d	none	Continuous	172 g	87 × 23 mm
400		50 mL hydraulic		preset 1.0 and 6.0 mL/d	none	Continuous	208 g	87 × 28 mm[+]
(Single and Dual Catheters)							249 g (Dual)	94 × 28 mm[+]
Infusaid 500	Self-contained	25 mL hydraulic	none	preset 1.0 and 6.0 mL/d	none	Continuous	165 g	87 × 20 mm
Infusaid 1000 (Investigational Device) (Shiley Infusaid Inc.)	Microprocessor	22 mL hydraulic	yes	programmable 0–0.5 mL/hr	unknown	Continuous bolus, KVO,* Multiple rates	272 g	90.2 × 27 mm
Medtronic 8610H/8611H Microprocessor (Medtronic) (Investigational Device)		18 mL	Lithium	2.0–200 mL/d	LB; LF; PE*	Continuous, bold	185 g	70 × 28 mm

+Excluding sideport
*Abbreviations: KVO = keep vein open; LB = low battery; LF = low fluid; PE = program error
Adapted from: Lawson and Finley 1988, p. 7. Reprinted with permission

Both the pump and the catheter are sutured into place, including closing the pocket containing the pump. Pump placement and flow rate must be checked before the pump is used (Dangel 1985).

Accessing the pumps should be done according to institutional policy and procedure. Aseptic technique must be maintained throughout the procedure. Often at the time of insertion, a small dye marker is placed on the skin above the pump's access port. The Infusaid pumps are accessed with special Huberlike needles, but a 22-gauge needle can be used for the Medtronic pump (Hagle 1987). There are many steps to this procedure and it is beyond the scope of this book to present them here. Resources are available from both Shiley Infusaid, Inc. and Medtronics, Inc. that outline the correct procedures for their equipment.

CONCLUSION

There are many innovative products available to deliver the complex chemotherapeutic protocols of today. Each day it seems there is a new product being introduced that is somehow better than all of the others. Education of the health care staff and the patients is essential. Only staff competent in the product technique should use or teach its use to others. Before a patient is sent home with a particular device, it is important to make sure the community support services are also familiar with it. Product companies and their representatives are probably the best resource available, especially concerning a new product.

BIBLIOGRAPHY

Brown J (1987) Chemotherapy, in Groenwald SL (ed): *Cancer Nursing Principles and Practice*. Boston, Jones and Bartlett

Camp LD (1988) Care of the Groshong catheter. *Oncology Nursing Forum* 15(6): 745–746

Catheter Technology Corportation (1988). *Advanced Performance CV Catheter with Groshong Valve*. Salt Lake City, Catheter Technology Corp

Crudi C, Larken M (1984) Scope of practice, in National Intravenous Therapy Association: *Core Curriculum for Intravenous Nursing*. Philadelphia, JB Lippincott

Dangel RB (1985) How to use an implantable pump. *RN*, Sept: 40–43

Davol Inc (1988) *How to Care for Your Hickman or Broviac Catheter*. Cranston, RI, Davol Inc

Dorr RT, Fritz W (1980) *Cancer Chemotherapy Handbook*. New York, Elsevier

Esparza DM, Weyland JB (1982) Nursing care for the patient with an ommaya reservoir. *Oncology Nursing Forum* 9(4): 17–20

Garvey EC (1987) Current and future nursing issues in the home administration of chemotherapy. *Seminars in Oncology Nursing* 3(2): 142–146

Goodman M (1988) External venous catheters: home management. *Oncology Nursing Forum* 15(3): 357–361

Goodman MS (1986) *Cancer: Chemotherapy and Care*. Evansville, Ind, Bristol Laboratories

Groenwald SL (ed) (1987) *Cancer Nursing Principles and Practice*. Boston, Jones and Bartlett, Inc

Groenwald SL (1990) The clinical evaluation of chemotherapeutic agents in cancer, in Macleod CM (ed): *Evaluation of Chemotherapeutic Agents*. New York, Columbia University Press

Hagle, ME (1987) Implantable devices for chemotherapy: access and delivery. *Seminars in Oncology Nursing* 3(2): 96–104

Harbor Medical Devices (1988) *S.E.A.–Port Implantable Access System Instruction Manual*. Boston, Harbor Medical Devices, Inc

Haskell C (1980) *Cancer Treatment*. Philadelphia, WB Saunders

Hoff ST (1986) Concepts in intraperitoneal chemotherapy. *Seminars in Oncology Nursing* 3(2): 112–117

Hubbard SM, Seipp CA (1982) Administration of cancer treatments: a practical guide for physicians and oncology nurses, in DeVita VJ, Hellmann S, Rosenberg SA (eds): *Cancer Principles and Practice of Oncology*. Philadelphia, JB Lippincott

Hughes CB (1986) Giving cancer drugs IV—some guidelines. *American Journal of Nursing*, January: 34–38

Johnston–Early A, Cohen MH, White KS (1981) Venipuncture and problem veins. *American Journal of Nursing*, September: 1626–1640

Johnston S, Pratt YZ (1981) Caring for the patient on intra-arterial chemotherapy . . . are you ready? *Nursing*, November: 108–112

Karnofsky DA, Burchenal JH (1949) The clinical evaluation of chemotherapeutic agents in cancer, in McLeod CM (ed): *Evaluation of Chemotherapeutic Agents*. New York, Columbia Univ Press, 191–205

Knobf T (1982) Intravenous therapy guidelines for oncology practice. *Oncology Nursing Forum* 9(2): 30–34

Lasley K, Ignoffo R (1981) *Manual of Oncology Therapeutics*. St. Louis, CV Mosby Co

Lawson M, Finley RS (1988) Vascular access and drug administration systems, in Adria Laboratories: *Continuous Infusion and Chemotherapeutic Drugs*. Philadelphia, Miniscus Ltd

Lokich JJ (1978) *Primer of Cancer Management*. Boston, G K Hall Co

Milliam DA (1986) Performing IV procedures like an expert: 10 questions about IV therapy and the revealing answers. *Nursing Life*, Jan/Feb: 33–40

Miller SA (1980) Nursing actions in cancer chemotherapy administration. *Oncology Nuring Forum* 6(4): 8–16

Mioduszewski J, Zarbo AG (1987) Ambulatory infusion pumps: a practical view at an alternative approach. *Seminars in Oncology Nursing* 3(2): 106–111

Oncology Nursing Society (1988) *Cancer Chemotherapy Guidelines Module II. Recommendations for Nursing Practice in the Acute Care Setting*. Pittsburgh, ONS

Oncology Nursing Society (1988) *Cancer Chemotherapy Guidelines Module V. Recommendations for the Management of Extravasation and Anaphylaxis*. Pittsburgh, ONS

Peters PS (1987) Cancer incidence and trends, in Ziegfeld CR (ed): *Core Curriculum for Oncology Nursing*. Philadelphia, WB Saunders

Raaf JH (1985) Results from the use of 826 vascular access devices in cancer patients. *Cancer* 55: 1312–1321

Rahr V (1986) Giving intrathecal drugs. *American Journal of Nursing*, July: 829–831

Ratcheson RA, Ommaya AK (1968) Experience with the subcutaneous cerebrospinal fluid reservoir. *New England Journal of Medicine* 279(19): 1025–1031

Shiley Infusaid (1987) *Your Infusaid Pump. Information for the Patient*. Norwood, Mass, Shiley Infusaid, Inc

Simon RC (1987) Small-gauge central venous catheters and right atrial catheters. *Seminars in Oncology Nursing* 3(2): 86–95

Spross J (ed) (1982) Issues in chemotherapy administration. *Oncology Nursing Forum* 9(1): 50–54

Troutman J (1985) Step-by-step guide to trouble-free IV chemotherapy. *RN*, Sept: 32–34

Tenebaum L (1987) Nursing administration of chemotherapy, in Ziegfeld CR (ed): *Core Curriculum for Oncology Nursing*. Philadelphia, WB Saunders

Wainstock, JM (1987) Making a choice: the vein access method you prefer. *Oncology Nursing Forum* 14(1): 80–82 (Jan/Feb)

Wujcik D (1987) Chemotherapy administration. *Cancer Nursing* 10(1): 53–64

8

THE SAFE HANDLING OF CANCER CHEMOTHERAPEUTIC AGENTS

INTRODUCTION

Practitioners handling antineoplastic agents are exposed to potential health hazards in a variety of settings. Chemotherapy is given in many settings: hospitals, oncology clinics, cancer treatment centers, private oncologists' offices, and in the home. Potential exposure to antineoplastic agents on a regular basis exists through the preparation and handling of these substances and through the handling of the excreta of patients receiving the drugs. Issues regarding the safe handling of antineoplastic drugs have surfaced within the past several years. At present over forty agents have been approved by the Food and Drug Administration (FDA) for the sole purpose of treating neoplastic diseases (Muller 1988). The possible risks of antineoplastic drugs to health professionals have received increasing attention since they were first reported by Falck et al. in 1979. Reports have been cited about the effects of these agents on workers who have prolonged contact with them (Hirst et al. 1984). The health care workers who come into contact with these agents are nurses, pharmacists, physicians, nursing assistants, and housekeeping personnel. The purpose of this chapter is threefold:

- To discuss the actual and potential problems involved with the handling of chemotherapeutic agents
- To understand the action and toxic effects of these agents
- To recognize measures to reduce exposure to such agents

More research needs to be done in the area of occupational safety and the handling of antineoplastic drugs.

TOXICITY OF ANTINEOPLASTIC DRUGS

Since the effect of nitrogen mustard was discovered in the 1940s, many antineoplastic drugs (chemotherapeutic agents) have come into existence. Many of these drugs are known to be mutagenic, teratogenic, and carcinogenic in animals. These terms can be defined as follows:

Mutagenic—able to cause mutations. A mutation is an unusual change in genetic material occurring spontaneously or by induction. The alteration changes the original expression of the gene. Genes are stable units, but when a mutation occurs it is transmitted to future generations.

Teratogenic—able to cause development of abnormal structures in the embryo or fetus if the individual is exposed to that substance during pregnancy.

Carcinogenic—able to cause the development of a cancer (Gullo 1988).

Many antineoplastic drugs were known to be potent toxins prior to their initial therapeutic use in cancer patients. Their toxicity was quite often what prevented dose escalation in clinical trials. It is, therefore, not surprising that these agents' toxicity is not selective and is harmful to cancer cells and normal cells alike (see chapter 4).

Some cancer chemotherapeutic agents' benefits have far outweighed the risk of toxicities involved. For some patients with leukemia, lymphoma, and testicular cancers, chemotherapy has offered a cure to the disease. Certain of these drugs have been shown to induce second cancers (a second primary) in patients who receive them. Alkylating agents for patients with ovarian carcinoma, myeloma, and possibly breast cancer, result in an increased incidence of acute leukemia (Jones, Frank, and Mass 1983). Long-term oral use of cyclophosphamide is associated with an increased risk of bladder carcinoma (Jones, Frank, and Mass 1983).

Teratogenic effects from single-agent and combination chemotherapy have been reported. Single chemotherapeutic regimens are known to produce toxic damage to both sperm and ovum of treated patients (Schein et al. 1982). Table 8.1 summarizes the results of studies on the chemotherapeutic agents with regard to their potential for carcinogenicity, mutagenicity, and teratogenicity (Rogers 1986).

In addition to patient risk, health care workers who have been exposed to antineoplastic agents have expressed concern about the potential hazard involved. The risk of exposure arises during drug preparation and drug administration. Individuals handling the human or drug waste and those individuals who decontaminate the equipment used to prepare the drug also risk being exposed to antineoplastic agents.

Table 8.1 Experimental Testing of Antineoplastic Agents

Antineoplastic Agents	*In Vitro* Testing for Mutagenicity	*In Vivo* Animal Carcinogenicity	Testing for Teratogenicity
Actinomycin D	−	+	+
Adriamycin	+	+	
Ara-C	−	−	+
Azacytidine	+	+	
AZQ	+	NR	
BCNU	+	+	+
Bleomycin	+	NR	+
Busulfan	+	−	
CCNU	+	+	+
Chlorambucil	+	+	
Cisplatin	+	+	+
Cyclophosphamide	+	+	
Dacarbazine	+	+	+
Daunorubicin	+	+	+
Fluorouracil	−	−	+
Hydroxyurea	NR	±	+
Ifosfamide	+	+	
L-Asparaginase	−	NR	
Mechlorethamine	+	+	
Melphalan	+	+	+
6-Mercaptopurine	+	+	
Methotrexate	−	−	+
Mitomycin C	+	+	+
Prednisone	−	−	
Procarbazine	−	+	
Streptozocin	+	+	+
Thiotepa	+	+	+
Uracil Mustard	+	+	+
Vinblastine	−	NR	+
Vincristine	−	NR	+
VP16	+	NR	+
VM26	+	NR	+

NR—Not Reported
Source: Rogers 1986. Reprinted with permission.

REVIEW OF THE LITERATURE

Research has suggested that antineoplastic drugs pose a significant hazard to those who handle these agents routinely. Review of the literature reveals several research studies with conflicting results and inconclusive findings. Some findings were positive, while others were questionable regarding the effects of occupational exposure to antineoplastic agents. These studies investigated a variety of possible effects of exposure: mutagenicity in urine of nurses who routinely prepared and administered antineoplastic agents; sister chromatid exchange frequencies in lymphocytes of nurses who handled these agents; chromosomal alterations; and urine mutagenicity. The conclusion that can be drawn from these studies is that the risk associated with chronic low-level exposure to antineoplastic drugs is yet unknown. Studies often utilized the *Salmonella* or *E. coli*-microsome assay system (Ames, McCann, Yamasaki 1975) (Waksvik, Klepp, Brogger 1981)—a sensitive measure for the presence of mutagenic substances in urine of exposed subjects. These studies are fraught with methodological problems. Small sample size, lack of appropriate control groups, and failure to allow for other causes of urinary mutagens, such as smoking, drug or medication and alcohol use, or age differentials, are some examples of the lack of scientific method. Several of the studies report a decrease in urine mutagens after a weekend away from work. In 1981, Wilson and Solimando published a study noting the absence of any acute or apparent long-term side effects when handling chemotherapeutic agents safely. Their study reported negative results for mutagenicity of urine samples. This study did use properly ventilated preparation rooms, laminar flow hoods, and strict adherence to aseptic techniques (Wilson and Salimando 1981). Studies by Crudi (1980) and Ladik et al. (1980) have reported on a variety of somatic complaints from personnel handling antineoplastic agents.

EXPOSURE POTENTIAL

The primary routes of exposure during preparation and administration of antineoplastic agents are through inhalation of the aerosolized drug, direct skin contact, and less often through ingestion. The risks to personnel who handle these agents are a result of the level and duration of exposure to these toxic agents while at work.

The evidence outlined thus far in the chapter suggests that exposure to antineoplastic agents can result in systemic absorption and produce measurable effects. Guidelines for safe handling of these agents have been published in recent years. The Occupational Safety and Health Act of 1970 provides legislative authority for the Occupational Safety and Health Administration (OSHA) of the Department of Labor to set standards which most adequately assure that no employee will suffer material impairment of health or functional capacity. OSHA suggests precautions in handling blood, vomitus, excreta, and contaminated linens for 48 hours after drug administration. In the 1988 revision of ONS *Cancer Chemotherapy Guidelines*, the issue of safe handling of chemotherapeutic agents is included in all the modules for various practice settings.

Experts conclude that protective measures to reduce potential exposures are warranted. Protecting the health care worker from contamination is imperative. Reducing exposure begins with education about the chemotherapeutic agents and the routes of absorption, and training related to the cost effective implementation of 1986 OSHA Guidelines for the safe handling of antineoplastic agents.

PRACTICE IMPLICATIONS

Cloak, Connor, and Stevens (1985) identified work practices in their research that led to occupational exposure of nursing personnel to antineoplastic agents. Nursing tasks performed included:

- Administering an antineoplastic agent
- Administering an antineoplastic agent IV push
- Priming intravenous (IV) tubing with an antineoplastic agent
- Administering an antineoplastic agent (connecting IV bag with primed IV tubing to an infusion system)
- Disposing of an empty container used to administer an antineoplastic agent
- Loading an Autosyringe pump with a syringe containing an antineoplastic agent
- Correcting a Travenol infusor filled with an antineoplastic agent
- Priming an I-MED Volumetric Infusion Pump cassettte with an antineoplastic agent

There is evidence that personnel who prepare and administer these drugs are inconsistent in observing safe handling practices (Valanis and Shortbridge 1987). Recommendations for safe preparation of antineoplastic agents include appropriate engineering controls, such as a biological safety cabinet or use of a respirator with a high-efficiency filter. Because aerosolization is a major problem with chemotherapeutic agents, it is cautioned that the use of surgical masks does not protect against breathing in of aerosols. The use of personal protective equipment such as plastic face shields or splash goggles should be worn during mixing and in the event of a spill. Eyewash fountains should be available or a sink with fresh running water because studies show that if a spill occurs to the skin, washing immediately reduces the exposure and potential of the agent to fix to the skin surface. Long-sleeved cuffed gowns made of low permeability fabric and latex surgical gloves prevent exposure through the skin. Practicing aseptic techniques such as hand washing before and after gloving reduces any accidental exposure. Utilizing a clean technique while reconstituting the antineoplastic agents minimizes exposure. Table 8.2

lists recommendations to avoid exposure by inhalation, skin absorption, and ingestion. Table 8.3 lists items to include in a spill kit.

For more specific guidelines, the reader is referred to the ONS *Cancer Chemotherapy Guidelines* (1988). These guidelines discuss how to handle and dispose of chemotherapeutic agents in various practice settings, based on OSHA recommendations. Appendix 3 includes the Recommendations for Handling Cytotoxic Agents authored by the National Study Commission on Cytotoxic Exposure.

Personnel disposing excreta from patients receiving antineoplastic agents are another at-risk population to the hazards mentioned throughout this chapter. The research in this area of practice with this population is virtually absent.

When handling the waste products for patients on chemotherapy, nursing practice is based on pharmacokinetic principles. Some of these principles are:

- There is a relationship between the concentration of a drug and its effect. This relationship assists in determining administration schedules for many agents.
- Most drugs are eliminated from the body by first order kinetics. In first order kinetics, a constant fraction (or percent) of the drug is eliminated per unit of time. The rate of elimination is often described in terms of a drug's half-life. The half-life of a drug is the amount of time required for 50% of the drug to be eliminated from the body. The half-life of a drug is independent of the dose or concentration, if the drug follows first order kinetics.
- The drug concentrations initially fall off very quickly followed by a more prolonged decline. Simple calculations of half-life reveal that most of a drug is eliminated in four to five half-lives. For example: if half of the remaining drug is eliminated after two half-lives, then 75% of the total drug has been eliminated. After three half-lives 87.5% of the total drug has been eliminated (Cersosimo 1987).

Table 8.2   Recommendations to Avoid Exposure to Antineoplastic Agents

Recommendations to Avoid Exposure via Inhalation	Recommendations to Avoid Exposure via Ingestion (continued)

Recommendations to Avoid Exposure via Inhalation

1. Mix all antineoplastic drugs in an approved Class II Biologic Safety Cabinet using appropriate technique. Ideally, all IV bags containing chemotherapy drugs also should be primed under the hood. If this is impossible, a maintenance bag of normal saline or D_5W should be used to prime the tubing, and the chemotherapy bag should be added to the line afterwards.

2. Use a needle with a hydrophobic filter to remove the solution from vials when in home or office settings without a safety cabinet. (The OSHA guidelines recommended using a safety cabinet in all settings; however, home and office settings usually do not have this equipment.) The area should also be well ventilated and the pattern of preferred air flow should be examined to avoid air flow into the drug preparer's face.

3. Break ampules by wrapping a sterile gauze pad or an alcohol wipe around the neck of the ampul to decrease chances of droplet contamination.

4. Vent vials containing cytotoxic agents with a hydrophobic filter needle to equalize internal pressure or use negative pressure techniques.

5. Do not dispose of materials by clipping needles, breaking syringes, or removing needles from syringes.

6. Use a gauze pad when removing chemotherapy syringes and needles from IV injection ports. Gauze also should be used when removing spikes from IV bags of chemotherapy.

Recommendations to Avoid Exposure via Ingestion

1. Do not eat, drink, smoke, chew gum, or apply cosmetics in the drug preparation area.

2. Keep all food and eating items away from the mixing area.

3. Do not place food or drink in the same refrigerator as antineoplastic drugs.

Recommendations to Avoid Exposure via Ingestion (continued)

4. Wash hands before and after preparation or administration of chemotherapy drugs.

5. Avoid hand-to-eye or hand-to-mouth contact when handling antineoplastic drugs or body fluids.

Recommendations to Avoid Exposure via Absorption through Skin

1. Wear latex surgical gloves and a gown of low-permeability fabric with a closed front and cuffed long sleeves when mixing chemotherapy drugs.

2. Change gloves approximately every 30 minutes when working steadily with antineoplastic drugs. Gloves should be removed immediately after spilling drug solution on them or puncturing or tearing the glove.

3. Wash hands before putting on gloves and after gloves are removed.

4. Cover the work surface of the cabinet with a plastic-backed absorbent pad. This pad should be changed when the cabinet is cleaned or after a spill.

5. Clean all internal surfaces of the biological safety cabinet before and after drug preparation, using 70% alcohol and a disposable towel. Discard the towel into a leakproof chemical-waste container.

6. Use syringes and IV sets with Luer-Lock fittings.

7. Use an absorbent pad directly under the injection site to contain any accidental spillage.

8. Label all antineoplastic drugs with a chemotherapy hazard label.

9. In the event of skin contact with antineoplastic drugs, wash the area thoroughly with soap and water as soon as possible.

10. In the event of eye contact with antineoplastic drugs, immediately flush the eye with eye solution or clean water and seek medical attention.

11. Use spill kits for major spills on floor or work surface.

Source: Adapted from Gullo 1988. Reprinted with permission.

Table 8.3 Contents of an Antineoplastic Drug Spill Kit

Number	Item
1	Gown with cuffs and back closure (made of water non-permeable fabric)
1 pair	Shoe covers
2 pair	Gloves (double gloving recommended)
1 pair	Goggles
1	Mask
1	Disposable dust pan (to collect any broken glass)
1	Plastic scraper (to scoop materials into dust pan)
2	Plastic backed or absorbable towels
1	Container of desiccant powder or granules (to absorb wet contents)
2	Disposable sponges (one to clean up spill, one to clean up floor after removal of spill)
1	Puncture proof, leak proof container (to place all contents in). Should be marked Biohazard Waste
1	Container of 70% alcohol for cleaning spill area

Source: Gullo 1988. Reprinted with permission.

The principles of drug elimination can be used to determine length of time for drug elimination. Application of these principles to antineoplastic agents is of great importance. It has been determined that the elimination half-life of most antineoplastic agents is less than six hours, indicating that over 90% of a dose of these drugs will be eliminated within one day of administration (Cerrisumo 1987). Exceptions to this rule are lomustine and carmustine metabolites, cis-Platinum, dactinomycin, daunorubicin, doxorubicin, vinblastine, and vincristine. The longer half-lives of these agents indicate that they may not be completely eliminated for several days (Cersosimo 1987). OSHA suggests precautions in handling blood, vomitus, excreta, and contaminated linen be maintained for 48 hours after drug administration. With patients who have received drugs with longer elimination half-lives, the OSHA guidelines may need to be extended. Table 8.4 illustrates excretion patterns of antineoplastic drugs.

Research has not looked at self-protective practices of those handling the waste products of antineoplastic administration. Such things as IV tubing, unused portions of prepared agents, and syringes are only a few of the toxic wastes which, according to federal disposal regulations, can be dumped in landfill areas or incinerated.

Federal disposal regulations depend upon the category of hazardous waste. Barry and Booker (1985) note that a few antineoplastic agents are on the U list classified as toxic waste: chlorambucil, cyclophosphamide, Daunomycin, melphalan, mitomycin, streptozocin, and uracil mustard. Current regulations provide that small quantity generators—those facilities that produce less than a total of 1000 kg/month of toxic waste—are exempt from regulation. The reason for this exemption may be due to a perceived cost-benefit ratio. Many outpatient clinics, physicians' offices, and home health care agencies fall into this category (Barry and Booker 1985).

THE ONCOLOGIST'S OFFICE

In the oncologist's office often the nurse is responsible for preparing the cancer chemotherapeutic agents, in addition to administering these agents. The guidelines used in institutions may be impractical and costly for a small oncology office. Both the biological safety cabinet and gloves would appear to be minimal precautions. Barhamand (1986) states that there does not seem to be enough statistical support for the use of gowns or masks to compensate for their costliness and inconvenience in a small office situation.

The office setting needs to provide the minimum standards for safety. Legal clearance from potential health problems could be achieved by a

Table 8.4 Excretion Patterns of Antineoplastic Drugs

Drug	Excretion
Asparaginase (Elspar®)	Trace amounts appear in urine.
Azacitidine (5-Azacyt) (investigational drug)	90% excreted in urine in first 24 hours.
Bleomycin (Blenoxane®)	50% to 80% excreted as active drug in urine within 24 hours.
Carmustine (BCNU®)	Most of drug is excreted as metabolites in urine within 24 hours.
Chlorambucil (Leukeran®)	Less than 0.5% unchanged drug in urine after 24 hours.
Cisplatin (Platinol®)	27% to 34% of dosage excreted by kidneys; initially excreted as unchanged drug but with increasing time, the by-products are excreted.
Cyclophosphamide (Cytoxan®, Neosar®)	30% excreted in urine as unchanged drug.
Cytarabine (Ara C®, Cytosar®)	Less than 10% unchanged drug in urine after 24 hours.
Dacarbazine (DTIC®)	50% excreted as unchanged drug in urine.
Dactinomycin (Cosmegen®)	(only slightly metabolized) 30% excreted as unchanged drug in urine and feces within nine days.
Daunorubicin (Cerubidine®)	Extensively metabolized in the liver; 14% to 23% of drug and metabolites excreted via urine within 72 hours.
Doxorubicin (Adriamycin®)	Metabolized by liver; excreted primarily in bile. 10% to 20% excreted as metabolites in feces within 24 hours.
Etoposide, VP-16 (Vepesid®)	40% to 60% excreted in urine as unchanged drug and metabolites within 48 to 72 hours. 20% to 30% excreted in urine within 24 hours; 2% to 16% excreted in feces as unchanged drug or metabolites within 72 hours.
Fluorouracil (5-FU, Adrucil®)	15% of dose excreted in urine as intact drug within 6 hours.
Ifosfamide (Isophosphamide) (investigational drug)	62% excreted unchanged in urine with an additional 20% as metabolites.
Melphalan (Alkeran)	13% recovered as unchanged drug in urine after 24 hours; 50% of dosage excreted as drug or metabolites.
Mechlorethamine, HN$_2$ (Mustargen®)	Less than 0.01% excreted unchanged in urine.
Methotrexate, MTX (Mexate®, Folex®)	75% excreted unchanged in urine within eight hours.
Mithramycin (Mithracin®)	50% excreted in urine within 24 hours.
Mitomycin (Mutamycin®)	10% excreted in urine as active drug; small amount excreted in bile (rapidly metabolized by liver).
Plicamycin (Mithracin®)	50% excreted in urine within 24 hours.
Procarbazine (Matulane®)	70% excreted in urine (less than 5% unchanged).
Streptozocin (Zanosar®)	Extensively metabolized by liver. 60% to 70% excreted as metabolites within 24 hours.
Thioguanine (6-TG) (Thioguanine®)	85% excreted unchanged and as metabolites in urine; after one hour 70% of the drug is excreted intact; by 13 hours only 2% is excreted as intact drug.
Thiotepa (Thiotepa®)	Extensively metabolized; traces excreted unchanged in urine—60% excreted as metabolites in 24 hours.

Source: Gullo 1988. Reprinted with permission.

waiver of responsibility. A pre-employment waiver stating that the employee is knowledgeable about the chemotherapeutic agents and the fact that long-term exposure risks are not clear is one means of addressing the problem. Records of nursing compliance with the individual office policies and procedures is mandatory. Anything less would leave open the possibility of being liable for negligence (Barhamand 1986).

The EPA's regulations regarding toxic waste disposal include combining all contaminated supplies in leakproof, sealed containers for the purpose of incineration. This makes for different problems in the office setting.

A private office could store the waste in sealed containers and periodically transport them to a nearby hospital or EPA-approved incinerator. Prior arrangements must be made with the appropriate administrator. Private companies will dispose of the waste but this can be an expensive option.

In the office, additional costs for the handling of chemotherapeutic agents cannot be absorbed by the practice or billed to the patient. It is for this reason that practicality and safety should go together. Efforts should be taken to minimize exposure to these agents (Barhamand 1986) within the constraints of cost.

THE COMMUNITY

The growing emphasis on outpatient care for persons with cancer demonstrates the need to utilize safe handling guidelines in the community setting. These guidelines should reflect safety for the personnel who have frequent and long-term exposure to antineoplastic agents.

Consideration of the potential environmental and community hazards which these agents impose cannot be overlooked (Barry and Booker 1985). With larger volumes of drugs being handled in home care settings, appropriate cost-effective and practical means of preparation, administration, and safe handling of both human waste and mechanical equipment waste are necessary.

Table 8.5 gives guidelines for the preparation, administration, and disposal of parenteral antineoplastic agents in the community setting. To date no guidelines or model policies exist to direct or serve as a standard for preventing inadvertent exposure in the home setting (Stevens 1989).

Existing hospital practices must be extrapolated to the home settings. Recently the Joint Commission of the Accreditation of Healthcare Organization (JCAHO) established accreditation standards for home care services. The standard cited in Safety Management and Infection Control addresses education to minimize hazards related to handling and disposal of hazardous materials and wastes. The lessons learned regarding occupational exposure must be translated to the home management of the person with cancer. The family and the patient are at risk of exposure.

Barry and Booker, from their research, suggest that the OSHA guidelines and related recommendations reflect what is currently known about antineoplastic agents and what is not yet known as potential problems. The ONS *Cancer Chemotherapy Guidelines Module IV. Recommendations for Nursing Practice in the Home Care Setting* (1988, 4) state:

> To date there have been no recommendations made on handling cytotoxic drugs in the home. The recommendations made in this document are based on current practice trends.

The guidelines continue by stating that the practices recommended by ONS are deemed reasonable in the absence of definitive studies. Health care professionals who work with chemotherapeutic agents should remain current on new information as it becomes available. As various home care agencies adapt guidelines to meet their specific needs, adherence to safety principles is essential.

CONCLUSION

In a recent study on self-protective practices of nurses handling antineoplastic drugs, Valanis

Table 8.5 Guidelines for Preparation, Administration, and Disposal of Parenteral Antineoplastic Agents in the Community Setting

Preparation

1. The nurse is responsible for bringing what she needs to ensure her safety as well as that of the person with cancer and the family when working with antineoplastic agents within the home. Disposable chemotherapy kits have recently been marketed that contain all items necessary for preparation, administration, and disposal of antineoplastic agents. (Winfield: Chemotainer System™; BioSafety: Chemo Safety™). Cost effectiveness of these kits should be determined by individual agencies.

2. Antineoplastic agents should be prepared in advance if an appropriate work space is available within the agency. The work area should be adequate in size to decrease chance of exposure. A kitchen or bathroom counter should be used for preparation of the agent within the home.

3. Agents should be transported within a lined, leakproof punctureproof container. A cooler is recommended for this purpose as it also has the ability to maintain the temperature of the agents.

4. Individuals receiving agents which have been prepared in advance should be seen first whenever possible in order to ensure the stability of the drug in solution.

5. Reconstituted antineoplastic agents should not routinely be left in the client's refrigerator without a complete assessment of the family situation to prevent accidental exposure.

6. Ceiling fans, heating or cooling units, and humidifiers located in the immediate working area should be turned off during preparation.

7. Individuals working with antineoplastic agents should observe aseptic techniques.

8. The work area should be washed thoroughly before and after preparation of agents with soap and water or 70% alcohol and allowed to dry. The workspace should be free of food or other items which may become contaminated.

9. A disposable absorbent plastic-backed pad should be taped in place over the work surface to reduce the chance of droplet contamination or spills and to facilitate cleanup. A disposable diaper works well for this purpose.

10. The client and family members should not be in the immediate work area during the preparation of agents. The nurse should explain that this precaution will decrease their chance of contamination by droplet or aerosolization of the agent.

11. Hands should be washed before and after preparation and administration of the agents.

12. A disposable gown with elastic at the wrists or disposable sleeves should be worn during preparation and administration of the agents.

13. Latex surgical gloves or thick polyvinyl gloves should be worn during preparation and administration.

14. A surgical mask and goggles should be worn if there is a chance that aerosolization may occur during mixing or transfer of the agents.

15. Reconstituted drug vials should be vented to prevent positive pressure build-up within the vials, resulting in aerosolization of the drug. Dispensing pins and filters are available to prevent drug blowback (Millipore: Millex-FG™; Burton Medical: Chemo Dispensing Pin™). Agencies should determine cost-effectiveness of these items on an individual basis. If these items are not available, then negative pressure technique should be used.

16. Ampules should be broken by wrapping sterile gauze or an alcohol wipe around the neck to decrease chances of droplet contamination. Use a filter needle to remove solution.

17. The external surfaces of the drug bottle and syringe should be cleaned with an alcohol wipe after preparation.

18. A sterile gauze pad should be placed under the distal tubing of the IV or over the needle tip when priming or removing air bubbles. Do not remove needle caps with teeth.

19. Syringes and IV sets should have Leur-lok fittings to decrease the chance of leakage.

20. IVs and syringes should be identified with labels designating that they contain antineoplastic agents.

Administration

1. If the client has a Hickman, Broviac or other type of central line, follow specific agency policy for cleansing the site prior to administering the antineoplastic agent.

2. Remove gloves worn during preparation of agent prior to starting the IV. Wash hands.

3. Place a disposable absorbent plastic-backed pad under the client's arm in case of agent leakage during administration.

4. Select an appropriate site and start IV according to agency policy.

5. Reglove.

6. Administer the antineoplastic agent in accordance with accepted agency policy for safe administration of parenteral medications.

7. If antineoplastic agent comes in contact with skin, wash area with soap and copious amounts of water and follow instructions for specific agent as specified on drug package insert.

8. If spillage occurs, wipe with absorbent pads while wearing double latex surgical gloves or double thick polyvinyl chloride gloves.

(continued)

Table 8.5 *(continued)*

Disposal

1. Unused portions of antineoplastic agents should not be disposed of down the drain or the toilet. Contents should be left in the container and placed in a plastic ziploc bag lined with paper towels.
2. Contaminated needles and syringes are disposed of intact to prevent aerosolization contamination. These items should be placed in a leakproof, punctureproof container.
3. All gloves, vials, tubings, gowns, masks, and absorbent pads as well as the needle container and unused agent bag should be placed in a large sturdy garbage bag, tied, and labeled *CAUTION: CHEMOTHERAPY WASTE.*

4. The plastic bag is then taken with the nurse and placed in her car in a lined cardboard box which is labeled as in #3. At the end of the day, this box is sealed with tape and deposited at a designated area from where it will be taken for appropriate disposal.
5. Arrangements should be made with either a hospital that has appropriate incineration facilities or with a private waste management firm that has a license to dispose of toxic waste materials.
6. Personnel and family members should be cautioned to avoid skin contact with excreta of individuals treated with antineoplastic agents. Hands should be washed thoroughly and gloves worn when dispensing of excreta.

Source: Barry and Booker 1985. Reprinted with permission.

and Shortbridge (1987) demonstrate the increasing rise in the use of self-protective practices. These practices include admixing the agents under a vertical laminar flow hood and increasing use of gloves. Protective clothing may or may not be available but the common reasons given for lack of use relate to convenience, comfort for the nurse, belief that no personal hazard exists, and belief that use is inappropriate.

A convincing body of knowledge documenting health risks due to chronic low-dose exposure to antineoplastic drugs is beginning to evolve. It is hoped that the personnel at risk to exposure will utilize self-protective behaviors until the verdict comes in on the mutagenicity, teratogenicity, and carcinogenicity of antineoplastic agents. Current guidelines are based on what is known about these drugs, what is not known, and what is suspected based on studies. The resolution of unanswered questions rests with future scientific research and nursing practice based on sound principles.

BIBLIOGRAPHY

Ames BN, McCann J, Yamaski E (1975) Carcinogens are mutagens: a simple test system. *Mutational Research* 33: 27–28

Anderson RW, Puckett WH, Dana WJ, Nguen TV, Theiss JC, Matney TS (1982) Risk of handling injectable antineoplastic agents. *American Journal of Hospital Pharmacy*, 39(11): 1881–1887

American Society of Hospital Pharmacists (1985) ASHP technical assistance bulletin on handling cytotoxic drugs in hospitals. *American Journal of Hospital Pharmacy* 42: 131–137 (Jan)

——— (1983) Procedures for handling cytotoxic drugs. Bethesda, Md, American Society of Hospital Pharmacists

Antineoplastic policies stress education, safety precautions. (1986) *Hospital Employee Health* (newsletter) 5(2): 17–19 (Feb)

Barhamand B (1986) Difficulties encountered in implementing guidelines for handling antineoplastics in the physician's office. *Cancer Nursing* 9(3): 138–143

Barry LK, Booker RB (1985) Promoting the responsible handling of antineoplastic agents in the community. *Oncology Nursing Forum* 12(5): 41–46 (Sept/Oct)

Cersosimo RJ (1987) Pharmacokinetic principles in the handling of antineoplastics. *Oncology Nursing Society—Boston Chapter Newsletter* 6(1): 1–3 (Sept/Oct)

Cloak MM, Connor TH, Stevens KR (1985) Occupational exposure of nursing personnel to antineoplastic agents. *Oncology Nursing Forum* 12(5): 33–39

Crudi CB (1980) A compounding dilemma: I've kept the drug sterile but have I contaminated myself? *NITA* 3: 77–78

Crudi CB, Stephens BL (1981) Antineoplastic agents: an occupational hazard? *NITA* 4: 233–234

Davis MR (1981) Guidelines for safe handling of cytotoxic drugs in pharmacy departments and hospital wards. *Hospital Pharmacy* 16: 17–20

de Werk A, Wadden RA, Chiou WL (1983) Exposure of hospital workers to airborne antineoplastic agents. *American Journal of Hospital Pharmacy* 40: 597–601

Dunne C (1989) Safe handling of antineoplastic agents; self-learning module. *Cancer Nursing* 12(2): 120–127 (April)

Education protects hospital workers who handle toxic cancer drugs. (1982) *Hospital Employee Health* 1: 154–156

Falck K, Grohn P, Sorsa M, Vainio H, Heinonen E, Holstil LR (1979) Mutagenicity in urine of nurses handling cytostatic drugs. *Lancet* 1:1250–1251

Fischer DS (1978) *Some guidelines to use of parenteral antineoplastic drugs*. November (booklet). Monsanto Co

Gross H, Johnson BJ, Bertino JR (1981) Possible hazards of working with cytotoxic agents. *Oncology Nursing Forum* 8: 10–12

Gullo S (1988) Safe handling of antineoplastic drugs: translating the recommendations into practice. *Oncology Nursing Forum* 15(5): 595–601 (Sept/Oct)

Harrison BR (1981) Developing guidelines for working with antineoplastic drugs. *American Journal of Hospital Pharmacy* 38: 1686–1691

Hirst M, Tse S, Mitts DG, et al. (1984) Occupational exposure to cyclophosphamide. *Lancet* 1: 186–188

Hoffman DM (1980) The handling of antineoplastic drugs in a major cancer center. *Hospital Pharmacy* 15(6): 302–304

Jeffrey L, Anderson R, Barker L, et al. (1983) *Recommendations for Handling Cytotoxic Agents*. Providence, RI, National Study Commission of Cytotoxic Exposure

Jones R, Frank R, Mass T (1983) Safe handling of chemotherapeutic agents: a report from the Mount Sinai Medical Center. *CA—A Cancer Journal for Clinicians* 33(5): 258–263 (Sept/Oct)

Knowles R, Virden T (1980) Handling of injectable antineoplastic agents. *British Medical Journal* 281: 589–591 (August 30)

Ladik CF, Storhr GP, Maurer MA (1980) Precautionary measures in the preparation of antineoplastics. *American Journal of Hospital Pharmacy* 37: 1184–1186 (September)

Laidlaw J, Connor T, Theiss J, Anderson RW, Matney TS (1984) Permeability of latex and polyvinyl gloves to 20 antineoplastic drugs. *American Journal of Hospital Pharmacy* 41(12): 2618–2623 (Dec)

Laidlaw J, Connor T, Theiss J, Anderson RW, Matney T (1985) Permeability of four disposable protective-clothing materials to seven antineoplastic drugs. *American Journal of Hospital Pharmacy* p. 42 (Nov)

Le Roy ML, Roberts MJ, Teisen JA (1983) Procedures for handling antineoplastic injections in comprehensive cancer centers. *American Journal of Hospital Pharmacy* 40: 601–603

Macek C (1982) Hospital personnel who handle anticancer drugs may face risks. *JAMA* 247(1): 11–12 (Jan 1)

Matia MA, Blake SL (1983) Hospital hazards: Cancer drugs. *American Journal of Nursing* 83: 759–762

Miller SA (1980) Nursing actions in cancer chemotherapy administration. *Oncology Nursing Forum* 7: 8–16

Muller RJ (1988) Handling antineoplastic agents—focus on the ambulatory setting. *Outpatient Chemotherapy* 3(1): 1–3

National Institute of Health, Division of Safety (1983) *Recommendation for the safe handling of parenteral antineoplastic drugs*. Bethesda Md, U.S. Department of Health and Human Services, Public Health Services, NIH Publications No. 83-2621

Ngugen TV, Theiss JC, Matney TS (1982) Exposure to pharmacy personnel to mutagenic antineoplastic drugs. *Cancer Research* 42(11): 4792–4796

Oncology Nursing Society (1988) *Cancer Chemotherapy Guidelines*. Pittsburgh, ONS

OSHA (1986) *Work Practice Guidelines for Personnel Dealing with Cytotoxic (Antineoplastic) Drugs*. Office of Occupational Medicine, Directorate of Technical Support, OSHA, USL, January 29

Parrish RH (1983) Antineoplastic drug—use process at a rural hospital. *Hospital Pharmacy* 18: 250–256

Power LA, Stolar MH (1984) *Safe Handling of Cytotoxic Drugs*. Bethesda, Md, American Society of Hospital Pharmacists

Rogers B (1986) Antineoplastic agents: actions and toxicities. *AAOHN Journal* 34(11): 530–538 (Nov)

Schein PS, Winoker S, McDonald JS, et al (1982) Long-term complications of cytotoxic and immunosuppressive chemotherapy, in Holland JF, Frei E (eds.): *Cancer Medicine*. Philadelphia, Lea & Febiger, 759–774

Simonowitz J (1983) *Guidelines for Preparation and Administration of Antineoplastic Drugs*. San Francisco, State of California Division of Occupational Safety and Health, June 17

Simple, economical means to help reduce cancer drug exposure. (1983) *Hospital Employee Health* 2(newsletter): 132–134

Stolar MH, Power LA (1983) The 1983–1984 ASHP practice spotlight: safe handling of cytotoxic drugs. *American Journal of Hospital Pharmacy* 40: 1161–1171

Stevens KR (1989) Safe handling of cytotoxic drugs in home chemotherapy. *Seminars in Oncology Nursing* 5(2): 15–20

Stolar MH, Power LA, Viele CS (1983) Recommendations for handling cytotoxic drugs in hospitals. *American Journal of Hospital Pharmacy* 40: 1163–1170

VA releases guidelines for handling antineoplastic drugs. (1985) *Hospital Employee Health* 4(9)(newsletter): 109 (Sept)

Valanis B, Shortbridge L (1987) Self-protective practices of nurses handling antineoplastic drugs. *Oncology Nursing Forum* 14(3): 23–27 (May/June)

Wilson JP, Solimando DA (1981) Aseptic technique as a safety precaution in the preparation of antineoplastic agents. *Hospital Pharmacy* 16: 575–581

Waksvik H, Klepp O, Brogger A (1981) Chromosome analyses of nurses handling cytostatic agents. *Cancer Treatment Reports* 65(7–8): 607–610

Willcox GS, Mahoney CD, Welch DW, Louis BS, Jeffrey LP (1983) A comparison of laminar air flow cabinetry. *Cancer Chemotherapy Update* 1: 1–3

Zellmer WA (1981) Reducing occupational exposure to potential carcinogens in hospitals. *American Journal of Hospital Pharmacy* 38: 1679

Zimmerman PF, Larsen RK, Barkley EW, Gallelli JF (1981) Recommendations for the safe handling of injectable antineoplastic drug products. *American Journal of Hospital Pharmacy* 38: 690–695 (November)

APPENDICES

Appendix 1: National Cancer Institute's Common Toxicity Criteria
Appendix 2: Chemotherapeutic Acronyms
Appendix 3: Recommendations for Handling Cytotoxic Agents: OSHA Guidelines
Appendix 4: Cancer Chemotherapeutic Agents Compatibility Chart: Oncology Drug Compatibilities
Appendix 5: Nomograms for Determination of Body Surface Area from Height and Weight (Adults)
Appendix 6: Table of Standard Body Weights

Appendix 1: National Cancer Institute's Common Toxicity Criteria

	Toxicity	Grade				
		0	1	2	3	4
Blood/Bone Marrow	WBC	≥4.0	3.0–3.9	2.0–2.9	1.0–1.9	<1.0
	PLT	WNL	75.0–normal	50.0–74.9	25.0–49.9	<25.0
	Hgb	WNL	10.0–normal	8.0–10.0	6.5–7.9	<6.5
	Granulocytes/ Bands	≥2.0	1.5–1.9	1.0–1.4	0.5–0.9	<0.5
	Lymphocytes	≥2.0	1.5–1.9	1.0–1.4	0.5–0.9	<0.5
	Hemorrhage (clinical)	none	mild, no transfusion	gross, 1–2 units transfusion per episode	gross, 3–4 units transfusion per episode	massive, >4 units transfusion per episode
	Infection	none	mild	moderate	severe	life-threatening
Gastrointestinal	Nausea	none	able to eat reasonable intake	intake significantly decreased but can eat	no significant intake	—
	Vomiting	none	1 episode in 24 hrs	2–5 episodes in 24 hrs	6–10 episodes in 24 hrs	>10 episodes in 24 hrs, or requiring parenteral support
	Diarrhea	none	increase of 2–3 stools/day over pre-Rx	increase of 4–6 stools/day, or nocturnal stools, or moderate cramping	increase of 7–9 stools/day, or incontinence, or severe cramping	increase of ≥10 stools/day or grossly bloody diarrhea, or need for parenteral support
	Stomatitis	none	painless ulcers, erythema, or mild soreness	painful erythema, edema, or ulcers, but can eat	painful erythema, edema, or ulcers, and cannot eat	requires parenteral or enteral support
Liver	Bilirubin	WNL	—	$<1.5 \times N$	$1.5–3.0 \times N$	$>3.0 \times N$
	Transaminase (SGOT, SGPT)	WNL	$\leq 2.5 \times N$	$2.6–5.0 \times N$	$5.1–20.0 \times N$	$>20.0 \times N$
	Alkaline Phosphatase or 5' nucleotidase	WNL	$\leq 2.5 \times N$	$2.6–5.0 \times N$	$5.1–20.0 \times N$	$>20.0 \times N$
	Liver—clinical	no change from baseline	—	—	precoma	hepatic coma

Appendix 1: National Cancer Institute's Common Toxicity Criteria *(continued)*

	Toxicity	Grade				
		0	1	2	3	4
Kidney, Bladder	Creatinine	WNL	$< 1.5 \times N$	$1.5–3.0 \times N$	$3.1–6.0 \times N$	$> 6.0 \times N$
	Proteinuria	no change	1+ or <0.3 g% or <3 g/L	2–3+ or 0.3–1.0 g% or 3–10 g/L	4+ or >1.0 g% or >10 g/L	nephrotic syndrome
	Hematuria	neg	micro only	gross, no clots	gross + clots	requires transfusion
	Alopecia	no loss	mild hair loss	pronounced or total hair loss	—	—
	Pulmonary	none or no change	asymptomatic, with abnormality in PFTs	dyspnea on significant exertion	dyspnea at normal level of activity	dyspnea at rest
Heart	Cardiac dysrhythmias	none	asymptomatic, transient, requiring no therapy	recurrent or persistent, no therapy required	requires treatment	requires monitoring; or hypotension, or ventricular tachycardia, or fibrillation
	Cardiac function	normal	asymptomatic, decline of resting ejection fraction by less than 20% of baseline value	asymptomatic, decline of resting ejection fraction by more than 20% of baseline value	mild CHF, responsive to therapy	severe or refractory CHF
	Cardiac—ischemia	none	nonspecific T-wave flattening	asymptomatic, ST and T-wave changes suggesting ischemia	angina without evidence of infarction	acute myocardial infarction
	Cardiac—pericardial	none	asymptomatic effusion, no intervention required	pericarditis (rub, chest pain, ECG changes)	symptomatic effusion; drainage required	tamponade; drainage urgently required
Blood Pressure	Hypertension	none or no change	asymptomatic, transient increase by greater than 20 mm Hg (D) or to >150/100 if previously WNL. No treatment required	recurrent or persistent increase by greater than 20 mm Hg (D) or to >150/100 if previously WNL. No treatment required	requires therapy	hypertensive crisis
	Hypotension	none or no change	changes requiring no therapy (including transient orthostatic hypotension)	requires fluid replacement or other therapy but not hospitalization	requires therapy and hospitalization; resolves within 48 hrs of stopping the agent	requires therapy and hospitalization for >48 hrs after stopping the agent

Appendix 1:   National Cancer Institute's Common Toxicity Criteria *(continued)*

			Grade		
Toxicity	**0**	**1**	**2**	**3**	**4**
Neurologic					
Neuro—sensory	none or no change	mild paresthesias, loss of deep tendon reflexes	mild or moderate objective sensory loss; moderate paresthesias	severe objective sensory loss or paresthesias that interfere with function	—
Neuro—motor	none or no change	subjective weakness; no objective findings	mild objective weakness without significant impairment of function	objective weakness with impairment of function	paralysis
Neuro—cortical	none	mild somnolence or agitation	moderate somnolence or agitation	severe somnolence, agitation, confusion, disorientation, or hallucinations	coma, seizures, toxic psychosis
Neuro—cerebellar	none	slight incoordination, dysdiadokinesis	intention tremor, dysmetria, slurred speech, nystagmus	locomotor ataxia	cerebellar necrosis
Neuro—mood	no change	mild anxiety or depression	moderate anxiety or depression	severe anxiety or depression	suicidal ideation
Neuro—headache	none	mild	moderate or severe but transient	unrelenting and severe	—
Neuro—constipation	none or no change	mild	moderate	severe	ileus >96 hrs
Neuro—hearing	none or no change	asymptomatic, hearing loss on audiometry only	tinnitus	hearing loss interfering with function but correctable with hearing aid	deafness not correctable
Neuro—vision	none or no change	—	—	symptomatic subtotal loss of vision	blindness
Skin	none or no change	scattered macular or papular eruption or erythema that is asymptomatic	scattered macular or papular eruption or erythema with pruritus or other associated symptoms	generalized symptomatic macular, papular, or vesicular eruption	exfoliative dermatitis or ulcerating dermatitis
Allergy	none	transient rash, drug fever <38 °C, 100.4 °F	urticaria, drug fever = 38 °C, 100.4 °F mild bronchospasm	serum sickness, bronchospasm, req parenteral meds	anaphylaxis

Appendix 1: National Cancer Institute's Common Toxicity Criteria *(continued)*

	Toxicity	Grade				
		0	1	2	3	4
	Fever in absence of infection	none	37.1–38.0 °C 98.7–100.4 °F	38.1–40.0 °C 100.5–104.0 °F	>40.0 °C >104.0 °F for less than 24 hours	>40.0 °C (104.0 °F) for more than 24 hrs or fever accompanied by hypotension
	Local	none	pain	pain and swelling, with inflammation or phlebitis	ulceration	plastic surgery indicated
	Weight gain/loss	<5.0%	5.0–9.9%	10.0–19.9%	≥20.0%	—
Metabolic	Hyperglycemia	<116	116–160	161–250	251–500	>500 or ketoacidosis
	Hypoglycemia	>64	55–64	40–54	30–39	<30
	Amylase	WNL	<1.5 × N	1.5–2.0 × N	2.1–5.0 × N	>5.1 × N
	Hypercalcemia	<10.6	10.6–11.5	11.6–12.5	12.6–13.5	≥13.5
	Hypocalcemia	>8.4	8.4–7.8	7.7–7.0	6.9–6.1	≤6.0
	Hypomagnesemia	>1.4	1.4–1.2	1.1–0.9	0.8–0.6	≤0.5
Coagulation	Fibrinogen	WNL	0.99–0.75 × N	0.74–0.50 × N	0.49–0.25 × N	≤0.24 × N
	Prothrombin time	WNL	1.01–1.25 × N	1.26–1.50 × N	1.51–2.00 × N	>2.00 × N
	Partial thromboplastin time	WNL	1.01–1.66 × N	1.67–2.33 × N	2.34–3.00 × N	>3.00 × N

Appendix 2: Chemotherapeutic Acronyms

Selected Combination Chemotherapy Regimens

The letter acronym and corresponding chemotherapy regime are given. Original references or medical texts should be consulted for full description of chemotherapy regime.

ACUTE MYELOGENOUS LEUKEMIA

CD $\{$ Cytosine Arabinoside 100 mg/m^2 CI* d1–7
Daunorubicin 45 mg/m^2 IV d1–3

—87% complete responses in patients <60 years old (induction)
—Ellison RR (1975), Management of acute leukemia in adults. *Med Pediatr Oncology* 1:149–158

CA $\{$ Cytosine Arabinoside 100 mg/m^2 CI* d1–7
Doxorubicin 30 mg/m^2 IV d1–3

—80% complete response (induction remissions)
—Priesler HD, *et al.* (1977), Adriamycin–cytosine arabinoside therapy for advanced acute myelocytic leukemia. *Ca Treatment Reports* 61:89–92

BREAST CANCER

AC $\{$ Doxorubicin 40 mg/m^2 IV d1 $\}$ q 21 days
Cyclophosphamide 1 g/m^2 IV d1

—Kennealey GT, *et al.* (1978), Combination chemotherapy for advanced breast cancer: two regimens containing adriamycin. *Cancer* 42:27–33

CAF $\{$ Cyclophosphamide 500 mg/m^2 IV d1
Doxorubicin 50 mg/m^2 IV d1 $\}$ q 21 days
5-Fluorouracil 500 mg/m^2 IV d1

—Smalley RV, *et al.* (1977), A comparison of cyclophosphamide, adriamycin, 5-fluorouracil (CAF) and cyclophosphamide, methotrexate, 5-fluorouracil, vincristine, prednisone (CMF-VP) in patients with metastatic breast cancer. *Cancer* 40:625–632

CMF $\{$ Cyclophosphamide 600 mg/m^2 IV d1
Methotrexate 40 mg/m^2 IV d1 $\}$ q 21 days
5-Fluorouracil 600 mg/m^2 IV d1

—Weiss RB, *et al.* (1987), Adjuvant chemotherapy after conservative surgery plus irradiation versus modified radical mastectomy. *Am J Med* 83:455–463

BLADDER CANCER

MVAC $\{$ Methotrexate 30 mg/m^2 IV d1, 15, 22
Vinblastine 3 mg/m^2 IV d2, 15, 22 $\}$ q 28 days
Doxorubicin 30 mg/m^2 IV d2
Cisplatin 70 mg/m^2 IV d2

—Sternberg CN, *et al.* (1985), Preliminary results of M-VAC for transitional cell carcinoma of urothelium. *J Urol* 133:403–407

CISCA $\{$ Cisplatin 100 mg/m^2 IV d2
Cyclophosphamide 650 mg/m^2 IV d1 $\}$ q 21–28 days
Doxorubicin 50 mg/m^2 IV d1
(Adriamycin)

—Samuels ML, *et al.* (1980), Cytoxan, Adriamycin, and cisplatin (CISCA) in metastatic bladder cancer. *Proc Am Assoc Cancer Res* 21:137

COLON CANCER

LF $\{$ Leukovorin 500 mg/m^2 in 2 hour
IV infusion $\}$ q wk × 6
5-Fluorouracil 600 mg/m^2 IVB 1 hour
after start of leukovorin

—Petrelli N, *et al.* (1987), A prospective randomized trial of 5-fluorouracil versus 5-fluorouracil and high-dose leukovorin versus 5-fluorouracil and methotrexate in previously untreated patients with advanced colorectal carcinoma. *J Clin Oncol* 5:1559–1565

GASTRIC CANCER

FAM $\{$ 5-Fluorouracil 600 mg/m^2 IV d1, 8, 29, 36
Doxorubicin 30 mg/m^2 IV d1, 29 $\}$ q 56 days
Mitomycin 10 mg/m^2 IV d1

—MacDonald JS, *et al.* (1980), 5-FU, doxorubicin, and mitomycin (*FAM*) combination chemotherapy for advanced gastric cancer. *Ann Intern Med* 93:533–536

HEAD AND NECK CANCER

CF $\{$ Cisplatin 100 mg/m^2 IV d1 $\}$ q 21 days
5-Fluorouracil 1000 mg/m^2 CI d1–5

—Decker DA, *et al.* (1983), Adjuvant chemotherapy with CDDP and 120 hour 5-FU in stage III and IV squamous cell carcinoma of the head and neck. *Cancer* 51:1353–1355

LUNG CANCER

Nonsmall Cell

CAP $\left\{\begin{array}{l}\text{Cyclophosphamide} \quad 400 \text{ mg/m}^2 \text{ IV d1} \\ \text{Doxorubicin} \qquad\quad 40 \text{ mg/m}^2 \text{ IV d1} \\ \text{Cisplatin} \qquad\qquad 60 \text{ mg/m}^2 \text{ IV d1}\end{array}\right\}$ q 28 days

—Egan RT, *et al.* (1979), Phase II trial of CAP by infusion in patients with adenocarcinoma and large cell carcinoma of the lung. *Cancer Treatment Reports* 64:1589–1591

Small Cell

ACE $\left\{\begin{array}{l}\text{Cyclophosphamide} \quad 1 \text{ g/m}^2 \quad\text{ IV d1} \\ \text{Doxorubicin} \qquad\quad 45 \text{ mg/m}^2 \text{ IV d1} \\ \text{Etoposide} \qquad\qquad 50 \text{ mg/m}^2 \text{ IV d1–5}\end{array}\right\}$ q 21 days

—Rudolph A, *et al.* (1983), CAE vs CAV in the treatment of small cell carcinoma of the lung. *Proc Am Soc Clin Oncol* 2:192

CAV $\left\{\begin{array}{l}\text{Cyclophosphamide} \quad 1000 \text{ mg/m}^2 \text{ IV d1} \\ \text{Doxorubicin} \qquad\quad 40 \text{ mg/m}^2 \text{ IV d1} \\ \text{Vincristine} \qquad\qquad 1 \text{ mg/m}^2 \text{ IV d1}\end{array}\right\}$ q 21 days

—Oldham RK, *et al.* (1978), Small cell lung cancer: a potentially curable neoplasm. *Proc Am Soc Clin Oncol* 19:361

LYMPHOMA

Hodgkin's Disease

MOPP $\left\{\begin{array}{l}\text{Nitrogen Mustard} \quad 6 \text{ mg/m}^2 \text{ IV d1, 8} \\ \text{Vincristine} \qquad\quad 1.4 \text{ mg/m}^2 \text{ IV d1, 8} \\ \text{Procarbazine} \qquad 100 \text{ mg/m}^2 \text{ PO d1–14} \\ \text{Prednisone} \qquad\quad 40 \text{ mg/m}^2 \text{ PO d1–14}\end{array}\right\}$ q 28 days

—DeVita, *et al.* (1970), Combination chemotherapy in the treatment of advanced Hodgkin's disease. *Annals of Internal Medicine* vol 73:881–895

ABVD $\left\{\begin{array}{l}\text{Doxorubicin} \quad 25 \text{ mg/m}^2 \text{ IV d1, 15} \\ \text{Bleomycin} \qquad 10 \text{ u/m}^2 \text{ IV d1, 15} \\ \text{Vinblastine} \qquad 6 \text{ mg/m}^2 \text{ IV d1, 15} \\ \text{Dacarbazine} \quad 375 \text{ mg/m}^2 \text{ IV d1, 15}\end{array}\right\}$ q 28 days

—Santoro A, *et al.* (1982), Salvage chemotherapy with ABVD in MOPP-resistant Hodgkin's disease. *Ann Intern Med* 96:139–143

Non-Hodgkin's Lymphoma

CHOP $\left\{\begin{array}{l}\text{Cyclophosphamide} \quad 750 \text{ mg/m}^2 \text{ IV d1} \\ \text{Adriamycin} \qquad\qquad 50 \text{ mg/m}^2 \text{ IV d1} \\ \text{Vincristine} \qquad\qquad 1.4 \text{ mg/m}^2 \text{ IV d1} \\ \text{Prednisone} \qquad\quad 100 \text{ mg/m}^2 \text{ IV d1–5}\end{array}\right\}$ 3 weeks

—McKelvey EM, *et al.* (1976) Adriamycin combination chemotherapy in malignant lymphoma. *Cancer* 38:1484–1493

M-BACOD $\left\{\begin{array}{l}\text{Methotrexate} \qquad 200 \text{ mg/m}^2 \text{ IV d 8, 15} \\ \text{Leukovorin} \qquad\quad 10 \text{ mg/m}^2 \text{ PO q} \\ \qquad\qquad\qquad\quad 6\text{h}\times 8 \text{ beginning 24 h} \\ \qquad\qquad\qquad\quad \text{after methotrexate} \\ \text{Bleomycin} \qquad\quad 4 \text{ u/m}^2 \text{ IV} \quad \text{d1} \\ \text{Adriamycin} \qquad\quad 45 \text{ mg/m}^2 \text{ IV d1} \\ \text{Cyclophosphamide} \; 600 \text{ mg/m}^2 \text{ IV d1} \\ \text{Vincristine} \qquad\qquad 1 \text{ mg/m}^2 \text{ IV d1} \\ \text{Dexamethasone} \quad 6 \text{ mg/m}^2 \text{ PO d1–5}\end{array}\right\}$ q 21 days

—Skarin AT, *et al.* (1983), MBACOD in advanced, diffuse histiocytic leukemia. *Proc Am Soc Clin Oncol* 2:220

MULTIPLE MYELOMA

MP $\left\{\begin{array}{l}\text{Melphalan} \qquad 10 \text{ mg/m}^2 \text{ PO d1–4} \\ \text{Prednisone} \qquad 60 \text{ mg/m}^2 \text{ PO d1–4}\end{array}\right\}$ q 6 weeks

—Southwest oncology group (1975), Southwest Oncology Group study: remission maintenance for multiple myeloma. *Arch Intern Med* 135:147–152

VAD $\left\{\begin{array}{l}\text{Vincristine} \qquad 0.4 \text{ mg/da CI d1–4} \\ \text{Doxorubicin} \qquad 9 \text{ mg/m}^2 \text{ da CI d1–4} \\ \text{Dexamethasone} \; 40 \text{ mg PO d1–4, 9-12, 17–20}\end{array}\right\}$ q 25 days

—Barlogie B, *et al.* (1984), Effective treatment of advanced multiple myeloma refractory to alkylating agents. *NEJM* 310(21):1353–1356

OVARIAN CANCER

CC $\left\{\begin{array}{l}\text{Cisplatin} \qquad\qquad 100 \text{ mg/m}^2 \\ \text{Cyclophosphamide} \; 100 \text{ mg/m}^2\end{array}\right\}$ q 21 days

—O'Mura GA (1989), A randomized trial of cyclophosphamide/cisplatin plus/minus doxorubicin in ovarian carcinoma: a gynecology-oncology group study. *J Clin Onc* 7(4):457–465

CP $\left\{\begin{array}{l}\text{Cyclophosphamide} \quad 600 \text{ mg/m}^2 \\ \text{Carboplatin} \qquad\qquad 300 \text{ mg/m}^2 \\ \text{(Paraplatin)}\end{array}\right\}$ q 21 days

—Edmonson JH (1989), Cyclophosphamide cisplatin versus cyclophosphamide/carboplatin in stage III-IV ovarian cancer. *JNCI* 81:1500–1504

TESTICULAR CANCER

PVB $\Big\{$
Cisplatin	20 mg/m^2 IV d1–5 q 3 wks × 3–4 cycles
Vinblastine	0.3 mg/kg IV d1 q 3 wks
Bleomycin	30 u IV q wk × 12

± Maintenance therapy: Vinblastine 0.3
mg/kg IV q 4 wks × 2 years

—Einhorn LH, Williams SD (1980), Chemotherapy of disseminated testicular cancer. *Cancer* 46:1339–1344

**ET
(salvage)** $\Big\{$
Etoposide	75 mg/m^2 IV d1–5	
Ifosfamide	1200 mg IV d1–5	q 21
Cisplatin	20 mg/m^2 IV d1–5	days × 4
Mesna	120 mg/m^2 IVB, *then*	
(or uroprotector)	1200 mg/m CI d1–5	

—Loehrer PJ, *et al.* (1986), VP-16 plus ifosfamide plus cisplatin as salvage therapy in refractory germ cell cancer. *J Clin
Oncology* 4:528–536

CI = continuous infusion; IV = intravenous;
IVB = intravenous bolus; PO = oral

Appendix 3: Recommendations for Handling Cytotoxic Agents. National Study Commission on Cytotoxic Exposure, Occupational Safety and Health Administration (OSHA), September 1987. Reprinted with permission.

PREAMBLE

The mutagenic, carcinogenic, and local irritant properties of many cytotoxic agents are well established and pose a hazard to the health of occupationally exposed individuals. These potential hazards necessitate special attention to the procedures utilized in the handling, preparation and administration of these drugs, and the proper disposal of residues and wastes. These recommendations are intended to provide information for the protection of personnel participating in the clinical process of chemotherapy. It is the responsibility of institutional and private health care providers to adopt and use appropriate procedures for protection and safety.

I. Environmental Protection

1. Preparation of cytotoxic agents should be performed in a Class II biological safety cabinet located in an area with minimal traffic and air turbulence. Class II Type A cabinets are the minimal requirement. Class II cabinets which are exhausted to the outside are preferred.

2. The biological safety cabinet must be certified by qualified personnel at least annually or any time the cabinet is physically moved.

II. Operator Protection

1. Disposable surgical latex gloves are recommended for all procedures involving cytotoxic agents.

2. Gloves should routinely be changed approximately every 30 minutes when working steadily with cytotoxic agents. Gloves should be removed immediately after overt contamination.

3. Protective barrier garments should be worn for all procedures involving the preparation and disposal of cytotoxic agents. These garments should have a closed front, long sleeves and closed cuff (either elastic or knit).

4. Protective garments must not be worn outside the work area.

III. Techniques and Precautions for Use in the Class II Biological Safety Cabinet

1. Special techniques and precautions must be utilized because of the vertical (downward) laminar airflow.

2. Clean surfaces of the cabinet using 70% alcohol and a disposable towel before and after preparation. Discard towel into a hazardous chemical waste container.

3. Prepare the work surface of the biological safety cabinet by covering it with a plastic-backed absorbent pad. This pad should be changed when the cabinet is cleaned or after a spill.

4. The biological safety cabinet should be operated with the blower on, 24 hours per day—seven days a week. Where the biological safety cabinet is utilized infrequently (e.g. 1 or 2 times weekly) it may be turned off after thoroughly cleaning all interior surfaces. Turn on the blower 15 minutes before beginning work in the cabinet.

5. Drug preparations must be performed only with the view screen at the recommended access opening. Professionally accepted practices concerning the aseptic preparation of injectable products should be followed.

6. All materials needed to complete the procedure should be placed into the biological safety cabinet before beginning work to

avoid interruptions of cabinet airflow. Allow a two to three minute period before beginning work for the unit to purge itself of airborne contaminants.

7. The proper procedures for use in the biological safety cabinet differ from those used in the horizontal laminar hood because of the nature of the airflow pattern. Clean air descends through the work zone from the top of the cabinet toward the work surface. As it descends, the air is split, with some leaving through the rear perforation and some leaving through the front perforation.

8. The least efficient area of the cabinet in terms of product and personnel protection is within three inches of the sides near the front opening, and work should not be performed in these areas.

9. Entry into and exit from the cabinet should be in a direct manner perpendicular to the face of the cabinet. Rapid movements of the hands in the cabinet and laterally through the protective air barrier should be avoided.

IV. Compounding Procedures and Techniques

1. Hands must be washed thoroughly before gloving and after gloves are removed.

2. Care must be taken to avoid puncturing of gloves and possible self-inoculation.

3. Syringes and I.V. sets with Luer-lock fittings should be used whenever possible to avoid spills due to disconnection.

4. To minimize aerosolization, vials containing cytotoxic agents should be vented with a hydrophobic filter to equalize internal pressure, or utilize negative pressure technique.

5. Before opening ampules, care should be taken to insure that no liquid remains in the tip of the ampule. A sterile disposable sponge should be wrapped around the neck

of the ampule to reduce aerosolization. Ampules should be broken in a direction away from the body.

6. For sealed vials, final drug measurement should be performed prior to removing the needle from the stopper of the vial and after the pressure has been equalized.

7. A closed collection vessel should be available in the biological safety cabinet or the original vial may be used to hold discarded excess drug solutions.

8. Cytotoxic agents should be properly labeled to identify the need for caution in handling (e.g., "Chemotherapy: Dispose of Properly").

9. The final prepared dosage form should be protected from leakage or breakage by being sealed in a transparent plastic container labeled "Do Not Open if Contents Appear to be Broken."

V. Precautions for Administration

1. Disposable surgical latex gloves should be worn during administration of cytotoxic agents. Hands must be washed thoroughly before gloving and after gloves are removed.

2. Protective barrier garments may be worn. Such garments should have a closed front, long sleeves and closed cuff (either elastic or knit).

3. Syringes and I.V. sets with Luer-lock fittings should be used whenever possible.

4. Special care must be taken in priming I.V. sets. The distal tip or needle cover must be removed before priming. Priming can be performed into a sterile, alcohol-dampened gauze sponge. Other acceptable methods of priming such as closed receptacles (e.g., evacuated containers) or back-filling of I.V. sets may be utilized. Do not prime sets or syringes into the sink or any open receptacle.

VI. Disposal Procedures

1. Place contaminated materials in a leakproof, puncture-proof container appropriately marked as hazardous chemical waste. These containers should be suitable to collect bottles, vials, gloves, disposable gowns and other materials used in the preparation and administration of cytotoxic agents.

2. Contaminated needles, syringes, sets and tubing should be disposed of intact. In order to prevent aerosolization, needles and syringes should not be clipped.

3. Cytotoxic drug waste should be transported according to the institutional procedures for hazardous material.

4. There is insufficient information to recommend any preferred method for disposal of cytotoxic drug waste.

   4.1 One acceptable method for disposal of hazardous wase is by incineration in an Environmental Protection Agency (EPA) permitted hazardous waste incinerator.

   4.2 Another acceptable method of disposal is by burial at an EPA permitted hazardous waste site.

   4.3 A licensed hazardous waste disposal company may be consulted for information concerning available methods of disposal in the local area.

VII. Personnel Policy Recommendations

1. Personnel involved in any aspect of the handling of cytotoxic agents must receive an orientation to the agents, including their known risks, and special training in safe handling procedures.

2. Access to the compounding area must be limited to authorized personnel.

3. Personnel working with these agents should be supervised regularly to insure compliance with procedures.

4. Acute exposures must be documented, and the employee referred for medical examination.

5. Personnel should refrain from applying cosmetics in the work area. Cosmetics may provide a source of prolonged exposure if contaminated.

6. Eating, drinking, chewing gum, smoking or storing food in areas where cytotoxic agents are handled should be prohibited. Each of these can be a source of ingestion if they are accidentally contaminated.

VIII. Monitoring Procedures

1. Policies and procedures to monitor the equipment and operating techniques of personnel handling cytotoxic agents should be implemented and performed on a regular basis with appropriate documentation. Specific methods of monitoring should be developed to meet the complexities of the function.

2. It is recommended that personnel involved in the preparation of cytotoxic agents be given periodic health examinations in accordance with institutional policy.

IX. Procedures for Acute Exposure or Spills

1. ACUTE EXPOSURE

   1.1 Overtly contaminated gloves or outer garments should be removed immediately.

   1.2 Hands must be washed after removing gloves. Some cytotoxic agents have been documented to penetrate gloves.

   1.3 In case of skin contact with a cytotoxic drug product, the affected area should be washed thoroughly with soap and water. Refer for medical attention as soon as possible.

1.4 For eye exposure, flush affected eye with copious amounts of water, and refer for medical attention immediately.

2. SPILLS

2.1 All personnel involved in the clean-up of a spill should wear protective barrier garments (e.g. gloves, gowns, etc.). These garments and other materials used in the process should be disposed of properly.

2.2 Double gloving is recommended for cleaning up spills.

Approved by the National Study Commission on Cytotoxic Exposure
September 1987

POSITION STATEMENT

The handling of cytotoxic agents by women who are pregnant, attempting to conceive, or breast feeding.

There are substantial data regarding the mutagenic, teratogenic and abortifacient properties of certain cytotoxic agents both in animals and humans who have received therapeutic doses of these agents. Additionally, the scientific literature suggests a possible association of occupational exposure to certain cytotoxic agents during the first trimester of pregnancy with fetal loss or malformation. These data suggest the need for caution when women who are pregnant, or attempting to conceive, handle cytotoxic agents. Incidentally, there is no evidence relating male exposure to cytotoxic agents with adverse fetal outcome.

There are no studies which address the possible risk associated with the occupational exposure to cytotoxic agents and the passage of these agents into breast milk. Nevertheless, it is prudent that women who are breast feeding should exercise caution in handling cytotoxic agents.

If all procedures for safe handling, such as those recommended by the Commission are complied with, the potential for exposure will be minimized.

Personnel should be provided with information to make an individual decision. This information should be provided in written form and it is advisable that a statement of understanding be signed.

It is essential to refer to individual state right-to-know laws to insure compliance.

Appendix 4: Cancer Chemotherapeutic Agents Compatibility Chart: Oncology Drug Compatibilities

Part A: Oncology Drug with Oncology Drug

Oncology Drug A	Oncology Drug B	Solution	Concentration of Drugs	Stability and Compatibility Comments
Bleomycin	Cisplatin and Cytarabine	Sodium chloride 0.9%	0.12 units/mL and 0.2 mg/mL and 1.05 mg/mL	Stable for 24 hours at 25°C
	Cytarabine and Cisplatin	Sodium chloride 0.9%	0.12 units/mL and 1.05 mg/mL and 0.2 mg/mL	Stable for 24 hours at 25°C
	Fluorouracil	Sodium chloride 0.9%	0.02–0.03 units/mL and 1 mg/mL	Stable for 7 days at 4°C. May adsorb onto plastic
	Methotrexate	Sodium chloride 0.9%	0.02–0.03 units/mL and 0.25–0.5 mg/mL	Drug decomposes within 7 days at 4°C
	Mitomycin	Sodium chloride 0.9%	0.02–0.03 units/mL and 0.01–0.05 mg/mL	Drug decomposes within 7 days at 4°C
	Vinblastine	Sodium chloride 0.9%	0.02–0.03 units/mL and 0.01–0.1 mg/mL	Stable for 7 days at 4°C. May adsorb onto plastic
	Vincristine	Sodium chloride 0.9%	0.02–0.03 units/mL and 0.05–0.1 mg/mL	Stable for 7 days at 4°C. May adsorb onto plastic
Carmustine	Cisplatin	Manufacturer's package inserts	1.4 mg/mL and 0.86 mg/mL	Both drugs stable for 3 hours at 23°C
Cisplatin	Bleomycin and Cytarabine	Sodium chloride 0.9%	0.2 mg/mL and 0.12 units/mL and 1.05 mg/mL	Stable for 24 hours at 25°C
	Carmustine	Dextrose 5%	0.86 mg/mL and 1.4 mg/mL	Both drugs stable for 3 hours at 23°C
	Carmustine	Sodium chloride 0.9%	0.86 mg/mL and 1.4 mg/mL	Both drugs stable for 3 hours at 23°C
	Cytarabine and Bleomycin	Sodium chloride 0.9%	0.2 mg/mL and 1.05 mg/mL and 0.12 units/mL	Stable for 24 hours at 25°C
	Etoposide	Sodium chloride 0.9%	0.2 mg/mL and 0.2–0.4 mg/mL	Stable for 24 hours at 25°C
	Etoposide	Dextrose 5% and sodium chloride 0.45%	0.2 mg/mL and 0.2–0.4 mg/mL	Stable for 24 hours at 25°C
Cyclophosphamide	Doxorubicin	Sodium chloride 0.9%	0.67 mg and 11.7 mg/mL	Both drugs stable for 7 days at 25°C
Cytarabine	Bleomycin and Cisplatin	Sodium chloride 0.9%	1.05 mg/mL and 0.12 units/mL and 0.2 mg/mL	Stable for 24 hours at 25°C
	Cisplatin and Bleomycin	Sodium chloride 0.9%	1.05 mg/mL and 0.2 mg/mL and 0.12 units/mL	Stable for 24 hours at 25°C
	Daunorubicin and Etoposide	Dextrose 5%	200 mg and 25 mg and 300 mg	All drugs stable for 72 hours at 20°C
	Daunorubicin and Etoposide	Sodium chloride 0.45%	200 mg and 25 mg and 300 mg	All drugs stable for 72 hours at 20°C
	Etoposide and Daunorubicin	Dextrose 5%	200 mg and 300 mg and 25 mg	All drugs stable for 72 hours at 20°C
	Etoposide and Daunorubicin	Sodium chloride 0.45%	200 mg and 300 mg and 25 mg	All drugs stable for 72 hours at 20°C
	Fluorouracil	Dextrose 5%	0.4 mg/mL and 0.25 mg/mL	Both drugs stable for 8 hours at 25°C; no significant UV spectra changes
	Methotrexate	Dextrose 5%	0.4 mg/mL and 0.2 mg/mL	Both drugs stable for 8 hours at 25°C; no significant UV spectra changes
	Methotrexate	Dextrose 5%	30–50 mg/12 mL and 12 mg/12 mL	Hydrocortisone Sodium Succinate 15–25 mg/12 mL; all drugs stable for 24 hours at 25°C

For further information regarding stability and compatibility of oncology drugs, phone (800) CETUS-RX. Please consult complete prescribing information for any drug mentioned.
Source: © 1988 Cetus Corporation. Cetus is pleased to grant reprint privileges for "Stability and Compatibility of Intravenous Oncology Drugs—1988 Reference Guide for Your Practice."

Appendix 4: Cancer Chemotherapeutic Agents Compatibility Chart (*continued*)

Part A: Oncology Drug with Oncology Drug

Oncology Drug A	Oncology Drug B	Solution	Concentration of Drugs	Stability and Compatibility Comments
Cytarabine—cont'd	Methotrexate	Elliot's B solution	30–50 mg/12 mL and 12 mg/12 mL	Hydrocortisone Sodium Succinate 15–25 mg/12 mL; all drugs stable for 24 hours at 25°C
	Methotrexate	Lactated Ringer's	30–50 mg/12 mL and 12 mg/12 mL	Hydrocortisone Sodium Succinate 15–25 mg/12 mL; all drugs stable for 24 hours at 25°C
	Methotrexate	Sodium chloride 0.9%	30–50 mg/12 mL and 12 mg/12 mL	Hydrocortisone Sodium Succinate 15–25 mg/12 mL; all drugs stable for 24 hours at 25°C
	Vincristine	Dextrose 5%	0.016 mg/mL and 0.004 mg/mL	Both drugs stable for 8 hours at 25°C; no significant UV spectra changes
Daunorubicin	Cytarabine and Etoposide	Dextrose 5%	25 mg and 200 mg and 300 mg	All drugs stable for 72 hours at 20°C
	Cytarabine and Etoposide	Sodium chloride 0.45%	25 mg and 200 mg and 300 mg	All drugs stable for 72 hours at 20°C
	Etoposide and Cytarabine	Dextrose 5%	25 mg and 300 mg and 200 mg	All drugs stable for 72 hours at 20°C
	Etoposide and Cytarabine	Sodium chloride 0.45%	25 mg and 300 mg and 200 mg	All drugs stable for 72 hours at 20°C
Doxorubicin	Cyclophosphamide Fluorouracil	Sodium chloride 0.9%	11.7 mg/mL and 0.67 mg/mL	Both drugs stable for 7 days at 25°C
		Dextrose 5%	0.01 mg/mL and 0.25 mg/mL	Precipitates; color change
	Vinblastine	Sodium chloride 0.9%	0.5–1.5 mg/mL and 0.075–0.15 mg/mL	May be stable for 10 days at 8 to 32°C, however, HPLC erratic
	Vincristine	Dextrose 2.5% and sodium chloride 0.45%	1.4 mg/mL and 0.033 mg/mL	Both drugs stable for 14 days at 25°C
	Vincristine	Sodium chloride 0.9%	1.4 mg/mL and 0.033 mg/mL	Both drugs stable for 14 days at 25°C
	Vincristine	Sodium chloride 0.45% and Ringer's	1.4 mg/mL and 0.033 mg/mL	Both drugs stable for 1 and 7 days, respectively, at 25°C
Etoposide	Cisplatin	Dextrose 5% and sodium chloride 0.45%	0.2 mg/mL and 0.2 mg/mL	Stable for 24 hours at 25°C
	Cisplatin	Dextrose 5% and sodium chloride 0.45%	0.4 mg/mL and 0.2 mg/mL	Mannitol 1.875% and Potassium Chloride 0.02 mEq/mL; stable for 24 hours at 25°C
	Cisplatin	Sodium chloride 0.9%	0.2–0.4 mg/mL and 0.2 mg/mL	Stable for 24 hours at 25°C
	Cytarabine and Daunorubicin	Dextrose 5%	300 mg and 200 mg and 25 mg	All drugs stable for 72 hours at 20°C
	Cytarabine and Daunorubicin	Sodium chloride 0.45%	300 mg and 200 mg and 25 mg	All drugs stable for 72 hours at 20°C
	Daunorubicin and Cytarabine	Dextrose 5%	300 mg and 25 mg and 200 mg	All drugs stable for 72 hours at 20°C
	Daunorubicin and Cytarabine	Sodium chloride 0.45%	300 mg and 25 mg and 200 mg	All drugs stable for 72 hours at 20°C

			Concentration	Remarks
Fluorouracil	Bleomycin	Sodium chloride 0.9%	1 mg/mL and 0.02–0.03 units/mL	Stable for 7 days at 4°C; may adsorb onto plastic
	Cytarabine	Dextrose 5%	0.25 mg/mL and 0.4 mg/mL	Both drugs stable for 8 hours at 25°C; no significant UV spectra changes
	Doxorubicin	Dextrose 5%	0.25 mg/mL and 0.01 mg/mL	Precipitates; color change
	Methotrexate	Dextrose 5%	0.25 mg/mL and 0.2 mg/mL	Both drugs decompose within 1 hour at 25°C; altered UV spectra
	Methotrexate	Fluorouracil (as diluent)	500 mg/10 mL and 50 mg/10 mL	Both drugs stable for 24 hours at 25°C
	Vincristine	Dextrose 5%	0.01 mg/mL and 0.004 mg/mL	Both drugs stable for 8 hours at 25°C; no UV spectra changes
Methotrexate	Bleomycin	Sodium chloride 0.9%	0.25–0.5 mg/mL and 0.02–0.03 units/mL	Drug decomposes within 7 days at 4°C
	Cytarabine	Dextrose 5%	12 mg/12 mL and 30–50 mg/12 mL	Hydrocortisone Sodium Succinate 15–25 mg/12 mL; all drugs stable for 24 hours at 25°C
	Cytarabine	Sodium chloride 0.9%	12 mg/12 mL and 30–50 mg/12 mL	Hydrocortisone Sodium Succinate 15–25 mg/12 mL; all drugs stable for 24 hours at 25°C
	Cytarabine	Lactated Ringer's	12 mg/12 mL and 30–50 mg/12 mL	Hydrocortisone Sodium Succinate 15–25 mg/12 mL; all drugs stable for 24 hours at 25°C
	Cytarabine	Elliot's B solution	12 mg/12 mL and 30–50 mg/12 mL	Hydrocortisone Sodium Succinate 15–25 mg/12 mL; all drugs stable for 10 hours at 25°C
	Cytarabine	Dextrose 5%	0.2 mg/mL and 0.4 mg/mL	Both drugs stable for 8 hours at 25°C; no UV spectra changes
	Fluorouracil	Fluorouracil (as diluent)	50 mg/10 mL and 500 mg/10 mL	Both drugs stable for 24 hours at 25°C
	Fluorouracil	Dextrose 5%	0.2 mg/mL and 0.25 mg/mL	Both drugs decompose within 1 hour at 25°C; altered UV spectra
	Vincristine	Dextrose 5%	0.008–0.1 mg/mL and 0.004–0.01 mg/mL	Both drugs stable for 8 hours at 25°C; no UV spectra changes
Mitomycin	Bleomycin	Sodium chloride 0.9%	0.01–0.05 mg/mL and 0.02–0.03 units/mL	Drug decomposes within 7 days at 4°C
Vinblastine	Bleomycin	Sodium chloride 0.9%	0.01–0.1 mg/mL and 0.02–0.03 units/mL	Stable for 7 days at 4°C; may adsorb onto plastic
	Doxorubicin	Sodium chloride 0.9%	0.075–0.15 mg/mL and 0.5–1.5 mg/mL	May be stable for 10 days at 8 to 32°C, however, HPLC erratic
Vincristine	Bleomycin	Sodium chloride 0.9%	0.05–0.1 mg/mL and 0.02–0.03 units/mL	Stable for 7 days at 4°C, may adsorb onto plastic
	Cytarabine	Dextrose 5%	0.004 mg/mL and 0.016 mg/mL	Both drugs stable for 8 hours at 25°C; no significant UV spectra changes
	Doxorubicin	Sodium chloride 0.9%	0.033 mg/mL and 1.4 mg/mL	Both drugs stable for 14 hours at 25°C
	Doxorubicin	Dextrose 2.5% and sodium chloride 0.45%	0.033 mg/mL and 1.4 mg/mL	Both drugs stable for 14 hours at 25°C
	Doxorubicin	Sodium chloride 0.45% and Ringer's	0.033 mg/mL and 1.4 mg/mL	Both drugs stable for 7 and 1 days, respectively, at 25°C
	Fluorouracil	Dextrose 5%	0.004 mg/mL and 0.01 mg/mL	Both drugs stable for 8 hours at 25°C; no UV spectra changes
	Methotrexate	Dextrose 5%	0.004–0.01 mg/mL and 0.008–0.1 mg/mL	Both drugs stable for 8 hours at 25°C; no UV spectra changes

Appendix 4:   Cancer Chemotherapeutic Agents Compatibility Chart (*continued*)

B: Oncology Drug with Other Drugs

Oncology Drug	Other Drug	Solution	Concentration of Drugs	Stability and Compatibility Comments
Bleomycin	Amikacin sulfate	Sodium chloride 0.9%	0.02–0.03 units/mL and 1.25 mg/mL	Stable for 7 days at 4°C
	Aminophylline	Sodium chloride 0.9%	0.02–0.03 units/mL and 0.25 mg/mL	Drug decomposes within 7 days at 4°C
	Ascorbic acid	Sodium chloride 0.9%	0.02–0.03 units/mL and 2.5–5 mg/mL	Drug decomposes within 7 days at 4°C
	Carbenicillin disodium	Sodium chloride 0.9%	0.02–0.03 units/mL and 4–12 mg/mL	Drug decomposes within 7 days at 4°C
	Cefazolin sodium	Sodium chloride 0.9%	0.02–0.03 units/mL and 1 mg/mL	Drug decomposes within 7 days at 4°C
	Cephalothin sodium	Sodium chloride 0.9%	0.02–0.03 units/mL and 2–5 mg/mL	Drug decomposes within 7 days at 4°C
	Cephapirin sodium	Sodium chloride 0.9%	0.02–0.03 units/mL and 3 mg/mL	Stable for 7 days at 4°C; may adsorb onto plastic
	Dexamethasone sodium phosphate	Sodium chloride 0.9%	0.02–0.03 units/mL and 0.05 mg/mL	Stable for 7 days at 4°C; may adsorb onto plastic
	Diazepam	Sodium chloride 0.9%	0.02–0.03 units/mL and 0.05–0.1 mg/mL	Physically incompatible
	Diphenhydramine	Sodium chloride 0.9%	0.02–0.03 units/mL and 0.1 mg/mL	Stable for 7 days at 4°C; may adsorb onto plastic
	Gentamicin sulfate	Sodium chloride 0.9%	0.02–0.03 units/mL and 0.01–0.6 mg/mL	Stable for 7 days at 4°C; may adsorb onto plastic
	Heparin sodium	Dextrose 5%	0.02–0.03 units/mL and 10–1,000 units/mL	Stable for 24 hours; may adsorb onto plastic
	Heparin sodium	Sodium chloride 0.9%	0.02–0.03 units/mL and 10–200 units/mL	Stable for 7 days at 4°C; may adsorb onto plastic
	Hydrocortisone sodium phosphate	Sodium chloride 0.9%	0.02–0.03 units/mL and 0.1–2 mg/mL	Stable for 7 days at 4°C; may adsorb onto plastic
	Hydrocortisone sodium succinate	Sodium chloride 0.9%	0.02–0.03 units/mL and 0.3–2.5 mg/mL	Drug decomposes within 7 days at 4°C
	Nafcillin sodium	Sodium chloride 0.9%	0.02–0.03 units/mL and 2.5 mg/mL	Drug decomposes within 7 days at 4°C
	Penicillin G sodium	Sodium chloride 0.9%	0.02–0.03 units/mL and 2,000–5,000 units/mL	Drug decomposes within 7 days at 4°C
	Phenytoin sodium	Sodium chloride 0.9%	0.02–0.03 units/mL and 0.5 mg/mL	Stable for 7 days at 4°C; may adsorb onto plastic
	Streptomycin sulfate	Sodium chloride 0.9%	0.02–0.03 units/mL and 4 mg/mL	Stable for 7 days at 4°C; may adsorb onto plastic
	Terbutaline sulfate	Sodium chloride 0.9%	0.02–0.03 units/mL and 0.0075 mg/mL	Drug decomposes within 7 days at 4°C
	Tobramycin sulfate	Sodium chloride 0.9%	0.02–0.03 units/mL and 0.5 mg/mL	Stable for 7 days at 4°C; may adsorb onto plastic
Carmustine	Sodium bicarbonate	Dextrose 5%	0.1 mg/mL and 0.1 mEq/mL	Drug decomposes within 1 hour at 25°C
	Sodium bicarbonate	Sodium 0.9%	0.1 mg/mL and 0.1 mEq/mL	Drug decomposes within 1 hour at 25°C
Cisplatin	Metoclopramide	Manufacturer's package inserts	173 mg and 10–160 mg	Use immediately
Cyclophosphamide	Metoclopramide	Manufacturer's package inserts	560 mg and 10–160 mg	Physically compatible for 24 hours at 25°C
Cytarabine	Cephalothin sodium	Dextrose 5%	0.8 mg/mL and 1 mg/mL	Both drugs stable for 8 hours at 25°C
	Methylprednisolone sodium succinate	Dextrose 5% and sodium chloride 0.9%	0.36 mg/mL and 0.25 mg/mL	Physically compatible for 24 hours
	Methylprednisolone sodium succinate	Dextrose 10% and sodium chloride 0.9%	0.36 mg/mL and 0.25 mg/mL	Physically compatible for 24 hours

Drug	Additive	Solution	Concentration	Comment
Cytarabine—cont'd	Methylprednisolone sodium succinate	Sodium chloride 0.9%	0.36 mg/mL and 0.25 mg/mL	Physically compatible for 24 hours
	Methylprednisolone sodium succinate	Ringer's	0.36 mg/mL and 0.25 mg/mL	Physically incompatible
	Methylprednisolone sodium succinate	Sodium lactate ⅙ molar	0.36 mg/mL and 0.25 mg/mL	Physically incompatible
	Metoclopramide	Manufacturer's package inserts	50–500 mg and 10–160 mg	Physically compatible for 48 hours at 25°C
	Prednisolone sodium phosphate	Dextrose 5%	0.4 mg/mL and 0.2 mg/mL	Both drugs stable for 8 hours at 25°C
	Sodium bicarbonate	Dextrose 5%	0.2–1 mg/mL and 0.05 mEq/mL	Stable for 7 days at 8 and 22°C in glass or PVC
	Sodium bicarbonate	Dextrose 5% and sodium chloride 0.225%	0.2–1 mg/mL and 0.05 mEq/mL	Stable for 7 days at 8 and 22°C in glass or PVC
Dacarbazine	Heparin sodium	Sodium chloride 0.9%	10 mg/mL and 100 units/mL	Precipitates in IV line
	Hydrocortisone sodium phosphate	Not specified	Not specified	Physically compatible
	Hydrocortisone sodium succinate	Not specified	Not specified	Precipitates
	Lidocaine hydrochloride	Not specified	Not specified and 1% or 2%	Physically compatible
	Metoclopramide	Manufacturer's package inserts	140 mg and 10–160 mg	Physically compatible for 8 hours at 25°C
Daunorubicin	Dexamethasone sodium phosphate	Not specified	Not specified	Precipitates
	Heparin sodium	Dextrose 5%	0.2 mg/mL and 4 units/mL	Physically incompatible
	Hydrocortisone sodium succinate	Dextrose 5%	0.2 mg/mL and 0.5 mg/mL	Physically compatible
Doxorubicin	Aminophylline	Not specified	Not specified	Color change
	Cephalothin sodium	Not specified	Not specified	Precipitates
	Dexamethasone sodium phosphate	Not specified	Not specified	Precipitates
	Diazepam	Not specified	Not specified	Precipitates
	Furosemide	Manufacturer's package inserts	2 mg/mL and 10 mg/mL	Precipitates
	Heparin sodium	Manufacturer's package inserts	2 mg/mL and 1000 units/mL	Precipitates
	Hydrocortisone sodium succinate	Not specified	Not specified	Precipitates
	Metoclopramide	Manufacturer's package inserts	103.8 mg and 10–160 mg	Physically compatible for 24 hours at 25°C

Appendix 4: Cancer Chemotherapeutic Agents Compatibility Chart (*continued*)

B: Oncology Drug with Other Drugs

Oncology Drug	Other Drug	Solution	Concentration of Drugs	Stability and Compatibility Comments
Etoposide	Metoclopramide	Manufacturer's package inserts	86.5 mg and 10–160 mg	Physically compatible for 48 hours at 25°C
	Morphine sulfate	Not specified	Not specified and 50 mg/mL	Stable for 24 hours
	Potassium chloride	Sodium chloride 0.9%	0.2–0.4 mg/mL and 0.04 mEq/mL	Physically compatible for 8 hours
	Potassium chloride	Dextrose 5%	0.2–0.4 mg/mL and 0.04 mEq/mL	Physically compatible for 8 hours
	Potassium chloride	Lactated Ringer's	0.2–0.4 mg/mL and 0.04 mEq/mL	Physically compatible for 8 hours
	Potassium chloride	Mannitol 10%	0.2–0.4 mg/mL and 0.04 mEq/mL	Physically compatible for 8 hours
Floxuridine	Heparin sodium	Sodium chloride 0.9%	2.5–12 mg/mL and 200 units/mL	Stable for 4 days at 37°C
Fluorouracil	Cephalothin sodium	Dextrose 5%	0.5 mg/mL and 1 mg/mL	Both drugs stable for 8 hours at 25°C; no UV spectra changes
	Diazepam	Not specified	Not specified	Precipitates
	Droperidol	Manufacturer's package inserts	50 mg/mL and 2.5 mg/mL	Precipitates
	Metoclopramide	Manufacturer's package inserts	840 mg and 10–160 mg	Physically incompatible
	Prednisolone sodium phosphate	Dextrose 5%	0.25 mg/mL and 0.2 mg/mL	Both drugs stable for 8 hours at 25°C; no UV spectra changes
Mechlorethamine	Methohexital	Dextrose 5%	0.04 mg/mL and 2 mg/mL	Drug decomposes within 3 hours
	Methohexital	Sodium chloride 0.9%	0.04 mg/mL and 2 mg/mL	Drug decomposes within 3 hours
Methotrexate	Cephalothin sodium	Dextrose 5%	0.4 mg/mL and 1 mg/mL	Both drugs stable for 8 hours at 25°C; no UV spectra changes
	Droperidol	Manufacturer's package inserts	25 mg/mL and 2.5 mg/mL	Precipitates
	Metoclopramide	Manufacturer's package inserts	50–200 mg and 10–160 mg	Use immediately
	Prednisolone sodium phosphate	Dextrose 5%	0.2 mg/mL and 0.2 mg/mL	Both drugs decompose within 1 hour at 25°C; UV spectra changes
	Sodium bicarbonate	Dextrose 5%	0.75 mg/mL and 0.05 mEq/mL	Stable for 7 days at 5°C or for 72 hours at 25°C when exposed to light
Mitomycin	Heparin sodium	Sodium chloride 0.9%	5–15 mg/30 mL and 1000–10,000 units/30 mL	Stable for 48 hours at 25°C
Vinblastine	Furosemide	Manufacturer's package inserts	1 mg/mL and 10 mg/mL	Precipitates
	Heparin sodium	Sodium chloride 0.9%	1 mg/mL and 200 units/mL	Decomposes within 24 hours at 37°C
	Metoclopramide	Manufacturer's package inserts	9.5 mg and 10–160 mg	Physically compatible for 48 hours at 25°C
Vincristine	Furosemide	Manufacturer's package inserts	1 mg/mL and 10 mg/mL	Precipitates
	Metoclopramide	Manufacturer's package inserts	2.4 mg and 10–160 mg	Physically compatible for 48 hours at 25°C

Appendix 5:   Nomograms for Determination of Body Surface Area from Height and Weight (Adults)[1]

Height	Body surface area	Weight
cm 200 — 79 in 78 195 — 77 76 190 — 75 74 185 — 73 72 180 — 71 70 175 — 69 68 170 — 67 66 165 — 65 64 160 — 63 62 155 — 61 60 150 — 59 58 145 — 57 56 140 — 55 54 135 — 53 52 130 — 51 50 125 — 49 48 120 — 47 46 115 — 45 44 110 — 43 42 105 — 41 40 cm 100 — 39 in	2.80 m^2 2.70 2.60 2.50 2.40 2.30 2.20 2.10 2.00 1.95 1.90 1.85 1.80 1.75 1.70 1.65 1.60 1.55 1.50 1.45 1.40 1.35 1.30 1.25 1.20 1.15 1.10 1.05 1.00 0.95 0.90 0.86 m^2	kg 150 — 330 lb 145 — 320 140 — 310 135 — 300 130 — 290 125 — 280 120 — 270 115 — 260 110 — 250 105 — 240 100 — 230 95 — 220 90 — 210 85 — 200 80 — 190 75 — 180 70 — 170 65 — 160 60 — 150 55 — 140 50 — 130 45 — 120 40 — 110 105 100 95 90 85 80 35 — 75 70 kg 30 — 66 lb

[1]From the formula of DuBois and DuBois. *Arch. micrn. Med.* 17.863 (1916): S = W$^{0.696}$ × H$^{0.726}$ × 71.84, or log S = log W × 0.425 + log H × 0.725 + 1.8564 (S = body surface in square centimeters. W = weight in kilograms. H = height in centimeters).

The body surface area results by the point of intersection on the middle scale when a straight line joins the height and weight scale (e.g. Patient A weighs 109 Kg and the height is 171 cm. The patient's BSA(m^2) is 2.2)

(*Source:* Hubbard SM, Seipp CA: Administration of Cancer Treatments: Practical Guide for Physicians and Oncology Nurses, in DeVita VJ, Hellman S, Rosenberg SA: *Cancer Principles and Practices of Oncology.* JB Lippincott Co., Philadelphia 1982 p. 1785.)

Appendix 5: Nomograms for Determination of Body Surface Area from Height and Weight (Adults)[1]

Height	Body surface area	Weight

[1]From the formula of DuBois and DuBois. *Arch. micrn. Med.* 17.863 (1916): S = W$^{0.696}$ × H$^{0.726}$ × 71.84, or log S = log W × 0.425 + log H × 0.725 + 1.8564 (S = body surface in square centimeters. W = weight in kilograms. H = height in centimeters).

The body surface area results by the point of intersection on the middle scale when a straight line joins the height and weight scale (e.g. Patient A weighs 109 Kg and the height is 171 cm. The patient's BSA(m^2) is 2.2)

(*Source:* Hubbard SM, Seipp CA: Administration of Cancer Treatments: Practical Guide for Physicians and Oncology Nurses, in DeVita VJ, Hellman S, Rosenberg SA: *Cancer Principles and Practices of Oncology.* JB Lippincott Co., Philadelphia 1982 p. 1785.)

Appendix 5: Nomograms for Determination of Body Surface Area from Height and Weight (Adults)[1]

Height	Body surface area	Weight

```
Height                     Body surface area          Weight

cm 200 — 79 in             — 2.80 m²            kg 150 — 330 lb
        78                                         145 — 320
  195   77                 — 2.70                  140 — 310
        76                                         135 — 300
  190   75                 — 2.60                  130 — 290
        74                                         125 — 280
  185   73                 — 2.50                  120 — 270
        72                                             — 260
  180   71                 — 2.40                  115 — 250
        70                 — 2.30                  110 — 240
  175   69                                         105 — 230
        68                 — 2.20                  100 — 220
  170   67
        66                 — 2.10                   95 — 210
  165   65                                          90 — 200
        64                 — 2.00
  160   63                 — 1.95                   85 — 190
        62                 — 1.90                       — 180
  155   61                 — 1.85                   80
        60                 — 1.80                   75 — 170
  150   59                 — 1.75                       — 160
        58                 — 1.70                   70
  145   57                 — 1.65                       — 150
        56                 — 1.60                   65
  140   55                 — 1.55                       — 140
        54                 — 1.50                   60
  135   53                 — 1.45                       — 130
        52                 — 1.40                   55
  130   51                 — 1.35                       — 120
        50                 — 1.30                   50
  125   49                 — 1.25                       — 110
        48                 — 1.20                       — 105
  120   47                 — 1.15                   45 — 100
        46                                             — 95
  115   45                 — 1.10                       — 90
        44                 — 1.05                   40
  110   43                 — 1.00                       — 85
        42                 — 0.95                       — 80
  105   41                                         35  — 75
        40                 — 0.90                       — 70
cm 100  39 in              — 0.86 m²          kg 30 — 66 lb
```

[1]From the formula of DuBois and DuBois. *Arch. micrn. Med.* 17.863 (1916): S = $W^{0.696} \times H^{0.726} \times 71.84$, or log S = log $W \times 0.425 + \log H \times 0.725 + 1.8564$ (S = body surface in square centimeters. W = weight in kilograms. H = height in centimeters).

The body surface area results by the point of intersection on the middle scale when a straight line joins the height and weight scale (e.g. Patient A weighs 109 Kg and the height is 171 cm. The patient's BSA(m²) is 2.2)

(*Source:* Hubbard SM, Seipp CA: Administration of Cancer Treatments: Practical Guide for Physicians and Oncology Nurses, in DeVita VJ, Hellman S, Rosenberg SA: *Cancer Principles and Practices of Oncology.* JB Lippincott Co., Philadelphia 1982 p. 1785.)

Appendix 6: Table of Standard Body Weights (Pounds—Kilograms)

MEN

Height		Age													
Feet	Inches	25–29		30–34		35–39		40–44		45–49		50–54		55 up	
		Lbs.	Kgs.	Lbs.	Kgs.	Lbs.	Kgs.	Lbs.	Kgs.	Lbs.	Kgs.	Lbs.	Kgs.	Lbs.	Kgs.
4	11	122	55.5	125	56.8	127	57.7	130	59.1	132	60.0	133	60.5	134	60.9
5	0	124	56.4	127	57.7	129	58.6	132	60.0	134	60.9	135	61.4	136	61.8
	1	126	57.3	129	58.6	131	59.5	134	60.9	136	61.8	137	62.3	138	62.7
	2	128	58.2	131	59.5	133	60.5	136	61.8	138	62.7	139	63.2	140	63.6
	3	131	59.6	134	60.9	136	61.8	139	63.2	141	64.1	142	64.5	143	65.0
	4	134	60.9	137	62.3	140	63.6	142	64.6	144	65.5	145	65.9	146	66.4
	5	138	62.7	141	64.1	144	65.5	146	66.4	148	67.3	149	67.7	150	68.2
	6	142	64.5	145	65.9	148	67.3	150	68.2	152	69.1	153	69.5	154	70.0
	7	146	66.4	149	67.7	152	69.1	154	70.0	156	70.9	157	71.4	158	71.8
	8	150	68.2	154	70.0	157	71.4	159	72.3	161	73.2	162	73.6	163	74.1
	9	154	70.0	158	71.8	162	73.6	164	74.6	166	75.5	167	75.9	168	76.4
	10	158	71.8	163	74.1	167	75.9	169	76.8	171	77.7	172	78.2	173	78.6
	11	163	74.1	168	76.4	172	78.2	175	79.5	177	80.5	178	80.9	179	81.4
6	0	169	76.8	174	79.1	178	80.9	181	82.3	183	83.2	184	83.6	185	84.1
	1	175	79.5	180	81.8	184	83.6	187	85.0	190	86.4	191	86.8	192	87.3
	2	181	82.3	186	84.5	191	86.8	194	88.2	197	89.5	198	90.0	199	90.5
	3	187	85.0	192	87.3	197	89.5	201	91.4	204	92.7	205	93.2	206	93.6

WOMEN

Height		Age													
Feet	Inches	25–29		30–34		35–39		40–44		45–49		50–54		55 up	
		Lbs.	Kgs.	Lbs.	Kgs.	Lbs.	Kgs.	Lbs.	Kgs.	Lbs.	Kgs.	Lbs.	Kgs.	Lbs.	Kgs.
4	11	116	52.7	119	54.1	122	55.5	126	57.3	129	58.6	131	59.6	132	60.0
5	0	118	53.6	121	55.0	124	56.4	128	58.2	131	59.5	133	60.5	134	60.9
	1	120	54.5	123	55.9	126	57.3	130	59.1	133	60.5	135	61.4	137	62.3
	2	122	55.5	125	56.8	129	58.6	133	60.5	136	61.8	138	62.7	140	63.6
	3	125	56.8	128	58.2	132	60.0	136	61.8	139	63.2	141	64.1	143	65.0
	4	129	58.6	132	60.0	136	61.7	139	63.2	142	64.5	144	65.5	146	66.4
	5	132	60.0	136	61.8	140	63.6	143	65.0	146	66.4	148	67.3	150	68.2
	6	136	61.8	140	63.8	144	65.5	147	66.8	151	68.6	152	69.1	153	69.6
	7	140	63.6	144	65.5	148	67.3	151	68.6	155	70.5	157	71.4	158	71.8
	8	144	65.5	148	67.3	152	69.1	155	70.5	159	72.3	162	73.6	163	74.1
	9	148	67.3	152	69.1	156	70.9	159	72.3	163	74.1	166	75.5	167	75.9
	10	152	69.1	155	70.5	159	72.3	162	73.6	166	75.5	170	77.3	173	78.6
	11	155	70.5	158	71.8	162	73.6	166	75.5	170	77.3	174	79.1	177	80.5
6	0	159	72.3	162	73.6	165	75.0	169	76.8	173	78.6	177	80.5	182	82.7

Occasionally drug doses are calculated on the basis of a person's standard or ideal body weight.
Determine the patient's standard weight from above, and compare this with the patient's actual weight. Whichever of these two numbers is lower should be used to determine the patient's dosage.

INDEX

ABVD (adriamycin, bleomycin, vinblastine, dacarbazine), 41–42
  plus MOPP, 41–42
  side effects of, 88
Achromatic microscope, 5
Acrindinyl anisidide, 141–144
Actinomycin D, 37
  nursing care plan for, 203–207
  side effects of, 81
Active immunotherapy, 40
Acute cerebellar syndromes, 123, 124–125
Acute leukemia, 44, 426
Acute nonlymphocytic leukemia (ANLL), 39
Adenine, 35
Adjuvant chemotherapy. *See* Chemotherapy
Administration of chemotherapy, 375–395
  ambulatory settings, 376–378
  anaphylactic reaction, 387–395
  assessment, 378, 379
  chemotherapy checklist, 376, 377
  controversial issues, 406–407
  dose calculations and modifications, 407–408
  extravasation reaction, 383–387, 400–401
  guidelines, 433–434
  home settings, 376–378
  hypersensitivity reaction, 387–395
  qualifications for, 375
  routes of, 397–400
  technical expertise, 12
  See also Drug delivery systems
Adoptive immunotherapy, 40
Adrenal steroid inhibitor, 149–152
Adrenocorticoids, 39, 145–148
Adriamycin, 42, 384, 387
  nursing care plan for, 213–217
Adrucil, 238–241
Aerosolization, 428
Akathesia, 100
Alcohol abuse, history of, 94
Alkeran, 280–284
Alkylating agents, 34–35, 41
  common, 35
  nursing care plans for specific drugs, 169, 171, 179, 183, 188,

197, 218, 244, 256, 270, 273, 280, 295, 332, 343
  side effects of, 35, 52, 53, 84, 87, 88, 124, 526
Allergic reaction
  to platelet transfusion, 61
  see also Hypersensitivity reaction
Allopurinol, 120, 121
Alopecia, 84–85
  nursing care plan for, 86
Altretamine, 244–246
Ambulatory care settings, 376–378
  chemotherapeutic agents used in, 378
  continuous infusion systems, 416–422
Amenorrhea, 35, 61, 87
American Cancer Society (ACS), 5, 9, 13, 23
American Nurses Association, Code for Nurses, 22–23
Amethopyerin, 290–294
Aminoglutethimide, 149–152
AMSA, 141–144
ANA and ONS: Standards of Oncology Nursing Practice (ANA), 12
Anagen, 84
Anaphylactic reaction, 39, 378, 387–395
  management of, 393
  nursing care plan for, 394–395
Anaphylactoid reaction, 387
Anaphylaxis, 387
Anaphylaxis kit, 379
Androgens, 38, 39
  nursing care plan for, 153–155
Anemia, 61–62
  bone marrow depression and, 61–62
  degrees of, 63
Anesthesia, early use of, 5
Antecubital fossa, 406, 407
Anthracenediones, 313
Anthracycline antibiotics, 37
  nursing care plan for, 208, 213
  side effects of, 105
Antiandrogens, 242
Antibiotics, 7, 37
  anthracycline (*see* Anthracycline antibiotics)

antitumor (*see* Antitumor antibiotics)
  common, 37
  nursing care plan for, 322–325
  side effects of, 37, 52, 69, 84
Anticipatory nausea and vomiting (ANV), 89, 93–94, 101
Antidotes
  for doxorubicin, 384
  for mechlorethamine, 383
  for vesicant/irritant drugs, 385–386
Antiemetics, 95
  pharmacology of, 96–99
  research, 101
  side effects of, 97–101
Antiemetic treatment, 93, 94–101
  designing, 94
  extrapyramidal reactions, 100–101
Antiestrogens, 38, 39, 337
Antifols, 6
Antifungal treatment, 70
Antihistamines, 99–100
Antihormone agents, 268, 310
Antimetabolites, 31, 35–37
  common, 37
  and neurotoxicity, 124
  nontoxicity of, 87
  nursing care plans for specific drugs, 193, 233, 238, 247, 285, 290, 340, 346
  side effects of, 37, 52, 53, 69, 84
Antineoplastic agents. *See* Chemotherapeutic agents
Antisepsis, 5
Antitumor antibiotics, 37, 53
  nursing care plans for specific drugs, 163, 203, 251, 305, 313
Appetite, increased, 38
Arabinosyl cytosine, 193–196
Ara-C, 193–196, 399
Arachnoiditis, 121, 123
Arsenic, 4
Asparagine, 39
Aspirin-containing drugs, 58, 59–60
Assessment
  for ambulatory and home chemotherapy, 378
  in clinical trials, 20
  for dosage, 407–408
  of extravasion, 390

Assessment (*cont.*)
  nursing, 11
  risk/benefit, 20, 22
  post-chemotherapy, 378–383
  pre-chemotherapy, 378–383
Ativan, 98
Atrabilis, 4
Audiograms, 127
Auditory loss, 127
Autologous BMT, 7
  complications, 45, 112
  phases of, 44–45
Autonomic neuropathy, 127
Autonomy, principle of, 22
Azacytidine, 156
Aziridinylbenzaquinone (AZQ), 159–162
Azospermia, 35, 87, 88

Bacilli, 5
Bacterial infections, 51, 70, 72
  decrease in neutrophils and, 54–55
Bands, 50–51, 54
Basophils, 51
B-cells, 51
BCG, 40
BCNU, 35, 120, 175–178
"Belmont Report," 21
Benadryl, 99, 100
Beneficence, principle of, 21, 22
Benzamides, 97
Benzodiazepines, 98
BiCNU, 35, 175–178
Biochemical approach, 40
Biological response modifiers (BRMS), 7, 40
Birth control practices, 88
Black bile, 3–4
Bladder cancer, 35, 46, 426
Bleeding. See Hemorrhage
Blenoxane, 163–168
Bleomycin, 31, 37
  administration of, 399
  nursing care plan for, 163–168
  side effects of, 37, 69, 84, 106–111, 120, 387–388
Blood cells
  life span of, 51
  red, 61
Blood clotting dysfunction, 37
Blood pressure, decreased, 89
Blood urea nitrogen (BUN), 112, 114
Body surface area determination, 408
Bone marrow, 50
Bone marrow depression (BMD), 37, 38, 50–62
  and anemia, 61–62
  expected time of drug nadirs, 52
  factors affecting degree of, 54

and neutropenia, 55–56
  nursing care plan for, 64–68
  nursing management with, 53–58
  physiological and psychological changes with, 59–60
  and thrombocytopenia, 58–61
Bone marrow transplantations (BMT), 6, 7–9
  allogeneic, 7
  autologous, 44–45
  complications, 45, 112
Bradycardia, 89
Breast cancer, 5, 6, 35, 44, 105
Burkitt's lymphoma, 6
Busulfan, 35
  nursing care plan for, 169–170
  side effects of, 106, 112
Butyrophenones, 97

Cancer(s)
  earliest evidence of, 3
  secondary, 35, 426
  theory of, 4
Cancer cells
  cycles of, 32
  with multidrug resistance, 42–43
Cancer chemotherapeutic drugs. See Chemotherapeutic agents
Cancer Chemotherapy National Service Center (CCNSC), 15
Cancer Drug Development Program, 6
Cancer therapy
  history of, 3–5
  new frontiers in, 7
  see also Chemotherapy
Candida albicans, 56, 70
Candida aspergillus, 56
Cannabinoids, 99, 101
Carboplatin, 171–174
Carcinogenic, 5, 426
Carcinogenicity, 426, 434
  of specific chemotherapeutic agents, 426
Cardiomyopathy, 49, 105–106
  factors increasing risk of, 105
Cardiotoxicity, 37, 105–108
  degrees of, 105
  drugs associated with, 107–108
Care planning. See Nursing care plans
Carmustine, 35
  nursing care plan for, 175–178
  side effects of, 106, 112
Catheters, 398
  external, 398
  Foley, 398
  long-term use of, 409
  silastic, 409–412, 420–422
  subclavian intravenous, 411
CCNU, 35

nursing care plan for, 270–272
  side effects of, 120
CDDP, 183–187
CeeNU, 270–272
Cell cycle
  of cancer cells, 32
  and chemotherapy, 31, 32–34
  importance of, 29–31
  mitosis, 30
Cell cycle phase-specific agents, 31–32, 33, 38, 41
Cell cycle phase-nonspecific agents, 32, 33, 35, 37, 41
Cell cycle-specific agents, 31
Cell cycle time, 32
Cell kill hypothesis, 33, 41
Central nervous system (CNS) toxicity, 121–125
Cerebrospinal fluid reservoir, 397, 398
Cerubidine, 208–212
Chemical Warfare Service, 5, 6
Chemoreceptor trigger zone (CTZ), 92–93, 95
Chemotherapeutic agents
  for ambulatory settings, 376, 378
  carcinogenic, mutagenic and teratogenic, 426
  cardiac toxicities and, 107–108
  and cellular activity, 31
  classification of, 31, 34–40
  earlist, 4
  emetic potential of, 95
  excretion patterns of, 431
  hepatotoxity and, 113
  mechanism of action of major, 36
  medications and, 408–409
  nephrotoxicity and, 115–119
  neurotoxicity and, 123, 124–125
  nursing care plans, 12, 139–369
  preparation, administration and disposal guidelines, 433
  pulmonary toxicity and, 109
  resistance to (see Drug resistance)
  safe handling of, 425–434
  sexual and reproductive dysfunction and, 90–91
  time sequence of discovery, 7–8
  vesicant, irritant and nonvesicant, 384
Chemotherapeutic regimens, 32
  designing, 33
Chemotherapy (cancer)
  adjuvant, 6, 20
  advances in, 7–9
  and cell kinetics, 32–34
  history of, 4, 5–6
  regimens, 32
  see also Administration of

chemotherapy; Combination chemotherapy; Single-agent chemotherapy
Chemotherapy checklist, 376, 377
Childhood acute leukemia, 6
Chlorambucil, 35, 430
  nursing care plan for, 179–182
Chlorotriarisene, 223–226
Cholinergic receptors, 100
Choriocarcinomas, 6
Chromatin, 38
Chronic leukemia, 4, 44
Cisplatin, 35
  nursing care plan for, 183–187
  side effects of, 81, 112, 113, 114, 120, 125, 126–217
Cis-Platinum, 183–187
Citrovorum factor, 266–267
Clinical experience, 375
Clinical trials, 16–17
  disease-oriented approach, 19–20
  dosage schedule, 19–20
  drug-oriented approach, 19
  ethical issues, 20–22
  federal guidelines, 21
  informed consent, 17, 21, 22
  interpretable data, 16
  nonrandomized study, 20
  patient selection, 17, 20, 22
  phases of, 17–20
  protocol components, 16–17
  randomized study, 20
  toxicities, 19–20, 25
Clinical nurse specialist (CNS), 23–24
Clinical research nurse, 23, 24
Clinical specialist, 23
Clowes, George, 5
Code for Nurses (ANA), 22–23
Colony stimulating factors (CSFs), 46
Combination chemotherapy, 6, 7
  and nadirs, 53
  teratogenic effects of, 426
  versus single-agent therapy, 40–41
Community, hazards to, 432–434
Compassionate use, 39
Confidentiality, 22–23
Congestive heart failure, 105, 106
  signs and symptoms of, 106
Conjugated equine estrogen, 223–226
Constipation, preventing, 127
Continuous infusion systems, 416–422
  external pumps, 417–418, 419
  implantable pumps, 418–422
Cooley's toxins, 5
Corticosteroids, 38
Cortisone, 145–148
Cosmegan, 203–207
Cranial nerve damage, 127

Creatinine, 114
Cushingoid features, 38
Cyclophosphamide, 40, 45, 430
  nursing care plan for, 188–192
  side effects of, 35, 44, 84, 94, 112, 120, 125, 426
Cytadren, 149–152
Cytarabine, 31, 37
  nursing care plan for, 193–196
Cytokinetic approach, 40
Cytosar-U, 193–196
Cytosine arabinoside, 31, 33, 35
  administration of, 399
  nursing care plan for, 193–196
  side effects of, 112, 122, 124
Cytostatic agents, 33
Cytotoxic agents, 33
Cytotoxic compounds, 34
Cytoxan, 188–192

Dacarbazine, 32, 35, 40
  nursing care plan for, 197–202
Dactinomycin, 37
  nursing care plan for, 203–207
  side effects of, 84
Data
  gathering process, 11
  interpretable, 16
Daunomycin, 37, 430
  nursing care plan for, 208–212
  side effects of, 81
Daunorubicin, 37
  nursing care plan for, 208–212
  side effects of, 84, 105, 106, 387
DCF, 318–321
DDMP, 37
Debulking, 41
Decadron, 99
Delivery systems. See Drug delivery systems
Department of Health, Education and Welfare (HEW), 21
Department of Health and Human Services, 17
Depo-Provera, 330–331
Desacetylvinblastine, 360–364
Dexamethasone, 98, 99, 101
  nursing care plan for, 145–148
Diagnosis, 11–12
  categories, 11
  nursing, 10, 11, 140
  terminology, 11–12
  see also Assessment
Diaphoresis, 89
Diarrhea, 37, 63, 81–84
  defined, 81
  medications for, 84
  nursing care plan for, 82–83
  sequelae of, 81

Didactic component, 375
Diethylstilbestrol (DES), 223–226
Diethystilbestrol diphosphate, 223–226
Diffusion capacity (DLCO), 111
Diphenhydramine, 99, 100
Direct patient care, 24
Disease-oriented approach, 19–20
Disposal, waste, 428–430, 433–434
DMDR, 251–255
DMSO, 384
DNA (deoxyribonucleic acid), 29, 35
Dopamine receptors, 100
Dosage
  calculations and modifications, 407–408
  in clinical trials, 19–20
  drug package inserts, 140
  patient assessment for, 407–408
  standard versus clinical trials, 407
  see also names of drugs
Doxorubicin, 41
  antidote for, 384
  nursing care plan for, 213–217
  side effects of, 37, 49, 69, 81, 84, 105, 106, 387
Droperidol, 97
Drug delivery systems, 397–422
  ambulatory continuous infusion systems, 416–422
  external pumps, 417, 419
  implantable pumps, 418–422
  implantable venous access ports (VAPs), 411–416
  intra-arterial (IA), 397, 398
  intracavitary (IC), 397, 398–399
  intramuscular (IM), 397, 399
  intrathecal (IT), 397–398
  intravenous (IV), 397, 400–406
  oral (PO), 397, 400
  silastic catheters, 409–412, 415–416
  subcutaneous (SQ), 397–399
  topical (TOP), 397, 399
  see also Administration of chemotherapy
Drug interactions, 408–409
Drug-oriented approach, 19
Drug resistance, 33
  current research on, 43
  mechanism of, 41–43
Drugs. See Chemotherapeutic agents
DTIC-Dome, 197–202
Dystonic reactions, 100

Education
  for administering chemotherapy, 375
  for clinical specialization, 23
  patient, 60, 61, 140, 376, 418
  self-care, 376, 418

Efudex, 238–241
Ehrlich, Paul, 4, 5
EISPAR, 261–265
EKG abnormalities, 105
Eldisine, 360–364
Electrolyte imbalance, 120
Elipten, 149–152
Embryonal rhabdomyosarcomas, 6
Emcyt, 218–222
Emergency home care kits, 379
Emetic drugs, 95
Emetine, 4
Emotional instability, 38
Empirical approach, 41
Encephalopathies, acute and chronic, 122–123
Endomyocardial biopsy, 105
Endoxan, 188–192
Endoxana, 188–192
Environmental carcinogens, 5, 432
Environmental Protection Agency (EPA), 432
Enzymes, 261–265
Eosinophils, 51
Erythrocytes, 61
Erythropoietin, 45
Escherichia coli, 56, 70
Esophogeal tears, 89
Esophagitis, 63, 74
  signs and symptoms of, 74
Estinyl, 223–226
Estracyte, 218–222
Estramustine, 35
  nursing care plan for, 218–222
Estrogens, 5, 38, 39
  nursing care plan for, 223–226
Ethical guidelines, 22
Ethical issues
  in chemotherapy administration, 378
  in clinical trials, 20–22
Ethinyl estradiol, 223–226
Etoposide
  nursing care plan for, 227–232
  side effects of, 38, 84
Eulexin, 242–243
Evaluation, 13. *See also* Assessment
Ewing's sarcoma, 6
Excretion patterns, 428–430, 431
Exposure to agents. *See* Safe handling of chemotherapeutic agents
External catheter, 398
External pumps, 417–418, 149
Extrapyramidal reactions, 100–101
  symptoms of, 100
Extrapyramidal tracts, 100
Extravasation, 378, 383–387, 389
  antidotes, 383–384
  intravenous route and, 400–401
  management of, 388

nursing assessment of, 390
nursing care plan for, 391–392
prevention of, 387, 400–401
treatment of, 383–384
Extravasation kit, 379
Eyewash fountains, 428

Farber, Sydney, 6
Fetal development, alterations in, 90
Fever
  hyperpyrexia, 387
  and infections, 56
  masking of, 38
Fidelity, principle of, 23
First order kinetics, 33
5AZ, 156–158
5-Azacytidine, 156–158
5-fluoro-2'-doxyuridine, 233–237
5-fluorouracil, 69
  nursing care plan for, 238–241
  side effects of, 37, 81, 84, 124
5-FUDR, 233–237
Flare reaction, 387, 400
Floxuridine
  administration of, 420
  nursing care plan for, 233–237
  side effects of, 37
Fluid retention, 38
Fluoropyrimidines, 37
Fluorouracil, 238–241
Fluoxymesterone, 153–155
Flutamide (Eulexin), 242–243
Folate antagonists, 37
Folex, 290–294
Folic acid antagonists, 290
Folinic acid, 266–267
Food and Drug Administration (FDA), 18, 39, 425
4-Demethoxydaunorubicin, 251–255
Fowler's solution, 4
FUDR, 233–237, 420
Fungal infections, 70, 72

Gated blood pool scans (GBPS), 106
G-CSF, 45
Generation time, 30
GI toxicity, 37
Glucocorticosteroids, 98–99
Glycoproteins, 42
Gompertzian growth curve, 32
Gonadal dysfunction, 35, 85–89
Government, federal
  drug development appropriations, 6
  nursing education grants, 9
  regulations on toxic wastes, 430
G phase, 29–31
Granulocyte-Macrophage colony Stimulating Favor (GM-CSF), 56–58

Granulocytes, 50
Growth fraction, 32
Guanine, 35

Hair follicles, 84
Hair loss, 84–85
Hair preservation techniques, 84–85
Haldol, 97
Halflives of agents, 428–430
Haloperidol, 97
Halotestin, 38
  nursing care plan for, 153–155
Handling of drugs. *See* Safe handling of chemotherapeutic agents
Health hazards. *See* Safe handling of chemotherapeutic agents
Hearing loss, 127
Heavy metal agents, 171, 183
Helsinki Declaration of 1964, 21
Hematopoietic growth factors. *See* Colony stimulating factors
Hemorrhage
  BMT and, 45
  cause of death, 7
  platelet count and, 58
  thrombocytopenia and, 60–61
Hemorrhagic cystitis, 44
Hepatic dysfunctions, 37
Hepatitis, 112
Hepatotoxicity, 112, 113
Hexamethylmelamine
  nursing care plan for, 244–246
  side effects of, 125
High-dose methotrexate (HDMTX) therapy, 120
Hirsutism, 38
Historical perspectives
  cancer research, 15
  cancer therapy, 3–5
  chemotherapeutic agents, 4
  chemotherapy, 4, 5–6
  clinical trials, 16
  medicine, 5
  oncology, 5
HN$_2$, 273–279
Hodgkin's disease, 6, 87, 88
  alkylating agents and, 35
  MOPP and, 41, 88
Home care kits, 379
Home settings, 376–378
  continuous infusion systems, 416–422
  exposure to drugs in, 432
Hormonal agents, 38–39
  common, 39
  nursing care plans for specific drugs, 145, 153, 223
  side effects of, 38
Hormones, 38–39

Hospitals for cancer, 4
Human Semen Cryobanks, 88
HXM, 244–246
Hydrea, 247–250
Hydrocortisone, 145–148
Hydroxyurea, 31
  nursing care plan for, 247–250
  side effects of, 37, 81, 84
Hyperglycemia, 38
Hyperpyrexia, 387
Hypersitivity reaction, 387–395
  management of, 393
  nursing care plan for, 394–395
Hypertension, 38
Hyperuricemic nephropathy, 120–121
Hyponatremia, 125
Hypothermia, and hair loss, 84–85

Idarubicin, 251–255
IFEX, 256–260
Ifosfamide, 35
  nursing care plan for, 256–260
IL-1, 45
Imidazole carboximide, 197–202
Immune system, 33
Immunotherapy, types of, 40
Implanted infusion ports, 411–415, 421
Implantable pumps, 398, 418–422
Inapsine, 97
Infection
  antibiotics and, 7
  bacterial, 51, 54–55, 70–72
  BMT and, 45
  common sites of, 56
  and death, 53
  fungal, 70, 72
  hormonal therapy and, 38
  long-term catheter use and, 409
  neutropenia and, 54–55, 70
  nosocomial sources of, 57
  viral, 70, 73
Informed consent, 17, 21, 22
Infusion method, 400
Institutional Review Boards (IRB), 21
Interferons, 40, 45, 399
Interleukins, 40
Intervention, 12
Intra-arterial (IA) route, 397, 398
Intracavitary (IC) route, 397, 398–399
Intramuscular (IM) route, 397, 399
Intrathecal (IT) route, 397–398
Intravenous (IV) administration, 397, 400–406
  adverse reactions to, 94, 400
  establishing new lines, 404
  methods of, 400
  needle selection, 401–402, 404
  preserving venous integrity, 402

techniques of, 401–404
"veinless" patients, 404–406
vein selection, 400–401, 402
Intravenous hydration, 120
Investigational agents, 39–40, 384
  nursing care plans for specific
    drugs, 141, 156, 159, 251, 295,
    299, 318, 346, 365
Investigational New Drug (IND)
  approval, 15–16, 18
Ipecac, 4
Irradiation, 45
Irritant agents, 384
  antidotes for 385–386

Joint Commission of the
  Accreditation of Healthcare
  Organization (JCAHO), 432
Justice, principle of, 21–22, 23

Karnovsky performance status scale,
  407
Kidneys, 120
Klebsiella pneumoniae, 56, 70

Lasix, 114
L-asparaginase, 39
  administration of, 399
  nursing care plan for, 261–265
  side effects of, 112, 125
Legal issues, 378
Leucovorin calcium, 266–267
Leukemias, 105
  acute, 44, 426
  acute nonlymphocytic (ANLL), 39
  childhood acute, 6
  chronic, 4, 44
  early treatment of, 4
  lymphatic, 38
  melphalan and, 35
Leukeran, 179–182
Leukocytes, 50, 55
Leukocytosis, 51
Leuprolide acetate, 268–269
Libido changes, 38
Limb distonia, 100
Liver, 112
Liver function tests (LFTs), 112
Lomustine, 35
  nursing care plan for, 270–272
Lorazepam, 94, 98, 100
Lumbar puncture, 397, 398
Lung cancer, 44
Lupron, 268–269
Lymphatic leukemias, 38
Lymphocytes, 51
Lymphomas, 6, 44, 126
  alkylating agents and, 35
  Burkitts, 6

malignant, 38
non-Hodgkin's, 6
Lysodren, 310–312

Macrophages, 40
Malignancies, secondary, 35, 426
M-AMSA, 141–144
Mandragora officinarum, 365
Mannitol, 114
Marijuana, 99
Mastectomy
  early records of, 4, 5
  radical, 5
Matulane, 326–329
Maximum tolerated dose (MTD), 19
MeCCNU, 120, 295–298
Mechlorethamine, 375
  antidote for, 383
  nursing care plan for, 273–279
  side effects of, 35
Medications
  for diarrhea, 84
  interfering with platelet function,
    59–60
  reaction with chemotherapeutic
    agents, 408–409
Medroxyprogesterone acetate,
  330–331
Megace, 330–331
Megakaryocytes, 58
Megestrol acetate, 330–331
Melanchole, 3
Melanomas, 40
Melphalan, 6, 430
  nursing care plan for, 280–284
  side effects of, 35, 84
Meningial irritation, 121–122
Menopause, premature, 87
Mesna, 288–289
Mesnex, 288–289
Metabolism. *See names of drugs*
Metabolites, 35
Methotrexate, 6
  administration of, 399
  nursing care plan for, 290–294
  side effects of 37, 69, 81, 112, 113,
    114–120, 122
Methyl-CCNU, 35
  nursing care plan for, 295–298
Methyl-G, 299–304
Methyl-GAG, 299–304
Methyl lomustine, 295–298
Methyl prednisolone, 99, 145–148
Methylprednisone, 145–148
Metoclopramide, 97, 98, 99, 101
Mexate, 290–294
Micrometastases, 6
Miscellaneous agents, 39, 247, 261
  common, 39

Miscellaneous agents (*cont.*)
  nursing care plan for specific
    drugs, 247, 261, 326
  side effects of, 39, 52
Misoprostol, 74
Mithracin, 322–325
Mithramycin, 37
  nursing care plan, 322–325
  side effects of, 122–120
Mitoguazone dihydrochloride, 299–304
Mitomycin, 32, 430
  nursing care plan, 305–309
  side effects of, 37, 84
Mitomycin C, 305–309
Mitosis, 30
Mitotane
  nursing care plan for, 310–312
  side effects of, 39, 125
Mitotic inhibitors. *See* Plant alkaloids
Mitoxantrone
  nursing care plan for, 313–317
  side effects of, 39, 84
Monoclonal antibodies, 7
Monocytes, 51
MOPP (mechlorethamine, vincristine,
    prednisone, procarbazine), 41
  and gonadal dysfunction, 88
  plus ABVD, 41–42
M phase, 30, 38
Mucositis, 37, 46, 62–84
  diarrhea, 63, 81–84
  esophagitis, 63, 74
  proctitis, 63
  sequelae of, 75
  stomatitis, 63–80
Multidrug resistance (MDR), 42–43
Multimodal therapy, 7
Multiple myeloma, 35, 44
Muscle wasting, 38
Mustargen, 273–279
Mutagenic, 87, 425–426
Mutagenicity, 426, 434
  of specific chemotherapeutic
    agents, 426
  urine, 427
Mutamycin, 305–309
Myeloma, 38
Myelosuppression, 35. *See also* Bone
    marrow depression
Myleran, 6, 169–170
Myofibril damage, 105

Nadirs, 51
  of specific drugs, 52
National Cancer Act, 9, 15
National Cancer institute (NCI), 6, 7,
    9, 13, 15, 23, 39, 50
  publications of, 378
National Commission for the

Protection of Human Subjects of
    Biomedical and Behavioral
    Research, 21
National Group for the Classification
    of Nursing Diagnosis. *See* North
    American Nursing Diagnosis
    Association
National Research Act, 21
Natulanar, 326–329
Nausea and vomiting, 12, 45, 89–101
  acute, 89
  anticipatory (ANV), 89, 93–95, 101
  antiemetic treatment of, 93, 94–101
  behavioral techniques with, 94
  causes other than drugs, 93
  complications of, 89
  delayed, 89
  nausea, 89
  nursing care plans for, 102–104
  physiology of, 93
  retching, 89
  sequelae of, 89, 92
  subacute, 89
  vomiting, 89
  vomiting center, 89, 93, 94
Neck dystonia, 100
Necrosis, 387
Necrotizing leukoencephalopathy, 122
Needles
  angiocath, 401
  butterfly, 401
  Huber, 411–413
  selection of, 401–402, 404
Neo-hombreol, 153–155
Neosar, 188–192
Nephrotoxicity, 112–121
  relative risks of chemotherapeutic
    agents, 115–119
Neuroblastoma, 44
Neuroleptics, 97
Neuropathies, 123, 126–131
  nursing care plan for, 128–131
Neurotoxicity, 38, 41, 121–131
  central nervous system toxicity,
    121–125
  neuropathies, 123, 126–131
  ocular toxicity, 126, 127
Neutropenia, 49
  and inflection, 54–55, 70
Neutrophils, 50, 51, 54–55
Nitrogen mustard, 32
  antidote for, 383
  earliest use of, 6, 375
  nursing care plan for, 273–279
Nitrosoureas (nitrosureas)
  nursing care plans for specific
    drugs, 175–178, 270–272, 295, 332
  side effects of, 35, 53, 81, 106, 113,
    120, 124

Nolvadex, 337–339
Nonmaleficence, principle of, 22
Nonrandomized study, 20
Nonseminomatous testicular cancer, 6
Nonspecific active immunotherapy, 40
Nonsteroidal antiinflammatory drugs
    (NSAIDs), 58
Non-vesicant agents, 384
North American Nursing Diagnosis
    Association (NANDA), 11
Novantrone, 313–317
Nucleid acids, 35, 36
Nuremberg Code, 20–21, 22
Nursing care plans
  for alopecia, 86
  for bone marrow depression, 56,
    64–68
  for diarrhea, 82–83
  for extravasation, 391–392
  for hypersensitivity and
    anaphylactic reaction, 394–395
  for minimizing toxicity of specific
    chemotherapeutic agents, 12,
    139–369
  for nausea and vomiting, 102–104
  for neuropathy, 128–131
  purposes for, 12, 13
  for sexual dysfunction, 91
  for stomatitis, 76–80
Nursing diagnosis, 10, 11–12, 140
Nursing process, 11–13

o,P'-DDD, 310–312
Occupational Safety and Health
    Administration (OSHA), 427, 432
Ocular toxicity, 126, 127
Oligogyric crisis, 100
Oligospermia, 35, 87
Ommaya reservoir, 397, 398
Oncologist's office, 430–432
Oncology, 5
Oncology clinical nurse specialist
    (OCNS), 23–24
Oncology nurse, 23, 24–25
  and research, 15–25
  role of, 9, 10–13, 375
Oncology nursing
  evolution of, 9
  qualifications, 375
  scope of practice, 15
Oncology Nursing Forum, 384
*Oncology Nursing Guidelines for Cancer
    Nursing Practice*, 71
Oncology Nursing Society (ONS), 13,
    23, 375
  guidelines for chemotherapy,
    391–392, 406–407, 427, 428, 432
  guidelines for extravasation,
    383–384

standards, 9–10
Oncovin, 355–359
1-PAM, 280–284
1-sarcolysin, 280–284
Opisthotonus, 100
Oral administration (PO), 397, 400
Oral care, 70, 71–74
Oral infections, 72–73
Ora-Testryl, 153–155
Oreton, 153–155
Osteoporosis, 38
Outpatient setting, 376–378
Ovarian cancer, 105

Package inserts, drug, 140
Pallace, 330–331
Paraplatin, 171–174
Parasthesia, 126, 127
Passive immunotherapy, 40
Patient advocacy, 25, 96
Patient education, 140
    for ambulatory and home settings,
        376, 418
    pre-chemotherapy, 60, 61
Patient protection, 17
Patient selection
    for clinical trials, 17, 20, 22
    for outpatient therapy, 376
Pentostatin, 318–321
Peripheral stem cell harvesting, 45
Perphenazine, 96
P-glycoprotein, 42–43
Pharmaceutical companies, 7, 16
Phase-nonspecific agents. See Cell
    cycle phase-nonspecific agents
Phase-specific agents. See Cell cycle
    phase-specific agents
Phenothiazines, 96–97, 101
Phenylalanine Mustard, 280–284
Phlebitis, 400
Piggyback (IVB) method, 400
Planning. See Nursing care plans
Plant alkaloids, 37–38
    common, 38
    nursing care plans for specific
        drugs, 227–232, 249, 355, 365
    side effects of, 69
Platelets, 58–61
    medications, interfering with
        count, 59–60
Platinol, 183–187
Platinum, 183–187
Plicamycin, 322–325
PLISSIT model for sexual
    rehabilitation, 88–89
Pneumonitis, 37, 110
Podophyllotoxins, 52
Postchemotherapy assessment,
    378–383

Postmenopausal breast cancer, 6
Potassium arsenite, 4
Prechemotherapy assessment,
    378–383
Prednisolone, 145–148
Prednisone, 99, 145–148
Preleukemic states, 44
Premarin, 223–226
Preservative-free, drug and diluent, 122
Procarbazine
    nursing care plan for, 326–329
    side effects of, 39, 125
Prochlorperazine, 96
Proctitis, 63
Progestational agents, 330–331
Progesterones, 38, 39
Proprioceptive losses, 127
Prostaglandins, 93
Prostate cancer, 5
Protective clothing/equipment, 428,
    434
Proteus, 70
Protocols, 16, 39
    essential components, 16–17
Provera, 330–331
Pseudomonas aeruginosa, 56
Psychosocial needs, patient, 45
Public Health Service, U.S., 15
Pulmonary fibrosis, 106–110
Pulmonary toxicity, 106–111
    acute, 106, 111
    drugs associated with, 109
Pumps
    choosing a system, 418
    external, 417–418, 419
    implantable, 398, 418–422
    portable infusion, 398–399
Purine antagonists, 37
Purinethol, 285–287
Push intravenous (IVP), 400
Pyramidal tracts, 100
Pyrimidine antimetabolites, 238

Quinine, 4

Radiation therapy, 5, 44, 122
Radionuclide angiography, 105, 106
Randomized study, 20
Rate of cell loss, 32
Recruitment cell, 33–34
Red blood cells (RBC), 61
Regimens. See Chemotherapeutic
    regimens
Reglan, 97, 98
Renal dysfunction, 37
Renal toxicity, 112, 114, 120
Reproductive dysfunction, 85, 87, 90,
    378, 379
Research

advances in chemotherapy, 7–9
    on drugs, 6, 7–9
    governmental guidelines and
        support of, 6, 21
    history of, 15–25
    on new therapies, 7
    oncology nursing and, 15–25
    on side effects, 9
    on toxicities, 18
    see also Clinical trials
Resistance to chemotherapy. See Drug
    resistance
Respect for persons, principle of, 21
Respiration, and vomiting, 89
Restorative immunotherapy, 40
Retching, 89
Reticulocytes, 62
Risk-benefit ratio, 20, 22, 426
Risks, of exposure. See Safe handling
    of chemotherapeutic agents
RNA (ribonucleic acid), 29, 30, 35
Rubex, 213–217
Ruter, Frances, 23

Safe handling of chemotherapeutic
    agents
    avoiding exposure, 429
    carcinogenicity, 426, 434
    in the community, 432–434
    disposal of drugs, 428, 430, 432
    guidelines for, 427, 428
    halflives of drugs, 428–430
    mutagenicity, 426, 434
    nursing tasks performed and,
        427–428
    in the oncologist's office, 430–
        432
    personal protective equipment,
        428, 434
    review of literature on, 427
    routes of exposure, 427, 429
    teratogenicity, 426, 434
    toxicity of drugs, 425–426
Scalp constriction, 85
Secondary malignancies, 35, 426
Secondary sexual characteristics,
    changes in, 38
Semustine, 295–298
Sensory-perceptual loss, 127
Serotonin antagonists, 101
Serum creatinine (Cr), 112
Sex hormone, 38
Sexual dysfunction, 35, 87, 90–91
    nursing care plan for, 91
Sexual fulfillment, altered, 90
Sexuality patterns, altered, 90
Sexual rehabilitation, 88–89
Shift to the left, 51
Sidearm method, 400

Side effects. *See* Toxicities; *names of drugs*
Silastic catheters, 409–412, 420–422
versus VAPs, 413–415
Single-agent therapy
teratogenic effects of, 426
versus combination therapy, 40–41
6-mercaptopurine, 37
nursing care plan for, 285–287
6-MP, 285–287
6-TG, 340–342
6-thioguanine, 37
nursing care plan for, 340–432
Skin toxicity, 37
Sloan-Kettering Institute for Cancer Research, 6
Socium thiosulfate, 383
Solu-Medrol, 99
Specialization, 23
Specific active immunotherapy, 40
Spermatogenesis, 88
S phase, 29, 32
Spill kits, 428, 430
Stabs, 51
Staphyloccus aureas, 56
Staphyloccus epidermidis, 56
Sterility, 88
Stilbestrol diphosphate, 223–226
Stilphostrol, 223–226
Stomatitis, 37, 45, 63–74
degrees of, 63–69
incidence of, 69
nursing care plan for, 76–80
nursing interventions, 70–74
oral infections and, 70–73
Streptococcal infection, 70, 73
Streptococci, 5
Streptomyces plicatus, 322
Streptomyces verticullus, 163, 203
Streptozocin, 35, 430
nursing care plan for, 332–336
side effects of, 120
Streptozotocin, 332–336
Subcutaneous intravenous port, 398
Subcutaneous (SQ) route, 397, 399
Sucralfate suspension, 74
Sulfydryls, 288
Supportive therapy, 7
Suppressor cells, 40
Survival statistics, 6, 7
Synchronization, principles of, 33
Syndrome of Inappropriate Antidiuretic Hormone (SIADH), 125

Tabloid, 340–342
Tace, 223–226
Tachycardia, 89

Tactile changes, 127
Tamoxifen citrate, 337–339
Taste changes, 69–70, 127
T-cells, 40, 51
Telogen, 84
Tendon reflexes, loss of, 126
Teniposide, 38, 365–369
Teratogenic, 87, 426
Teratogenicity, 426, 434
of specific chemotherapeutic agents, 426
Teslac, 153–155
Testicular cancer, 6, 41
Testolactone, 153–155
Testosterone propionate, 153–155
Tetrahydrocannabinol, 101
Thioguanine, 340–342
Thiophosphoramide, 343–345
Thiopurine antimetabolite, 340
Thiotepa, 35
nursing care plan for, 343–345
Thrombocytopenia, 58–61
patient instructions for, 61
T-lymphocytes, 39
Tongue protrusion, 100
Topical (TOP) administration, 397, 399
Toxicities
and alopecia, 84–85
antibiotic, 37
antibodies and, 7
antimetabolite, 37
and bone marrow depression, 50–62
cardiac, 105–108
with combination therapy, 41
common, classification of, 49–50
and gonadal dysfunction, 85–89
to health care workers, 425–426
hepatotoxicity, 112, 113
minimizing, nursing care plans for, 139–369
and mucositis, 62–84
and nausea and vomiting, 89–101
nephrotoxicity, 112–121
neurotoxicity, 121–131
to normal cells, 50–89
to organs attracting chemotherapeutic agents, 101–131
pulmonary, 106–111
research testing on, 18, 19–20, 25
Toxic wastes, 428–430, 432
Treatment. *See* Assessment; Nursing care plans; Nursing diagnosis
Triethylene, 343–345
Trimetrexate, 37
nursing care plan for, 346–348

Trismus, 100
Tumor doubling time, 32, 33
Tumor lysis syndrome (TLS), 121
nursing protocol for, 122
Tumor resistance to drugs, 41
Tumors
clinical detection of, 33
growth of, 32–33, 38
solid, 6
2'-deoxycofomycin, 318–321

Ulcers, 38
Uremia, 120
Uric acid, 120
Urinary alkalinization, 121
Urine mutagenicity, 427
Utadren, 38

"Veinless" patients, 404–406
Vein selection, 400–402
Velban, 349–354
Veno-occlusive disease, 112
Venous access ports (VAPs), 411–415
versus silastic catheters, 413–416
Vepesid, 227–232
Veracity, principle of, 22
Vesicants, 383, 384, 387
antidotes for, 385–386
Vinblastine, 31, 38
nursing care plan for, 349–354, 360
side effects of, 38, 126
Vinca alkaloids, 31
nursing care plan for, 360
side effects of, 38, 52, 124, 125, 126, 127
Vinca rosea, 38, 349, 355
Vincristine, 31
nursing care plan for, 355–359
side effects of, 38, 84, 125, 126, 127
Vindesine
nursing care plan for, 360–364
side effects of, 126
Viral infections, 70, 73
Visual loss, 127
Vitamins, 266
VM-26, 365–369
Voice changes, 38
Vomiting, 89. *See also* Nausea and vomiting
VP-16, 227–232

Waste products, handling, 428–430
Wilm's tumor, 6
WR-2721, 127

X-rays, 5

Zanosar, 332–336